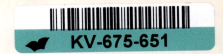
The Care of the Cancer Patient

L. G. CAPRA, D.M.R.T.

*Formerly Consultant Radiotherapist to Guildford and Godalming
Group Hospital*

*Cancer, created by life itself, exists within life,
Yet in the end make life untenable*

SECOND EDITION

MACMILLAN

First published 1972 by
William Heinemann Medical Books Limited, London

Second edition published 1986 by
MACMILLAN EDUCATION LTD
Houndmills, Basingstoke, Hampshire RG21 2XS
and London
Companies and representatives
throughout the world

Printed in Hong Kong

British Library Cataloguing in Publication Data
Capra, L. G.
The care of the cancer patient — 2nd ed.
1. Cancer — Treatment
I. Title
616.99'406   RC270.8
ISBN 0-333-38615-9
ISBN 0-333-38616-7 Pbk

Contents

From the nurse, patience and understanding,
From the doctor, skill and compassion,
From the patient, courage and endurance.

A young woman, dying of carcinoma of the ovary, could only be relieved by repeated paracenteses. This, my introduction as a student to cancer, made an indelible impression and led me into the field of radiotherapy. Today, such patients can be offered a wide range of treatment and analgesia. Often advances have been made because the patients and their families by their dignity and fortitude, have inspired doctors to continue in what seemed at times a hopeless task. Every nurse, whether she remains in the hospital service or takes a post outside it, will, sooner or later, have charge of a patient with malignant disease. The total care of such a patient is the task of a team of workers, but in the end its quality will depend upon the human relationship between the patient, the nurse, and the doctor. Any member of the cancer team can inadvertently destroy this delicate balance, through lack of knowledge or understanding, for the folk tales about malignant disease and its treatment are legion.

This book will, it is hoped, enable the nurse to take her full share in this exciting but exacting work.

Io Credo

Writing this book for nurses has been a privilege for they have taught me what it is they really want to know. If I have succeeded, I owe it to them. It has been my intention to include sufficient material to enlighten the beginner, expand the knowledge of the more experienced, and provoke thought and further reading by the advanced student or tutor.

Each profession has its own language, be it medicine, engineering, or law. While it is possible to explain and simplify for the uninitiated, it is impossible for members of a profession to do this continuously when they are discussing among themselves. Therefore although I have explained terms, once this has been done I have used them thereafter without explanation. A nurse must try to learn this language if she is to understand as she listens at the bedside.

Some readers may wonder at the amount of anatomy, physiology, and pathology included in each chapter, but without it understanding of the nature of the disease and the rationale of its treatment is almost impossible. All sections are meant however to serve only as a basis for thought and discussion, for the art and practice of radiotherapy is much more than a mere catalogue of treatment and dosages.

It is probable that many may find the descriptions of physiology conservative. This has been a deliberate policy. In many areas facts are still unknown and mechanisms the subject of much debate. It would be reasonable to expect doctors who have had a long training in the subject to weigh up the different opinions, but for a nurse, they could easily be confusing. Controversial matter has therefore been deliberately omitted, but I hope that the material which has been included will stimulate further reading.

There has been no attempt to outline every malignant condition, only those more usually encountered have been described. While acknowledging the debt of the specialist to the surgeon, full details of operations are not given, for these the nurse is referred to a textbook of surgery.

Theories of endocrinology and aetiology, even when speculative, have been given space although they may not always be relevant to current practice. In this way it is possible to give some evaluation of present thought and future research. The nurse will find in the text fairly lengthy descriptions of cytology and genetics, for these two areas of research are likely to yield developments which will affect all branches of medicine in the near future.

The radiation procedures are fairly standard and practised by most centres, although with some variations. My attitude to my work, to the disease, and to my patients, is my own, evolved over the number of years which I have spent in this branch of medicine. It is not one which I expect others to adopt unthinkingly, for all of us who work in this field must think for ourselves and formulate our own attitudes to the patient and his disease. For this reason I have not written a conventional textbook, but rather a philosophy of treatment which the nurse can read, discuss, and adopt or reject according to her own interpretation.

With a solid foundation of fact, and an understanding of the rationale of treatment and care, the nurse can begin to know something of the disease and of the mind and aims of the doctor. She can then take her part in the whole care of the patient and will no longer feel unable to cope with his very natural fears and anxieties.

Here at the beginning my readers may well ask what I regard as the most important aspect of the care of the patient with malignant disease. Research, investigation, treatment, all are important, but by the end of the book I hope the reader will know that for me, the patient and our response to his needs, fears and hopes represent the greatest challenge. Each day the problems are different, for not only will the disease and the patient's needs alter but also we ourselves will vary in our response. It is here in the interplay of human character that we are most completely the doctor or nurse, for at this point Nature presents us with the greatest enigma, for Man must here challenge Man, the unchallengeable.

January, 1971   L. G. C.

Second Thoughts
Preface to the
Second Edition

Since the first edition of this book many readers have been kind enough to write to me. There have been suggestions for expansion, and even contraction(!) of different sections. If it were possible to act on them all it is likely that this one volume would become either very large or turn into two or three. I can only hope that the changes which have been made will satisfy at least some of these requests. Others have been based on a misconception as to my purpose. It was never my intention to give a detailed account of nursing techniques. Where they are discussed it is either because they are an integral part of therapy, or because I have been asked by nurses about their importance or relevance. Similarly, those who look for detailed blueprints of regimes in various situations, will be disappointed. There are fundamental principles, but their application will vary from patient to patient, otherwise elements of rigidity and uniformity will enter. Care, for me, is not detailed schedules, but the integration of skill, knowledge, technique, personality, and humility, into the response to individual needs.

Although production costs must be kept as low as possible, I have retained basic anatomy, physiology, etc., but condensed some of the sections. If these are too concentrated I can only apologise, and suggest amplification from other books. Similarly many readers will find simple explanations of some complicated subjects inadequate, or conversely that they are too simple. Perhaps both groups will be stimulated to extend their reading. If they do this, they will find that in some of my text I have paid the penalty of attempting to convey scientific minutiae in broad terms — the loss of complete clarity.

Since the first edition there have been some technical changes, introduction of new drugs, changes in the definition and naming of biological or radiation units, and these I have tried to include. Some of my readers are working outside the United Kingdom, and with them in mind I have retained references to older techniques and machines. They may be situated in Units which are unable as yet to obtain more sophisticated apparatus, but even so neither they nor we should forget that very good work can be done with these tools.

Increasing knowledge of the human body induces in me no sense of familiarity, but rather an attitude of continuing wonder. For convenience we describe processes and actions as if they occurred in isolation, whereas in fact they take place not only simultaneously but in relation to each other. To consider those we know about in such a dynamic model is mind boggling, whether we are looking at the whole body or just one cell, and to add to the complexity we are continual increasing our pool of knowledge.

It has been my privilege to learn from all members of the cancer team, but above all from my patients. They have taught me much, not only about cancer, but also about how human beings cope with its effects on body, mind, and spirit, and of course they have taught me much about myself.

It is my profound hope that before too long my speciality will change fundamentally, or even become redundant. If that happens it will be because we understand both the disease and its treatment, and there is no longer any need to write books. What will not become redundant, is the care which we owe to every patient, whatever his disease.

1986   L. G. C.

Because we die, we acknowledge the past
Because we live, we honour the future,
But we honour the present because,
If we are forgotten, we are nothing.

Acknowledgements

I acknowledge, with grateful thanks, the kindness of all those who have allowed me to reproduce the following illustrations.

My colleagues of:

The Guildford and Godalming Group Hospitals.
The Atkinson Morley Hospital, Wimbledon.
St. George's Hospital, London.
The National Hospitals for Nervous Diseases, London.
The Hospital for Sick Children, Great Ormond Street, London.
St. Mark's Hospital, London.
The Westminster Hospital, London.
Chapter 1: Figs. 2a, 2b.
Chapter 4: Fig. 1.
Chapter 5: Figs. 2, 3.
Chapter 6: Figs. 3, 5.
Chapter 9: Figs. 4, 7a, 7b, 8, 9a, 9b, 10, 11, 12, 13, 14, 15.
Chapter 10: Fig. 3.
Chapter 11: Figs. 4, 5, 7, 8.
Chapter 12: Figs. 3, 4.
Chapter 13: Fig. 4.
Chapter 14: Figs. 2, 3, 9.
Chapter 15: Figs. 5, 8.
Chapter 16: Figs. 3, 6.
Chapter 17: Figs. 2, 3.
Chapter 18: Figs. 2, 3.
Chapter 19: Figs. 6, 7, 8, 9.
Chapter 20: Figs. 3, 4, 8, 9.
Chapter 22: Fig. 2.
Chapter 27: Figs. 6, 7.

Reproduced by kind permission of the President and Council of the Royal College of Surgeons of England:

Chapter 3: Fig. 1.
Chapter 14. Fig. 8.

My every sincere thanks are due to Mrs. Jessie Hunt, who not only typed the manuscript, but encouraged me by her fortitude and her refusal to accept defeat. Many patients and their friends have from time to time supported various projects of mine. In memory of his son Stephen, Mr. Glover still does so. In naming him I would also wish to acknowledge all those others who have been so kind and helpful.

Many of my friends and colleagues, too numerous to list, have assisted me with their constructive criticism and editorial advice. I ask them to accept this acknowledgement as a token of my gratitude.

In dreams and dreams only
Do we escape from reality.
So much to be known, so little known.

1 The Nature of the Disease

Cellular division is normal (mitosis); from the moment of conception onwards multiplication and replacement is an ordered process. The trophoblasts of the placenta invade the uterus but stop in response to some as yet unknown control. When I saw the dissection of a three-month embryo I realised with wonder that the foetus, though miniature, was complete and that from now on only growth, repair, and replacement would take place in an orderly sequence. Rapid replacement of tissues suffering wear and tear means cells are in a constant state of mitosis, skin layers are continually worn and replaced, red cells have a limited life and the population must be maintained, and epithelial cells of the gut are constantly shed and renewed. The hallmark of all this cellular activity is order and control maintaining a constant balance. The factors which initiate and terminate the whole process are as yet undiscovered. It is when one or more cells escape from this control that the process of malignancy starts. Growth becomes uncontrolled, disorderly, and invasive, and the normal equilibrium is disturbed.

Benign and Malignant Growth

Benign Growth

Excess growth is not in itself malignant. A benign tumour grows slowly, is usually confined within a capsule, and does not invade or spread to distant parts of the body. Any local damage is the result of pressure, but occasionally systemic effects may be produced, such as the production by a pituitary adenoma of hormones. In a few cases tumours can undergo malignant change, for example the intestinal polyp can become the malignant adenocarcinoma. Clinically the benign tumours are often symptomless and may be only an accidental finding at operation or autopsy, typical of this is the uterine fibroid. Seen under the microscope the cells have a normal pattern resembling the parent tissue, mitotic figures are few.

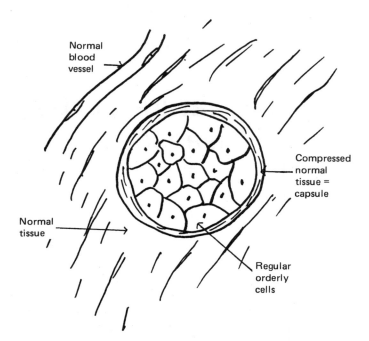

Normal blood vessel

Compressed normal tissue = capsule

Normal tissue

Regular orderly cells

Fig. 1.1a.   Benign growth

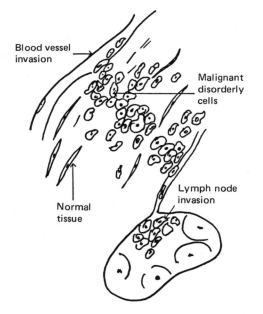

Blood vessel invasion

Malignant disorderly cells

Lymph node invasion

Normal tissue

Fig. 1.1b.   Malignant growth, showing invasion

Malignant Growth

By contrast, in malignant tissues the pathologist sees the following microscopical features.

1. Evidence of atypical growth; many abnormal mitotic figures, cells which are irregular in shape and staining, and tumour giant cells.
2. Atypical structure; the cells show a range from imperfect but recognisable parent tissue to a complete loss of pattern, i.e. dedifferentiation, anaplastic tumours.
3. Atypical blood vessels; the abnormality may lie in an increased number or in abnormality of the vessel walls.
4. Invasion of surrounding tissues, and offshoots outside the main tumour (metastases). No capsule.

Methods of Spread

Direct Invasion

The tumour not only expands in size but also infiltrates its cells as processes between the surrounding tissue cells. Hence the origin of the word 'cancer' meaning crab. Resistance to this infiltration varies, being less in the loose connective tissues but greater in bone or cartilage. The skin presents little barrier to the spread of a rodent ulcer on the nose, but invasion of the cartilage is slower and occurs much later.

Lymphatic Spread

Malignant cells invade the lymphatic vessels and are carried around to the lymph nodes. Here they are filtered out and settle down and grow. The node becomes hard, palpable, and eventually attached to the surrounding tissues. The flow of the lymph may be stopped or reversed, producing clinical signs such as peau d'orange of the breast or lymphoedema of the leg. Cells which escape beyond the nodes reach the thoracic duct, enter the blood stream, and so can be deposited in any part of the body. Certain tumours show a preferential lymphatic spread, e.g. tongue, cervix.

Blood-borne Spread

In addition to entering the blood stream from the lymphatics, tumour cells can invade vessels directly and be distributed throughout the body. They do not always produce metastases, but when they do they tend to occur in certain sites, lung, brain, bone, liver, and the site may be related to the type of tumour, prostate spreading to the bone, osteogenic sarcoma to the lung. The muscles are rarely involved, yet they form the bulk of the body tissue and have a rich blood supply. It has been postulated that constant movement does not allow the cells to settle and grow.

Implantation

This can occur naturally, cells can be spread or carried along a lumen (hollow tube) to a distant site, the medulloblastoma (brain tumour) cells can be carried by cerebrospinal fluid down the spinal canal giving rise to spinal metastases. At the time of surgery viable tumour cells may contaminate the wound giving rise to metastases later in the scar, as following cystectomy metastases from a bladder carcinoma in the abdominal scar.

Transcoelomic Spread

Coelom is the word used to describe a body cavity, peritoneal, pleural, pericardial space. Cells are shed from a tumour which has reached the surface of a viscus and implant on the lining of the cavity, e.g. lung tumour on the pleura. The lining membranes become studded with seedling tumours, and in response fluid is formed, pleural effusion or ascites. When this fluid is examined malignant cells are sometimes seen. Occasionally the tumour may spread from one structure to another across the space, as from carcinoma of the stomach to the ovary, the cells of the secondary deposit then have a characteristic signet ring appearance and are known as Krukenberg tumours.

Clinical Aspects

Malignant tumours do not show uniform progress, they may have periods of growth alternating with quiescence and may even regress spontaneously. Periods of quiescence may be so long that there is apparent cure, recurrence only occurring years later at another site. A prime example is carcinoma of the breast, the first metastasis has been recorded 40 years after the original growth, and 20 or 30 years is not uncommon.

Phasing of the Disease

In the early stage the cells are dividing but as yet no definite symptoms are produced. Screening procedures, such as the cervical smear, may reveal the presence of the disease. It is for this reason that so much research is being concentrated on such screening procedures.

As the cells continue to divide the phase is reached when symptoms are produced. These can be many and varied. A lump may be palpable, carcinoma of the breast; bleeding may occur, carcinoma of the bladder; a lesion of the bowel may alter bowel habits; persistent hoarseness may point to carcinoma of the larynx, and dysphagia to a lesion of the oesophagus. These are all local effects.

Interesting syndromes may be due to the production of hormones, or products of tumour metabolism. A tumour of the adrenal gland can give rise to obesity, osteoporosis, etc. (Cushing's syndrome), while carcinoma of the lung may produce changes in electrolyte balance or a peripheral neuropathy giving rise to weakness and sensory changes in the limbs. Some of these general effects are due to the excess production of hormones typical of the tumour's tissue of origin, others are due to ectopic formation of a hormone quite inappropriate to the tissue. The latter is typified by bronchial carcinoma which may secrete a variety of hormones including ACTH (adrenocortical hormone) and ADH (antidiuretic hormone). The other kind of tumour has been given the name apudoma, an example is an insulinoma, this is found in the Islets of Langerhans in the pancreas and secretes insulin. Other generalised effects are less easy to explain, pruritus, hyperviscosity of the blood (extra-thick blood), neuropathy (disturbance of nerve function), etc.

When metastases (secondaries) are present symptoms will vary according to their site. If in bone there will be pain and possibly pathological fracture, while those in the liver around the bile duct will produce jaundice. Rarely the first symptoms may be those of the secondary itself and only on biopsy is the presence of a primary suspected. A solitary cerebral secondary can mimic a primary brain tumour, and only when the section is examined is the histology found to be that of, for example, a carcinoma of the bronchus. Very occasionally although the histology is obviously that of a secondary deposit, despite searching clinical investigation the primary may only be found at autopsy.

While for clarity I have described these as discrete phases there is in fact a progression and often overlapping. For example on routine X-ray survey of a patient presenting for the first time with a small lump in the breast, lung or bone secondaries may be found.

Staging

There are two methods of staging, one based on clinical findings and the results of investigations such as lymphography, ultrasound, CATscan, the other is post-surgical and includes the histological findings. Staging is important for prognosis, treatment decisions, and the comparison of results in different centres with varying regimes. The actual recording system is only a classification, staging is based on an interpretation of these findings.

Clinical

This is based on clinical and investigation findings. The system has three components, T for initial tumour, N for regional lymph nodes, M for distant metastases. To each letter are assigned roman numbers indicating degrees of involvement. From this code a staging number may be derived. For example, for a breast tumour:

T. Tumour two centimetres in its greatest dimension. Skin not involved. No retraction of the nipple. No pectoral muscle fixation. No chest wall fixation = T.I.

N. Mobile axillary node on the same side = N.1.

M. No metastases = M.0.

The staging would be stage II (early version). Unfortunately, despite early enthusiasm, international acceptance has not been complete, and local variations of the TNM system have been developed. However if reference is made clearly to how the changes have modified the original, there can be some measure of comparison. Clinical staging gives an indication of prognosis and guides the clinician in his choice of treatment. Stage I carcinoma of the breast may be amenable to surgery whereas Stage IV carcinoma, advanced, is totally inoperable and must be dealt with by other means; the prognosis is more favourable in the former. Other letters may be added to the system, one for grading the pathology based on the microscopy findings of the degree and extent of infiltration, and another to designate the histological degree of malignancy.

Histological Findings

Well differentiated cells resemble closely the parent tissue and are less malignant. Gradually there is a loss of pattern, dedifferentiation, until finally the cell is completely atypical, anaplastic. When cells of this nature are found in a node which is the first manifestation of malignancy, it may be very difficult to suggest the tissue of origin. Classification is usually by numbers, I being well differentiated, and III or IV the anaplastic. Histology and clinical staging do not always agree, a clinical stage I tumour may be histologically IV, this of course modifies the favourable prognosis of the clinical staging. The radiosensitivity of the cell usually varies inversely with the differentiation.

In certain sites classification and staging have become universally accepted. A prime example is the staging of Hodgkin's lymphoma. When staging regimes have wide acceptance the details are given in the appropriate chapters.

While these two methods are adopted as a form of guide, other factors which cannot yet be evaluated play their part. The immune process, for example, the reaction between host and tumour, is believed to play its part in the modification

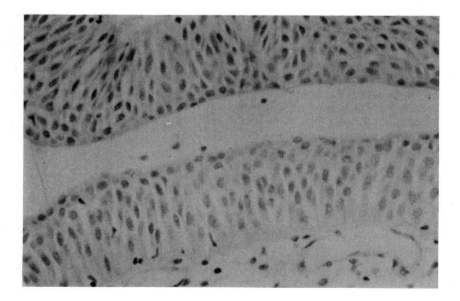

Fig. 1.2a.   Well-differentiated cell

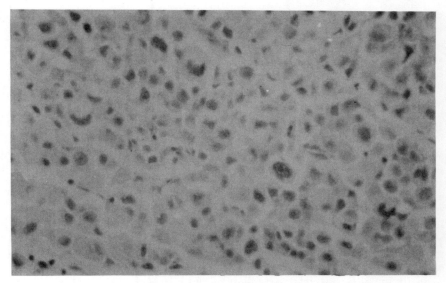

Fig. 1.2b.   Anaplastic cell

of tumour behaviour, but since it is not yet fully understood, nor yet capable of measurement, it finds no place in present staging systems.

Survival Figures

In order to compare results from different methods of treatment it is usual to quote survival figures. These are taken at three, five or ten years after either diagnosis or treatment. It is important not to misunderstand the term. It is merely a convenient reference figure. It does not mean that patients only survive for that period of time, many live much longer, others die in a much shorter time.

The wide expanse of desert
Must once have been
But a grain of sand.

2 Basic Principles, Physics and Biology

Introduction

X-rays were first described by Roentgen in 1895. All X-ray tubes are a development of his apparatus. The early workers did not realise the need to protect themselves against radiation and many of them developed dermatitis and some, malignant skin growths which caused their deaths. This sad discovery led doctors to wonder whether radiation might not also attack malignant tissue allowing natural healing to take place. So, from the very beginning, it was seen that radiation is a two-edged sword.

X-ray Tube

Electrons, negatively charged particles of the atom, are made to travel from the source (cathode), to strike the target (anode). The force required to speed these electrons across the vacuum is measured in thousands or millions of volts. The

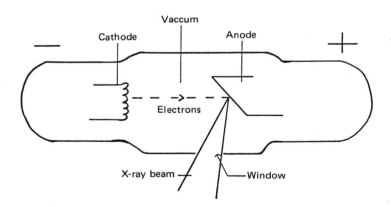

Fig. 2.1.   X-ray tube

sudden stopping of the electrons generates energy, 99% in the form of heat, the rest as X-rays. These bounce off the target and leave the tube through a special window. The heat is removed by a cooling system, usually oil. The greater the force used to push the electrons across to the target, the deeper will the X-rays penetrate into the patient. A machine generating X-rays of this greater penetration is the linear accelerator, but the method used to speed the electrons is different from that in the X-ray tube. Still greater penetration can be obtained from the betatron. Electrons are accelerated in a circle to very high energy and are then used to bombard the patient who becomes the target.

In a linear accelerator the electrons are passed along a line, receiving energy input at intervals to accelerate them before they either hit a target and emerge as X-rays, or are used as an electron beam.

For treating surface lesions such as eczema requiring penetration of a few millimetres, 10 kV (10,000 volts) would be used, but for a deeper tumour, e.g. cancer of the lung, possibly ten to fifteen centimetres deep, a force of 4 MV (4,000,000 volts) could be required. Radiation which penetrates a short distance is sometimes known as soft radiation. X-rays produced by a tube may be called conventional, and the more penetrating radiation can be described as mega- or supervoltage.

Radioactive Isotopes

A single substance is called an element. It is distinguished from other elements by the distinctive arrangement of the nucleus and circling electrons in its atoms. Each element is not in fact a single entity, but is made up of a number of different forms of the chemical. These behave chemically exactly like each other, but in each the nucleus of the atom is slightly different. These varying forms are called isotopes. Some of them are unstable and break down, decay, to form other elements. As they do so they give off energy as radiation and are therefore called radioactive.

Natural

These radioactive isotopes are found as naturally occurring substances on the earth.

Radium

This is a radioactive material found in certain rocks. Marie Curie was the first to isolate this element in 1898 from pitchblende. 'Radioactive' means that the radium is breaking down to reach its stable state (lead) and while it is breaking down it gives off radiation. Most of these rays are called gamma rays. Radium was once used in machines to provide radiation therapy, the radium bomb, and also in needles, gynaecological tubes and boxes.

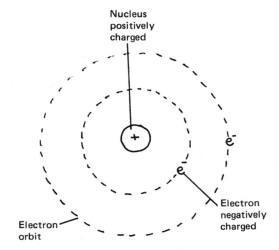

Fig. 2.2.   The atom

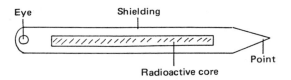

Fig. 2.3.   Radioactive needle

Artificial

Other elements can be made artificially radioactive by putting them in an atomic pile, they are also called radioactive isotopes. Like radium they break down and in doing so give off radiation; these rays may be alpha α, beta β and gamma γ.

Certain of these compounds are liquid and when given to a patient they are concentrated in target organs. The dose is very small. The radiation given off can be measured by instruments such as the Geiger counter. This process is called scanning. Lesions may show up as an absence or increase of activity. The pulses of activity are counted by the machine as the detector moves in a definite pattern over the area being surveyed. A pictorial record of the site and intensity of the activity is produced at the end of the scan, and so not only is a lesion detected, but also much information may be gained as to its location. Such knowledge is useful both to the surgeon and the radiotherapist.

Radioactive iodine is used to measure the activity of the thyroid gland. A high count in the first hours is found in thyrotoxicosis, while a low count may be found in myxoedema. Other radioactive isotopes which can be used for scans are technetium for the brain, iodine-labelled compounds for the kidney and phosphous for bone studies. There is a constant search for active isotopes which can be used to scan and treat other parts of the body.

Half Life

The term half life is used to describe the period of time taken for a radioactive isotope to lose half its initial activity (decay). The half life of cobalt-60 is 5.3 years, while that of iodine-131 is eight days. Therefore the former can be used in a machine as a source of radiation for a useful period of roughly four years, it will then need replacing as treatment times would after that become too prolonged; the latter is an example of those isotopes which can be left in the body as they decay rapidly, their residual activity becoming negligible in hours or days.

The radiation given off by an isotope can be used to treat malignancy inside the body. A high dose of radioactive iodine is used to destroy the thyroid gland. Radioactive phosphorus affects red bone marrow and is a form of treatment for polycythaemia vera. Other materials are placed in body cavities to treat seedling metastases (secondaries).

Other Rays

Alpha, α, rays penetrate a fraction of a millimetre in solids and the maximum amount of energy is absorbed when they come to rest; at the moment little therapeutic use has been found for them. Thorium is an element which gives off alpha rays. Beta rays are in fact electrons moving at a high speed. They can be given off by active isotopes such as yttrium, or they may be produced by machines, the linear accelerator and the betatron. Gamma rays are of the same nature as conventional X-rays, but they have greater energy and therefore greater penetration. The energy of gamma rays will vary according to the source, i.e. cobalt 1.17 and 1.33 MeV, radium mainly 0.55 and 1.65 MeV.

The gamma rays given off by cobalt and caesium radioactive isotopes are used in treatment machines. Unlike X-ray tubes which only generate radiation when switched on, cobalt and caesium sources are constantly active. The sources are therefore stored in protective chambers and only exposed in the head of the machine when treatment is being given.

The use of other particles of the atom to which a high energy can be given has been investigated. The particles are the neutron and the proton. The neutron reacts with the nucleus dislodging protons and heavy particles. These damage tissues irrespective of whether or not they are well oxygenated, this is in contrast to X- or gamma rays. Tissue in the centre of large tumour masses is often anoxic and more resistant to the latter more commonly used types of radiation. The machines producing neutrons are either very large machines like the cyclotron, or else smaller, cheaper machines which unfortunately rely on tubes which have to be replaced frequently. Neither type of machine is as yet in widespread use.

Ionisation

The atom can also be changed if electrons are detached from their orbits around the nucleus. The resulting structure is called an ion, and the radiation is known as ionising radiation. This is chemical damage, and to bring it about energy is required. This is supplied by the radiation and absorbed by the tissues. Other chemical structures called radicals may also be formed. These chemical products of radiation may be very active and cause further changes.

Measurement

The amount of radiation absorbed is measured in units now known as grays (formerly known as rads, 100 rads = 1 Gy). Instruments are placed in a block of material having the same absorption as the human body, and the amount of radiation reaching varying levels is measured. These points are plotted out on paper and a line is drawn through all the points having the same reading, this is the isodose curve.

From these charts it is possible to calculate the dose at any given point, the depth dose.

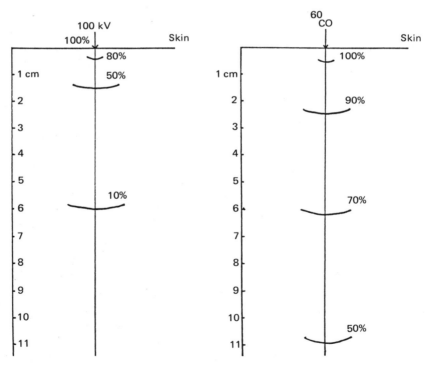

Fig. 2.4a.   100 kV depth dose   Fig. 2.4b.   Cobalt-60 depth dose

Applicators

X-rays, like light, spread out from a point. An applicator confines the radiation to the size and shape of the area to be treated, this area is called the field. On the lower voltage units applicators are fitted on to the machine. In higher voltage

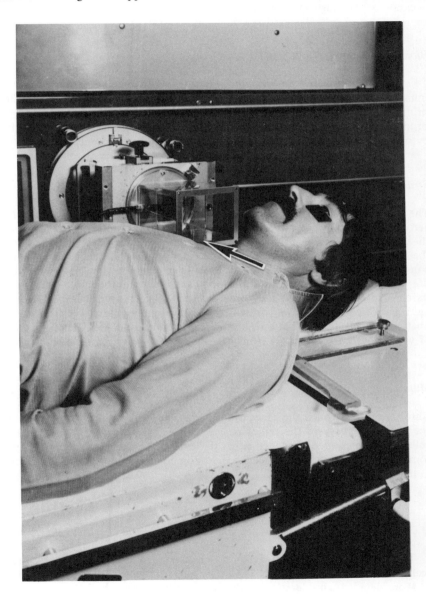

Fig. 2.5.   Applicator, betatron

machines the field is defined by moveable jaws. When the field to be treated is an irregular shape a lead cut-out may be placed directly on the patient when low voltage radiation is being used, or for higher voltages lead blocks are placed in a tray some distance above the patient. While the treatment is being set up a light shining along the same path as the radiation will take helps to ensure accurate positioning of the field.

Biological Effect of Radiation

Cells are more sensitive to radiation when they are dividing or when they are immature. Examples in the human body are the epithelial cells of the gut and the primitive precursors of the red cells in the bone marrow. Thus radiation may produce diarrhoea due to damage of the epithelial cells of the gut, and thrombocytopenia and anaemia due to its effect on the bone marrow.

Structure of the Cell

The human body is composed of millions of cells with varying functions and activities. Each cell may be regarded as a tiny world surrounded by its own wall, the membrane. Outside this world lies the extracellular fluid. Within the wall, the membrane, the cytoplasm is the workshop, and across the wall there is a constant two-way traffic, inwards materials necessary for the cell's continued life, and outwards its own waste products. The nucleus is the hub of this world, its chromosomes carry the code ordering the cell's life and division. Materials are transported to and from the cell by the surrounding blood vessels and lymphatics. All this activity has a rhythm which may be characteristic of the tissue of which the cell is a unit, or it may be varied by nervous or hormonal factors.

Mutation

Chromosomes, through the genes which lie along their length, carry the code for the orderly activity of the cell. This code is passed unchanged to the daughter cells at each division. A change in either the genes or the structure of the chromosomes alters the code and is called a mutation. Such a mutation causes a change in the cell which may:

1. Be lethal.
2. Lead to inability to divide.
3. Result in abnormalities which are reproduced in the daughter cells.

This process may be spontaneous or induced by radiation or cytotoxic drugs (cell poisons).

More detailed consideration of the cell, and its division cycle is reserved for the chapter on cytotoxic chemotherapy.

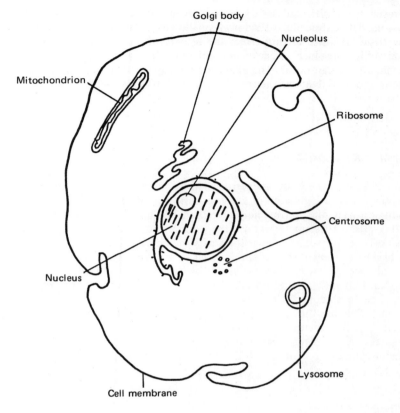

Fig. 2.6   The cell

Site of Action of Radiation

As we have seen when radiation passes through any material, part of its energy is absorbed and thereby the structure of the absorbing material is affected. The magnitude of the damage will depend upon the nature of the tissue and the amount of energy absorbed, the oxygenation of the cell, and whether it is resting or dividing. We must therefore consider action, (i) upon the cell, and (ii) upon the surrounding media.

Action on the Cell (Direct and Indirect)

Radiation can affect the membrane, the cytoplasm, or the nucleus. This is shown microscopically by swelling of the cell due to the damaged membrane allowing extra fluid to pass in, cloudiness of the cytoplasm indicating damage to its component structures, and fragmentation of the chromosomes and swelling of the nucleus. If persistent this leads to immediate cell death. Late cell death may result from initial sub-lethal damage giving rise to a cell mutation which is not viable. The extracellular fluid may be altered by damage to the blood vessels of the tissue, this will in turn affect the activity of the cell. So far we have considered only the local effects of radiation, but the body is an entity. Systemic effects can occur. The exact method by which they arise is unknown, but it is thought that by altering the overall biological balance, local damage may be worsened.

The Aim of Radiotherapy

Malignant cells in the body are surrounded by normal cells. Most of the malignant cells are in a high state of activity, dividing, and therefore more sensitive to radiation than the nearby normal cells. The aim of the radiotherapist is to deliver a dose sufficient to sterilise the tumour, but small enough to allow the normal cells to recover and repair the area affected by malignancy.

It has been shown that if an interval is left between treatments, normal cells will recover better than malignant cells, and a second dose of radiation given then kills more malignant cells but does less damage to the normal population. The total dose of radiation to be given is therefore split into doses, 'fractions'. This has the advantage of lessening some of the side effects of radiotherapy. Usually treatment is given once a day, three or five times a week, occasionally only weekly. Sometimes there is a break in the middle of the treatment course of one or two weeks, this is called 'split treatment'.

Localisation of Radiation

It is obvious that not only must the patient not move during treatment, but also each day the radiation must be given to exactly the same area, and normal tissues protected. The applicators, adjustable jaws in the machine, and light beam aid setting up, lead shields on the skin for low voltage work, and blocks in the beam for higher voltage work, all define the beam and treatment area. Sometimes the patient wears a plastics shell to ensure correct alignment, this is made specially for each individual. One of the most useful devices is a simulator. This mimics the characteristics of each type of radiation machine and shows on the viewing screen an X-ray of the area being treated with the field superimposed. This ensures accurate localisation and verification of the treatment field.

When more than one field is being used or the machine rotated round the patient, both methods of concentrating dosage at one point but giving less radiation to normal tissues, a plot of the isodose curves must be made. This ensures even dosage to the target area with no hot or cold spots. In the most sophisticated units, the treatment couch, simulator, and computer are all linked, so that planning, calculation of dose, and positioning of the patient are all done in one operation, and the results automatically stored for future use.

Improving Sensitivity to Radiation

Certain drugs have been shown to sensitise tumours to radiation and cytotoxic therapy. They are called sensitisers. The first to be used was the antibacterial metronizadole, but many more compounds have been developed and are being tested.

Since anoxic cells are less sensitive to radiation, it was a logical step to try and improve tissue oxygenation. Unfortunately the haemoglobin in the blood is almost at its maximum oxygen saturation at normal atmospheric pressure. To raise this and so oxygenate the tissues, oxygen must be given at several times normal atmospheric pressure, and this can only be done by putting the patient in a special pressure chamber. The associated problems have limited the use of the technique, and also varying reports of results have been given.

Immune Response

This is the body's response to foreign material known as antigen. While usually beneficial, it can on occasions be as it were 'overdone', resulting in pathological damage to the body, examples of this are anaphylaxis and serum sickness. There are two processes involved in an immune response, recognition and defence. Both these activities involve certain cells and tissue fluids, they are complex and interdependent, the final result is to trigger a system which should inactivate and eliminate the foreign material.

Recognition must be specific and capable of distinguishing minor differences between different materials, the potential of the system is therefore very great and indeed has a possibility of many millions of reactions. The defence mechanism is non-specific and involves cells such as macrophages which can ingest foreign material, and substances active in tissues or tissue fluid, one example being histamine.

The key role in recognition is played by antibody molecules and lymphocytes. The antibody, known as an immunoglobulin, is a molecule with a structure that allows it to combine with the antigen molecule, rather like two pieces of a jigsaw puzzle. The formation of this complex may cause some inactivation of the antigen, e.g. an exotoxin, but mostly the effect is to trigger the non-specific defence system.

Lymphocytes are divided into T and B types. B lymphocytes have antibody on the cell surface. This recognises a specific antigen. Following this stimulus, the B lymphocyte divides to form plasma cells which secrete antibody. T lymphocytes respond to antigenic stimulus by division into further T lymphocytes. Some of these interact with B lymphocytes either to help them proliferate and produce antibody, or to act as suppressor cells which regulate the B cells' response.

Immunoglobulins are divided into classes, the three main ones being IgM, IgG, and IgA. They are distinguished by a process known as immuno-electrophoresis. If the immunoglobulins are placed on to a strip, the ends allowed to dip into a special solution, and an electrical current passed through, the immunoglobulins tend to move, migrate towards one end of the paper. As each class of immunoglobulin is of a different weight, they all move at different speeds. When the strip is dried and a special stain used, the different classes show up as bands of varying position and width. More sophisticated processes are now available and quantitative estimation can be made of the serum concentrations of each immunoglobulin class present. In health and in certain diseases there are characteristic patterns.

Memory

When an antigen has stimulated the cell line, or clone, which is specific to it, it causes that cell line to produce more cells. This has the effect of causing a 'memory'. A second challenge by the same antigen then produces a much faster and efficient response. It is a well known fact that some illnesses result in life long immunity.

Auto-immunity

It is obviously important that the body should recognise its own protein and during the first days of an infant's life this 'self' recognition is established. Therefore when the immune system is mature, 'self' destruction does not take place. However in certain disease states the body does form antibodies to its own tissues and so destroys them, examples of such diseases are haemolytic anaemia and thyroiditis. Various theories have been advanced to explain the phenomenon including genetic predisposition.

Clones and Grafts

Each cell as it divides by mitosis produces daughter cells genetically exactly like itself. This cell line is called a clone. Such reproduction is asexual. In sexual reproduction, one chromosome of each chromosome pair in the resultant cell is derived from one parent, the other parent contributing the other chromosome. It is therefore genetically different from each parent. In humans this genetic dissimilarity means that tissues from one body will not be accepted by another body, because although both are human, the genetically determined human leucocyte antigen systems differ, they are not compatible. A perfect match can only be obtained from an identical twin. The aim of the tests to find a suitable donor for transplant surgery is to discover as close a match as is possible. To avoid rejection by the host, immuno-suppressive drugs must be used to prevent the host destroying (rejecting) the graft through reaction to the non-compatible fraction.

Polyclonal and Monoclonal Antibodies

Most antibody responses are made up of several different antibodies recognising different antigens on the foreign molecule. Each antibody is derived from a separate clone of cells. Such an antibody response is called polyclonal. If a single clone making one specific antibody is isolated, the antibody is then designated monoclonal.

It is now possible to fuse two cells together and maintain the resulting hybridoma. Myeloma tumours produce large quantities of immunoglobulins and proliferate rapidly. Mice injected with an antigen will develop antibody producing lymphocytes, each antibody specific for one antigenic site on the foreign molecule. Fusing these two types of cell gives rise to several different hybridoma cells, each secreting a specific antibody. These are separated and the individual clones maintained. If large quantities of the monoclonal antibodies they produce are required, they can be injected into animals or cultured.

Prostaglandins, Interferon

These are substances which form the subject of medical articles, and not infrequently figure in the lay press. There are several different types of prostaglandin. Increasingly they are being considered to be involved in immunological responses, they are capable of producing the classical features of inflammation.

Interferons are synthesised by leucocytes and fibroblasts. It is believed that interferons have a role in preventing viral infections and have an inhibitory effect on tumour cells. Interest in their role in cancer therapy has been stimulated because the substances can now be produced more easily. Formerly extracted from human cells the yield was low, but by inserting the necessary genetic information into bacteria or yeasts so that they produce the interferon, much higher yields have been obtained. One use to which monoclonal antibodies have been put is to purify interferon.

It is not possible to give either full details of some of these biological processes or to discuss all the fascinating possibilities. Many scientific papers have been written on each subject and the reader is advised to consult these and the appropriate textbooks. Their importance here is that in subsequent chapters these technical terms will be used from time to time.

Cancer is often described as unconquerable.
It poses many problems,
Its pattern of behaviour is unpredictable.
Its causation is variable,
Its spread is elusive,
Its treatment manifold.
Its understanding requires a lifetime,
A lifetime of thousands of men.

3   Yesterday, Today and Tomorrow

For centuries cancer has been a problem, a challenge to the intellect and imagination of Man. At times it has seemed unanswerable, yet despite failure the will to succeed never fails. The disease is as old as Man himself. The evidence survives in the remains of the old civilisations. Its treatment has been infinitely varied and at times bizarre. The ancient Egyptians trephined the skull to let out the evil spirits, when often the patient must have been suffering from a brain tumour. The theories concerning the cause of the disease have been equally varied, ranging from a belief that cancer was a retribution for sin to the evil influence of witches. Though the treatment offered for malignant disease has improved during the last few decades, the rapidity of its advance has not been fully matched by understanding of the basic process. The other fields of medicine have experienced explosive expansions of knowledge, but progress in the field of malignant disease has so far been slow and gradual. The minds and imaginations of many brilliant men have been turned upon the problem and there is continuing research into all its many aspects. The break will come, we shall then have the equivalent of penicillin or the transplanted kidney. The overall improvement has been the sum of many small advances either in diagnosis or in treatment.

From our simple diagram we can trace on broad lines the normal and abnormal patterns of cellular activity. On the one hand we have peaceful community activity resulting finally in ageing and death, on the other a state of anarchy resulting, if unchecked, in the death of local tissues and finally the host. The aim of all workers in this field is to resolve the question mark, to find out what causes the parent cell to take the path towards the malignant cellular state. Yet this question poses another: 'What causes the cell to follow a normal path?' Both states are living processes, eventually we find we are dealing with the question of life itself, and to define life humbles the greatest.

BIRTH

|
Parent Cell

Normal Cellular State   Malignant Cellular State

Normal Tissue Pattern   Loss of Tissue Pattern

Ordered Function and Control   Loss of Purpose and Function

Organisation   Disorganisation and
and Discipline = Peace   Loss of Control = Anarchy

Ageing = Natural Decline   Metastases and Invasion =
                                         War on Many Fronts

DEATH
The Diversion, to be Restored to Normal

The Problem

To every investigator, past, present, or future, the problem presents itself in many aspects; we shall define four, and then review what has been achieved, the work now being done, and possible future developments. These four headings are:

1. *Clinical*. The behaviour of the disease in patients.
2. *The disease process*. This involves all levels from gross anatomy to the activity of the cell and its constituents.
3. *Carcinogens*. The factors initiating malignant development.
4. *Treatment*. This may be further subdivided into prevention, detection, cure.

Clinical. The Past

The research worker must first be presented with the problem which the clinician has observed. The only tools for investigations which the doctor had until recently were his own senses. He could apply his ear to the chest or taste the urine for sugar, now he has a sophisticated battery of apparatus. He began with the stethoscope and progressed to the present electronic systems of analysis, yet it must not be forgotten that the cornerstone of research is still patient, careful, clinical observation.

Epidemiology

Epidemiology is a study which by surveying the history of patients suffering from the same disease, seeks to find a pattern of common factors which will explain its causation, its progress, and lead ultimately to its cure and perhaps its prevention. All doctors are to a certain extent epidemiologists, their observations can only be fully understood after laboratory investigation, but it is from what they have seen in patients that research advances have been made. Potts, in the last century, noted that there was a high incidence of carcinoma of the scrotum among chimney sweeps and concluded that soot was the causative agent. Laboratory work later isolated the carcinogen, adding to the growing body of evidence on the relation of chemical carcinogens and skin cancer. Realisation of the link between the radiation given off by radioactive materials, and the subsequent development of carcinoma, followed clinical observation; many uranium ore workers suffered from carcinoma of the lung, other workers noted that among girls who used radium to paint the dials of luminous watches malignant bone tumours were more common than in the normal population.

Remission and Regression

The progress of cancer is not always relentlessly downward, natural remissions and regressions occur. Often the careful clinician noting these has been able to suggest forms of treatment or theories of causation. Well documented cases of regression following an anaphylactoid type of illness stimulated an interest in the whole question of the body's immune response to malignancy. Observation of normal physiological processes has also led to advances. In 1896 Beatson wrote in *The Lancet* of his experience of a regression of breast carcinoma following oophorectomy. He had formulated a theory of the influence of the ovary on breast carcinoma after a study of lactation. From this beginning has grown the hormone therapy of breast carcinoma.

Genetics

Familial adenomatous polyposis of the colon is an inherited disease. In a high proportion of these patients one of the polyps undergoes malignant change. This strong familial tendency to carcinoma — the families concerned have been carefully studied has been one of the facts reviewed by workers looking into the possibility of an inherited, genetic basis for the development of cancer.

Radiation

Radiation itself has proved to be carcinogenic if given in excess of tolerance. We have already seen that many early workers paid the price of ignorance of this fact, and after the atomic bomb explosions the link between radiation and leukaemia became evident. Support to this theory was given by a study of the patients in Britain who had received high doses of radiation to the whole spine as a treatment for ankylosing spondylitis, the subsequent rate of development of leukaemia among them was higher than in the rest of the population.

Clinical. The Present

Epidemiology

At this time clinical observation has given an impetus to research into several carcinogens. The strong link between smoking and carcinoma of the lung, the larynx, and the bladder, was found after careful study of the clinical history of many patients. It has been noted that carcinoma of the nasopharynx appears to be more common among workers in the woodworking industry, research is now being carried out on precipitating factors and the possible role of wood dust as a carcinogen. Carcinoma of the cervix has been found to be very rare in virgins, and further work demonstrated a link between the disease, early age of first coitus and the social status of the patient. Now the role of the viral infections which cause clinical herpes and genital warts has come under scrutiny. This epidemiological work has directed further research. An outstanding example of observation leading first to surveys in the field, and then on to laboratory studies is the work of Denis Burkitt, a surgeon who was working in East Africa. Among his patients he had a large number of children suffering from lymphoma of the jaw. Plotting the incidence he discovered a geographical concentration of the disease, and was led to postulate the existence of an infection as a cause. Laboratory work showed the presence of a virus and it was suggested that infection might be spread by an insect vector. The position is complicated by the discovery of this same virus associated not only with other tumours but also non-malignant disease. Intensive laboratory work is going on to define the exact role of this agent.

Genetics

Interest in genetics is still strong. Patients suffering from breast carcinoma often have a family history of the disease. Animal experiments have shown a genetic

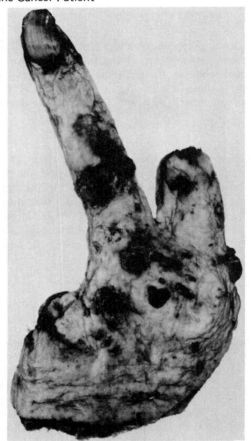

Fig.3.1.   Radiation dermatitis (pathological specimen).
Many progressed to carcinoma

link in mice with the same disease, but caution must be exercised in applying these results to humans, laboratory animals are the progeny from pure strain breeding, human beings most certainly are not. Clinical observation of the variation of the disease with the hormonal status of the women, pre- or post-menopausal, together with its familial tendency encouraged research into a screening test. This was based on the ratio between certain hormones excreted in the urine, such a hormone pattern might be inherited. Time must elapse before it is possible to know whether such a predictive test is valid.

Carcinogens

By clinical observation and animal experiments the link between certain factors and particular types of cancer has been proved, chemical, soot and cancer of the

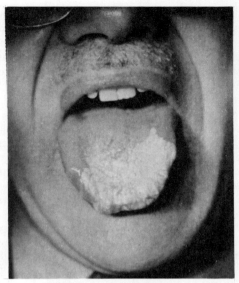

Fig. 3.2.   Leukoplakia of the tongue showing 'coat of paint'
appearance and fissuring

scrotum, physical, repeated burns and cancer of the skin, genetic, polyposis and
intestinal cancer. Other studies have been directed towards the relationship
between malignancy and factors such as leukoplakia, a pre-malignant condition
of the skin, syphillis and carcinoma of the tongue, iron deficiency anaemia and
pharyngeal carcinoma. Knowing how in the past so-called harmless substances
have been found to be carcinogenic, great vigilance is exercised over new products.
Artificial food flavourings have been banned on suspicion, and any widely used
drug, such as the oral contraceptive, is closely monitored.

Research was directed to discovering how these substances cause a cell to
become malignant, a change in the chromosome, in the protein synthesis, or
in some other cellular system? The theory was that carcinogens offered an
initial sensitising insult to the cell which was regarded as 'primed'. Since not
all such 'primed' cells become malignant, it was suggested that one, or maybe
several co-carcinogens (other unknown factors), may induce malignancy after a
latent period. At present research into the disease process itself has both modified and extended this theory.

The Disease Process

Research into the disease was for a long time limited by the comparatively crude
tools available. Naked-eye and microscopical observations were made on biopsy
and post-mortem material, chemical carcinogens were isolated and their causative role proved in animal experiments. However, the advent of the electron
microscope with its revelation of the cell's structure brought into the field many

workers who had previously been able to play little part. The biochemist with improved methods has been able to investigate the structure of the chromosomes, the nature of the genes, and protein synthesis within the cell. He is investigating the chemical differences between the normal and abnormal cell. Animal experiments are valuable, but the results cannot necessarily be applied to humans. The biologist who discovered a method of culturing mammalian cells made possible the study of living human tumours in the laboratory. The virologist has joined the research team and is looking at the role of viruses in malignant disease. The remissions which can occur naturally have led other biologists to study the immune reaction of the host to the tumour. From this has followed work, on the immune system as the source of the antibodies taking part in this immune reaction, and on the development of methods, such as anti-tumour vaccines, to enhance it. The epidemiologist can often save research time by pointing to the lines of enquiry most likely to yield results in treatment and prevention.

However a very fundamental discovery has altered our way at looking at all these different findings. We know that the way the cell behaves is governed by its genetic code carried in the genes on the chromosomes, but although a gene may be present it is not always active or 'expressed'. Two terms are used to describe these states, genotype for the basic potential, and phenotype for the actual expression (behaviour). It is known that there are many genes on the chromosomes which are never expressed. Why they are there we are not sure, they could be relics of our very distant developmental past, but they do by their presence have an effect on the position on the chromosome of 'active' genes. This spatial pattern may be significant in the control of the degree of activity of genes.

So far in looking for the initial change which sends a normal cell down the malignant path we have searched for qualitative differences, an actual change in the chemical composition of a cell. Now however it is known that the presence *in excess* of substances quite normally produced by a cell can confer on it malignant potential. The genes which code for the production of these substances are called oncogenes. Now some of the previously observed facts are capable of a slightly different interpretation. A virus which passes from one host to another may by chance pick up an oncogene from one, incorporate it in its own D.N.A. and 'infect' the new host by giving it an increased oncogene content. Some genes are promoters of the activity of others, a virus could by chance insert a promoter gene next to an oncogene causing overproduction of the normal substance coded by the host gene, as if the accelerator jammed. For such a rare chance event, continuous infection for a long time would be necessary, hence the long latent period between infection and the appearance of malignancy.

While the mutation of chromosomes caused by chemicals, radiation, etc., is a fact, its significance may lie in a possible enhancement of an oncogene. At the same time the carcinogen could be acting by altering the positioning of an oncogene on the chromosome again resulting in enhanced activity and over-production.

This initial change, if not deleted by the host's surveillance systems, will cause further stepwise changes in the cell leading to malignancy. It may be that familial or regional differences in cancer incidence lie in either the inherited surveillance capacity, or in the environmental co-carcinogens or carcinoma repressors. This means that epidemiological findings may become very relevant to prevention or even therapy. For instance could a natural constituent of a diet help to control cancer? A tribe in Kashmir is thought to have a very low incidence of cancer and to eat a diet rich in benzaldehyde, and benzaldehyde has been claimed to cause regression in some cancers.

Treatment

Prevention

It is not necessary to know how carcinogens act to prevent the development of cancer. Carcinoma of the scrotum among textile workers whose clothing was soaked by lubricating oil, was eliminated by proper measures. The recognition of the carcinogenic role of aromatic amines used in the rubber and cable industry led to industrial legislation, and to the periodic survey of workers at risk.

Exciting though basic research is, it has not yet pointed the way to any major breakthrough in treatment. Prevention must therefore be pursued even more energetically than in the past. Carcinoma of the lung is extremely difficult to treat but it is preventable. Where smoking has been reduced, as among British doctors, the incidence has fallen significantly. We have here a disease which is 90% preventable, but is not prevented because, despite wide publicity given to the facts, most people persist in smoking. We need detailed sociological studies to discover the reasons for this attitude.

Now that the dangers of excessive radiation are known a code of protection has been drawn up, the dosages to which both the public and workers in medicine and industry may be exposed have been decided, and the whole question kept constantly under review. As research provides more answers swift action must be taken to expand preventive measures.

Detection

Early Diagnosis and Education   For too long cancer has been veiled in mystery and superstition, for tumours are often inaccessible, are symptomless when small, and cannot be inspected. Therefore the patient is not alerted and often goes to the doctor when the disease is well advanced and little can be offered. A visible or palpable tumour is a late tumour in the biological sense. The clinician has a better chance in many cases if the tumour is treated in its early stages. This problem can be tackled by education and by improved methods of screening and investigation.

Education of the public should include both knowledge of early symptoms and the realisation that orthodox medicine can offer so much. If this work has been done well patients will come earlier and quack cures will fall into disrepute. The doctor too needs education. Patients may not be referred because there is no realisation of what can be done, or because signs and symptoms, which are commonplace to the specialist in malignancy, may be missed because they are vague or rarely seen. A vigorous programme needs to be followed both in medical schools and post-graduate centres. To ensure adequate coverage every aid should be employed, the film, the videotape, the film strip, television, and programmed learning. I hope this book may help.

Screening   There are signs that there is some change in the public attitude, certain women's organisations pressed very hard for the establishment of cervical screening clinics. To call them Well Woman Clinics was a sound psychological step, for those attending have thereby accepted more readily an examination of the breast, and the idea of returning periodically for routine checks. When carcinoma of the cervix is detected at this asymptomatic stage it can usually be cured, and a lump in the breast may be detected before the patient is even aware of it herself.

At present the technique of X-raying the breast, mammography, which can detect tumours before they are palpable, is usually used only for patients who have known or suspected disease.

A programme in which all women at risk are screened can generate many questions, and the conclusions drawn, as for example from the New York project, may be the subject of fierce debate. In the U.K. a pilot scheme to compare two comparable populations, one screened, the other not, may take longer but produce data less open to question.

In industry carcinogens cannot always be eliminated. Workers at risk must be protected and regularly screened. With the help of trained personnel officers it is often possible to get other screening unrelated to the industrial hazards accepted. It is often only by this approach that women at risk from cervical cancer can be contacted.

Investigations

Whatever the test, the aim is to see whether there is a change from normal, be it numerical, a raised white cell count, in the image produced, a difference in quality such as myeloma protein, or a changed reaction to a stimulus, as skin testing with antigens. If such a difference is found, the question must then be asked, is this due to malignant disease?

Imaging

Under this heading can now be grouped all the varying methods of producing an image which shows contrasts between normal tissues, and are sensitive enough to show up the abnormal. Such images may be static with pictures taken at set intervals, or dynamic with continuous recording and either a ciné or speeded up sequential display. Some or all of these investigations may be grouped in a department loosely labelled Radiology, in other hospitals separate departments deal with different techniques. Some procedures are as yet experimental, but will rapidly become part of the everyday investigation routines.

X-rays

To the plain X-ray and contrast studies have been added the CATscan, sub-traction radiography, lymphography, mammography, the list is constantly expanding. The CATscan, computerised axial tomography scan, was originally called the EMI scan after the firm that pioneered the method. A very narrow X-ray beam is moved in an arc around a patient. The emerging radiation at each point is registered by sensitive detectors on the opposite side of the patient. The amount of absorption in a grid pattern corresponding to the area of the beam is stored in a computer as a series of values. The thousands of readings obtained can then be used to make an X-ray picture. The tomogram represents a slice. By repeating the procedure at stated intervals up and down from the point of interest, not only can a series of horizontal pictures be produced, but also others for different planes.

Subtraction radiography is a technical manipulation of X-ray views of the same area with and without contrast medium. The effect is to ghost out the tissues which are not of immediate interest. The technique is of particular value when, even with contrast medium, there is little difference between adjacent tissues, as for example an artery containing contrast medium lying over bone.

Radioactive Isotopes

We have already discussed how radioactive isotopes can be used in diagnosis. The functioning secondaries of a thyroid tumour may not show up on con-ventional X-rays, but may be detected after the injection of radioactive iodine. Others can be used to assess function, as for example hippuran in the kidney. Now, short lived isotopes which emit particles called positrons are being used experimentally. The positrons travel only a few millimetres in tissue, and when they stop, their energy is transformed, given off in a definite pattern, and can be detected outside the body. If an isotope of oxygen is used, then not only is its location detected, but also as it enters into tissue metabolism its route and the extent of its uptake can be traced and measured, the route being oxygen in the lungs, oxyhaemoglobin, diffusion into the tissues, return to the blood in products of metabolism. That is of course a gross simplification of a very complex process. The technique is called positron emission tomography, PET.

Ultra-sound

There are sounds which are above the range of the human ear. We have all seen dogs respond to someone blowing an apparently silent whistle. We are also familiar with echoes, sound bounced back from some object so that we can hear it twice, the original followed by the echo. The two notes of a police car seem to change in pitch as it comes towards us and then goes away, this is called the Doppler effect. All these effects are exploited to produce images using ultra-sound. A pulse of ultra-sound is beamed into the patient, and the resultant echoes from the various tissues recorded and used to build an image. Sophisticated developments have enabled the diameter of blood vessels to be measured, and, utilising the Doppler effect, the speed of blood flow also. Ultra-sound can be used to visualise the foetus without harmful effects. In other situations it is also not only an alternative to X-rays, but can produce better diagnostic images.

The contrast in echoes, particularly in enclosed spaces such as the heart chambers, can be enhanced. The contrast medium is not iodine containing like the conventional media, but much more nearly physiological. Dextrose 5% can be used. It gives different echoes from blood and looks like tiny bubbles in the ultra-sound images. Ciné pictures of the heart after giving it as a bolus injection, show the flow patterns in the chambers.

Nuclear Magnetic Resonance (N.M.R.)

CATscans have now become part of the conventional radiology scene, it is likely that N.M.R. scanning will also rapidly become established. Anyone who has brought a magnet near a compass has seen the needle deflect, and then swing back to the original position when the magnet is taken away. Before settling back it does however waver. The nucleus of an atom has certain magnetic properties, and therefore if an external magnetic field is applied certain movements occur, these can be varied by applying in pulses another field at right angles. The resultant changes are characteristic for different atomic nuclei, the one usually studied is the proton, the hydrogen nucleus. Images depend upon the relative concentration of these protons in the tissues, and these will vary with disease and functional states.

Monoclonal Antibodies

These have been used experimentally both in diagnosis and therapy. If a monoclonal antibody specific to a tumour can be linked to a radioactive isotope, the antibody should concentrate in the tumour and its metastases, the radioactivity it carries can be then detected in the conventional way. Radioactive iodine has been used in most of the work done so far.

Exfoliative Cytology

Cells are constantly shed from epithelial surfaces and can be recovered from the body by suitable techniques. The sputum contains cells from the lungs, they may also be found in gastric washings; cervical or vaginal smears will contain those shed from the cervix. By using special stains the histologist can examine these specimens and detect cells which are dysplastic, that is abnormal but not frankly malignant, and those which are definitely malignant. This type of study is called exfoliative cytology. Its importance with regard to the cervical smear lies in its ability to detect malignancy in advance of symptoms, that is in the early stage when the disease is curable.

Biochemistry

Rapid strides have been made in the investigation of the chemistry of the cell. The structure of the nucleic acids has been discovered, the chemical processes of the cytoplasm are being slowly explored. Improved methods of analysis have enabled the biochemist to trace abnormal metabolites in body fluids. These markers are useful but are not generally sufficiently specific to be predictive. As work goes on, it becomes clear that the researches of the biochemist and the biologist overlap, and the distinction between their fields becomes blurred.

Therapy

Radiation

At first the only weapons were magic, incantations, bizarre ointments. Their uniting feature was their total ineffectiveness. More scientific but still with little success was haphazard surgery and cautery. Treatment only began to advance with the discovery of X-rays and radium in the last five years of the 19th Century, and the co-operation which then became possible between the surgeon and the radiotherapist. The early machines were used with little knowledge of either the hazards or the benefits of radiation. The penetration was poor, the limits of treatment not defined, and the protection of the operator non-existent. Some early workers developed dermatitis and subsequently cancer of the skin. There were no methods of measuring either the dose given or the total dose required; one woman who was given several treatments to epilate the skin of the face later developed a malignant growth at the same site. Today both the patient and operator are protected, the dosage is measured, the limits known. The machines range through the gamut of X-rays, radioactive isotope, and electron therapy. Radium, which was once the only source of contact therapy, has been joined by a sophisticated group of substances often tailored specifically to their purpose.

Oxygen Effect   One of the difficulties in treating a tumour is that parts of it are less well oxygenated, anoxic, this decreases the sensitivity of the cells to radiation. Such cells escape the full effect of treatment and may well become the nucleus of recurrence. To overcome this various methods have been employed.

1. By raising the oxygen tension of the body during radiation; this can only be done by putting the patient into an oxygen tank and raising the pressure to three or four times that of the ordinary air. This is tedious, often uncomfortable for the patient, and is not without its hazards.
2. By employing particles of the atom, neutrons, which have no electrical charge. The radiation they give is less influenced by oxygen tension, so far this method is in the experimental stage.
3. Sensitisers are chemicals which enhance the damage done by radiation or radio-mimetic cytotoxic drugs. This should help to overcome the anoxic effect. This work is still experimental, the first drug used, metronizadole, had to be given in doses which were toxic, and research is directed to discovering more effective, less toxic substances.

Surgery

At various stages improved surgical techniques have contributed much to the control and palliation of tumours. The surgeon can alter the hormonal environment by ablation procedures, hypophysectomy, adrenalectomy; where he is unable to remove the tumour he can for example often relieve raised intracranial pressure by a by-pass; by many other operations he can supplement the work of the radiotherapist. The instrument maker, by the use of flexible fibres which transmit light and magnification, has enabled the surgeon to view the pleural and peritoneal spaces, and photograph a viscus such as the stomach, and has also put into his hands the powerful laser.

Chemotherapy

Certain drugs have been found to mimic the effects of radiation and have therefore been called radio-mimetic drugs. Because they are poisonous to cells they are also called cytotoxic agents. They are used to treat malignant disease, either alone or as an adjunct to surgery or radiation. Their effect is most marked on dividing cells, and so they attack not only tumour cells but normal cells also, particularly those of the bone marrow. Treatment is often limited because of the effect on the bone marrow, a fall in white-blood-cell count giving rise to poor resistance to infection, and a fall in platelets resulting in spontaneous bruising and haemorrhage. Current research is directed towards finding new agents which will be effective anti-tumour drugs, more specific, and at the same time not depress the blood-cell count too dangerously.

Radioactive Isotopes

These are used as an established method of treatment, radioactive phosphorus to stop excessive red-cell formation (polycythaemia vera), radioactive iodine to destroy functioning thyroid tumour. Another use is for the palliation of pleural or peritoneal secondaries. An isotope emitting short-range radiation, such as yttrium, can be placed in the cavity after taking off a malignant effusion. In some cases this will destroy the seedling metastases and stop further fluid accumulating.

Monoclonal Antibodies

These have been used experimentally to destroy malignant cells. A necessary condition is that either the antigen to which the monoclonal antibody binds is specific, or, that if it is present on normal cells it should be in low concentration, or the normal cell one which will be replaced. So far success has been greater against circulating cells than tumour masses, perhaps because of poor penetration, changes in antigen, or a change in the cell's membrane.

A second possible use is to combine the antibody with another substance toxic to the malignant cells. Again experiments have shown that coupling it with a radioactive isotope can produce a concentrated lethal dose of radiation in malignant tissue. Similarly if linked to cytotoxics by a chemical bond which can be broken by enzymes in the cell, a far higher dose could be given locally than would be tolerated systemically. The use of powerful cell poisons such as ricin, or diphtheria toxin similarly linked, is another possibility.

The Role of the Oncologist

There are no diseases, only patients with disease.

The oncologist has progressed much since the early days. His machines are more sophisticated, his knowledge of their potentialities and dangers are greater. Yet his role still remains above all to care for the whole man. The patient first visits the doctor with what may seem a trivial complaint, his suspicion and anxiety mount as he is referred to the hospital, and finally to the oncologist. The first interview presents the therapist with the most difficult task of all. He must understand the patient's hopes and fears and remove his misconceptions. The trust established at this first meeting, enables him to leave the consulting room with a confidence in the doctor and the department which hopefully will persist throughout the whole of his treatment and after-care.

The Future

While efforts will continue to use radiation more effectively, overcome the effects of anoxia, use particles of the atom not yet in service, synthesise more specific cytotoxic drugs or develop the use of isotopes, logical advances in treatment will grow out of the emerging results of basic research into the process of carcinogenesis. Until now treatment has been empirical, that is to say it has been found to be effective, but the reasons for this have not been completely understood.

Detection and Early Diagnosis

The tests so far described still only detect established malignancy. What is needed are reliable sensitive tests to detect the cell at the point of deviation from normal, this would give the clinician a reasonable chance. Ideally if the cell carrying within itself the seeds of change could be discovered, treatment could then be preventive. The exciting discoveries concerning the nature of how a cancer cell differs from normal may offer us a means of realising such a hope.

Education

Prevention

As we have already seen a great effort must be made to eliminate carcinogens from our environment. To do this the educated co-operation of the public is required. Where it is possible to eradicate a carcinogen all modern means of communication must be used to reach the lay public. This is a gigantic task. We have to change habits, as with smoking, or even to alter a way of life. It will be impossible without the help of sociology and psychiatry.

Early Diagnosis

Unfortunately the discussion of cancer is still almost taboo. It is now regarded in the same way as tuberculosis was before the advent of effective drugs. Even doctors are often reluctant to face the problem with their patients. There is greater awareness of the need for discussion with relatives and with the patient if he wishes, but in turn this may lead to an opposite extreme, the thrusting of information on to people ill-prepared to deal with it and the belief that this traumatic outpouring of the truth is adequate and humane.

Patients must be encouraged to seek help early. In the civilised world, cancer, above all diseases, breeds a fear that paralyses action. It is more than apathy, it is an active fear of having a suspicion confirmed. It is common to all levels of society, a matter of the emotions rather than the intellect. The basis of this inertia may well be that it is not realised how much can be done to help, for, once the initial step has been taken there is relief at sharing the knowledge and often a new found confidence in facing the facts. Workers in this field must, despite pressure of work, devote time not only to talking to patients and relatives, but also to any groups of people prepared to listen.

Research

Communication

Communication is vital to research. Often contact between the research worker and the doctor in the field is small. Those who are working with patients can provide research with pointers to the most fruitful lines to follow, while in return the laboratory can ask for observations on theories formulated after experiments. Together far more can be achieved than by each working in iso-lation. How can this better communication be established? Conferences and meetings are valuable but they take up time and cannot be too frequent. Few can attend, and the papers delivered take time to be published, so that the results of current work are slow to circulate. Local meetings at hospital level increase local co-operation, but there is a need for rapid access to up-to-date information. Using computers, some agency is required that could store the results of world-wide work and release it to any enquirer. Yet this would still only be storage of facts emerging at the end of research programmes which could have stretched over years. Clinicians and researchers need to be able to discuss their current work, problems, and results. Telecommunication satellites could provide the means whereby face-to-face discussion could take place, and demonstrations of experiments be made, although the centres taking part might be thousands of miles apart, mobile links are beginning to be established to enable third world countries to have access to specialised diagnostic programmes in the developed world. Computers could store the information, keep it updated, and give a print-out whenever required.

The Questions

What are the questions to be answered?
WHY DOES THE CELL REMAIN NORMAL?
WHAT IS THE ROLE OF THE VIRUS, CARCINOGENS, AND HOW DO THEY ACT?
WHAT IS THE REACTION BETWEEN HOST AND TUMOUR?
Recent discoveries about the probable initial difference between normal and malignant cells at last gives some hope, not only of more specific therapy but even of reversing the malignant process. Malignant cells have the ability to migrate within the body, a return to the state of a unicellular organism. Is this due to the expression of genes long since suppressed in development, has a promoter gene been inserted close to them by the action of a virus or carcinogen? It is possible that substances naturally present in the diet or the environment prevent the step wise development of malignancy or reverse it. If so it is feasible that they should be used both to treat and prevent malignancy, the cytostatic approach. Some cancer cells seem to require growth factors in the tissue fluid around them in order to divide, some indeed produce these factors themselves, autostimulation. It may therefore be possible to synthesise substances which would preferentially occupy the sites to which these growth factors bind.

The clinician, the nurse, and the patient could well ask what is the relevance of all this research to the present situation. The answer must surely be that while it is not apparent today, it could well be tomorrow.

Hypotheses upon hypotheses of tumour formation have been formulated only to explode into myths like balloons at the prick of a pin. We have posed but a few of the questions, there are yet many more to be asked, but it may be that answering just one question, the right question, will be decisive.

Man in his experimental research,
May well have sacrificed animals on its altar.
Yet in the end,
Man himself must be the inevitable
And final experimental animal.

4 Cytotoxic Chemotherapy

AIMS

The target is the malignant cell and the aims of chemotherapy are the same as for any form of cancer treatment. They can be summarised as follows.

Action on the tumour:

1. Arrest of cellular growth and division.
2. Destruction.
3. Replacement by normal tissue.
4. No recurrence.

Action on the whole body:

1. No death or maiming.
2. No irreparable damage to normal tissue.
3. No initiation of change leading to future malignancy.

At once it becomes obvious that this is an ideal and that no present treatment meets all these requirements.

Before we can discuss the mode of action of these drugs, we must remind ourselves briefly of the structure and physiology of a cell.

Nucleus, Chromosome and Genes

When a cell reproduces itself normally by mitosis, the daughter cells have the same structure, and carry out exactly the same functions as the parent. A cell's activity is governed by the chromosomes in the nucleus. A chromosome is formed from a special nucleic acid called deoxyribonucleic acid, D.N.A. This is a long molecule consisting of two strands joined chemically at certain points, the double helix. Each chromosome carries genes along its length. The genes are made up of sequences of organic chemicals called bases. There are only four types of

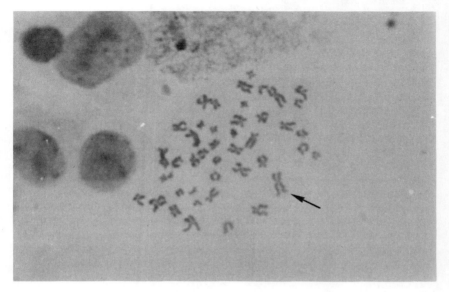

Fig. 4.1.   Normal chromosomes

base, the difference between the genes lies in the order in which these bases are arranged and in the number each contains. Each gene lies at a specific point (locus) along the chromosome, opposite the corresponding gene on the other chromosome of the pair. The total combination of genes is the code for all a cell's activities and structure. Each cell at division passes this genetic coding unchanged to the daughter cells. A dividing cell in the basal layer of the skin will produce daughter cells exactly like itself, behaving like skin cells and not for instance like cells of the stomach mucosa.

Mitosis (Replacement Division)

During replacement division the chromosomes split along their length and each forms two chromatids. Each pair thus forms two pairs, mirror images of each other. The cytoplasm of the cell divides and the mirror-image pairs separate into the two resultant cells. Each cell then has 46 chromosomes, 23 pairs.

Meiosis (Sexual Reproduction)

During sexual reproduction a male germ cell, spermatozoon, fuses with a female germ cell, ovum. This is fertilisation. If each germ cell contained 46 chromosomes the resultant fertilised ovum would contain 92 and the next generation 184. In fact a reduction takes place at the division, meiosis, in the gonads (sex organs) and the germ cell contains 22 chromosomes and one sex chromosome. Since the female sex pair is always XX all the ova contain X, but the male is XY,

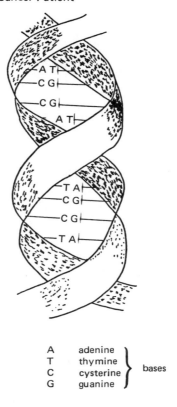

A	adenine	
T	thymine	
C	cysterine	} bases
G	guanine	

Fig. 4.2.   D.N.A. double helix

and the spermatozoa will contain either X or Y. The sex of the child is therefore always determined by the spermatozoon.

Cytoplasm

This cytoplasm is a workshop. It contains vast numbers of amino acids which are the building blocks for the protein molecules, nucleic acids which convey instructions from the nucleus, and enzymes to speed and ease chemical changes. Proteins are built up at a point called the ribosome.

A nucleic acid called messenger R.N.A. (ribonucleic acid) reads off the genetic code on the chromosome. After leaving the nucleus with the coding, messenger R.N.A. travels out through the cytoplasm to the ribosome. Here a second nucleic acid transfer R.N.A. sets to work. It brings up the protein building blocks to the ribosome, fitting them into the correct order according to the code of the messenger R.N.A. The product is a new protein molecule.

The raw materials of the building process are obtained from the food which enters the cell across the wall membrane. Unlike an ordinary factory the cell may have to break down the raw materials into smaller pieces before they can be used. This process is called digestion. It is carried out by the lysosome which contains enzymes. The function of these is to speed up and make easier the chemical changes. Many of these enzymes are contained in the cell. Every factory needs power and the cell obtains this from its store, the mitochondrium.

When the assembly process is complete, the finished product is either used or stored. In the cell the Golgi apparatus acts as a store.

In and Out

The membrane, wall of the cell, consists of layers of fats (lipids) and proteins. The molecules, the building blocks of these layers, are held together by links or bridges. Unlike any ordinary wall it is flexible and parts can break off, the wall on either side closing in to fill the gap. This is one way in which materials enter and leave the cell. A large molecule reaches the cell wall which enfolds it and then sinks down with it into the cytoplasm. This 'bubble' of wall and molecule is called a vacuole. The wall on either side of the gap fills it by closing in. The reverse process passes materials out.

Again, unlike an ordinary wall, the membrane is not solid, it has gaps and is more like a sieve. Very small molecules, like water, can pass through these gaps, so the membrane is called porous. Some of the gaps are large and are the entrances of canals which run through the cytoplasm, some of them reaching the nucleus. This is the endoplasmic reticulum and is another means for transporting materials in and out of the cell.

The membrane wall is selective. It will not allow certain things to pass, or having let them in they are immediately pushed out again. The blood cell is an example of this latter process. Sodium, one of the body's chemicals, can pass the blood-cell wall but it is immediately pushed out. This mechanism is called the sodium pump. It is rather as if the sodium went through a revolving door to reach the other side of the wall, but before it could enter the cell it was carried out again by the revolving door.

Relation of Structure to Chemotherapy

How does this simple account of a fascinating structure relate to the subject of our chapter? It provides us with some understanding of the various processes which our drug can affect. First, of course, it must reach the cell. To do this it must enter the body, oral, intramuscular or intravenous administration, and must then be transported by the blood or the lymph to the tissue fluid which surrounds the cell. Once there it must either break down the wall and so expose the inhabitants of this cellular world to an environment in which they cannot exist, or it must cross the membrane and exert its disruptive influence on one of the processes within the cell. Many of the drug actions can be paralleled in the world of antibacterials. We are all familiar with these processes and it will be probably helpful to bear them in mind, particularly when considering how tumours can become resistant to drugs.

Mode of Action

General

Following radiation, changes in the chromosomes of cells have been noted. A simple discussion of genetics can show us that a chromosome can be disrupted. Part of it may recombine incorrectly after mitosis, or a change can occur in a gene, point mutation. We have now to add to these changes the effects of radiation on the cytoplasm of the cell. This can be damaged by altering or destroying its components. Unless the cell is killed outright the damage only becomes obvious when the cell attempts to divide, mitosis. Since the changes found after using cytotoxic drugs are similar they are often called radio-mimetic.

It would be premature to state that we know how all these drugs work. We know some of the facts, but much of our usage of these agents is empirical, that is we base it on observed response for which as yet we can offer no complete explanation.

History of Chemotherapy

At the beginning of this book I remarked that cancer is as old as man himself and that many remedies have been tried, most of them being distinguished only by their ineffectiveness and their unpleasantness. Many of them were poisons, one of them, arsenic, still lingers on today in different forms. These treatments were enshrined in folklore and many of the materials were derived from plants.

The story of modern antitumour drugs begins with the development of the mustard gases. It is sad that we have had to wait for a war before we found the first true cytotoxic. Nor should we be too contemptuous of our ancestors. The 'wise women' of the past knew the benefits of an extract of foxglove long before the scientist isolated the active ingredient, digitalis. Extracts of the autumn crocus have been used to treat gout for over 1,000 years, but only in the last 30 years have we appreciated its antitumour properties. Sobered by these discoveries we have now embarked on a survey of these and other agents derived from plants and fungi. It is now customary to study any new chemical compound both for its antibacterial and antitumour properties.

True progress, both in therapy and in the synthesis of new drugs, has only been possible as research has uncovered the structure and biochemistry of the cell. Further progress is dependent upon the discovery of fundamental differences between the cancer cell and the normal. As yet chemotherapy is a crude blunderbuss attack. The ideal chemotherapeutic agent would react only with the cells of a specific tumour and leave all normal cells both of the organ and the body unharmed.

Cell Wall

Certain antibacterials act by making the walls of bacteria more permeable and so destroying their selectivity. Penicillin has this type of action. As yet none of the present antitumour agents has been found to possess this property.

Disruption of Assembly

The first antibacterial to be discovered was sulphonamide. In order to make nucleic acids a vitamin, folic acid, is required. This is subjected to a series of chemical changes called a cycle, and each step requires an enzyme for its completion. Sulphonamide disrupts the cycle by its similarity to one of the chemicals, metabolite, produced at one of these steps. It is taken into the cycle but cannot be changed into the next chemical in the chain and so halts the whole process, effectively blocking the use of folic acid. It is as if a nut looking the same as the usual one were put into a factory conveyor-belt process. It is accepted, but when it should be put on to the matching bolt it is found to be slightly different, jams, and so halts the whole assembly line.

Antimetabolites

Methotrexate used in the treatment of leukaemia and chorionepithelioma acts in this way. An enzyme takes up methotrexate in preference to the natural metabolite of folic acid, but because it is slightly different the chemical step cannot be completed. Drugs which act in this way are called antimetabolites. Other agents of this type are 6-mercaptopurine and 6-thioguanine, their clinical usage varies.

Chemical Numbers

Chemicals which form part of living organisms are called organic. The groups of atoms of which they are composed are often joined in a ring structure. To each of these groups can be added on a string of other groups. these are known as side chains. To make it easier to discuss changes, each group in the ring is numbered, and any significant change there, or in the attached side chain, is referred to the number. It is a form of shorthand, 5-fluorouracil is a short way of writing that in the uracil ring the chemical group at position 5 has been changed to fluorine.

Attacking D.N.A.

Any saboteur infiltrating an enemy position aims to do the most damage, and if he can destroy the headquarters he will probably achieve his objective. Similarly, a cytotoxic drug which acts directly on D.N.A. must affect the whole cell since it is the D.N.A. which regulates the cell's life. Several agents have this action although the exact method by which they achieve it is not always known.

Alkylating Agents

A large number of cytotoxic drugs belong to this group. Certain chemical groups have an affinity for each other, that is to say they react with each other and result in a new compound. One such group is called an alkyl radical and the groups with which it reacts are present in many body tissues. Since many of these drugs are unstable in solution attempts to modify them have been made.

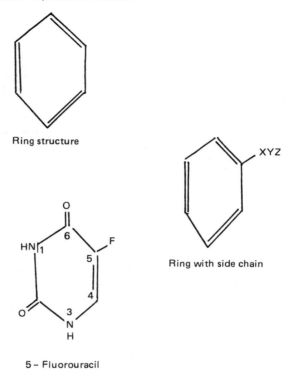

Ring structure

Ring with side chain

5 – Fluorouracil

Fig. 4.3.   Chemical ring structures

A change in the size of the molecule often resulted in the product being too big to cross the cell membrane. Alternative approaches were to attach the radical to a molecule which would be incorporated into a biochemical process, melphalan is an example of this type; or to make the drug inert until it was attacked by enzymes so releasing the active radical, cyclophosphamide represents this type.

Some of the alkylating agents are listed at the end of the chapter; the difference between them is partly the length of time the drug remains in the body.

The alkylating agents attack D.N.A. in various ways. D.N.A. is made up of two strands which are joined by links formed between certain chemical groups called bases. Each base pairs only with a specific base on the opposite strand. When each strand doubles before mitosis these links are broken. It is thought that one action of the alkylating radical is to provide an unbreakable link between the strands, normal replication before cellular division is thereby blocked. A change in a gene, mutation, can also be produced or the strand of D.N.A. may be so weakened that it breaks and replication is halted.

For the complete list of drugs, the nurse is referred to the table at the end of the chapter. The differences between them probably relate to the amount which reaches the cell and crosses into the cytoplasm. Further differences will result from the biochemical state within the cell itself.

The history of this patient will illustrate the use of the oldest member of this group, nitrogen mustard.

Mr. – was in his forties and suffering from Hodgkin's disease. Four years previously he had received radiation to glands in the neck and to the mediastinum and had remained well. He then developed recurrence in the radiated area, and signs of systemic involvement, fever and sweating. He was admitted for a course of nitrogen mustard. He experienced severe vomiting after the first injection, but the premedication was changed and he completed the course without any similar reaction. The fever subsided, the glands regressed, he returned to work and remained fit for a further 18 months. He then showed signs of enlarged mediastinal glands and had a further cytotoxic course. The effect on the glands could be seen from these X-rays taken before and after treatment.

Plant Extracts

The life of a cell is often spoken of as a cycle. The peak of its activity is during the process of mitosis and during much of the rest of the cycle it is said to be in a resting phase. The mitotic period is called the metaphase and it is during this part of the cycle that a cell is most vulnerable. The time taken for completion of a cycle varies with types of cells and within a tumour there may be several different cycle times. If the cells could be arrested in the metaphase not only would they be more vulnerable to attack by radiation or other chemical agents, it would also prevent the completion of mitosis and hence replication.

An extract of the autumn crocus, colchicine, will arrest cells in metaphase, the chromosomes replicate but mitosis fails. However this drug is now not used so frequently.

Substances derived from the periwinkle (*Vinca rosea*) are known as vinca alkaloids, they are vincristine and vinblastine. Vindesine is a drug synthesised from vinblastine. All interfere with metaphase, probably by disrupting the spindle elements to which the chromatids are attracted prior to the completion of mitosis.

Study of extracts from the plant *Podophyllum* led to the introduction of two drugs, etoposide and teniposide. They act as spindle poisons and also cause single strand breaks in D.N.A.

Antibiotics

Actinomycin D was the first drug in this group to be used widely. It forms a complex with D.N.A. which is irreversible. R.N.A. synthesis dependent on D.N.A. is thereby blocked. It is probable that doxorubicin and daunorubicin act similarly. Less is known of the mode of action of bleomycin, but it probably causes breaks in D.N.A. strands.

Enzymes

L-Asparaginase breaks down the circulating amino acid asparagine. This is needed by all human cells, but while normal cells of the bone marrow can make it, tumour cells cannot.

Other Drugs

There are many drugs which either do not fit neatly into one group, or whose mode of action is not yet completely understood. This is often more true of recently introduced drugs.

Toxic Effects of Chemotherapy

From a study of the mode of action of cytotoxic drugs it is obvious that it is the dividing cell which is vulnerable. Unfortunately, tumour cells are not necessarily dividing faster than those in the normal tissues of the body, and so cells of the bone marrow and the mucosa of the gastro-intestinal tract are also vulnerable. It must be emphasised however that signs and symptoms must not be assumed to be due to the cytotoxic drug, there can be other causes such as further extension of the tumour into bone marrow causing anaemia, or acquisition of new gut flora causing diarrhoea.

Bone Marrow

All the cells produced by the bone marrow are affected, but the specific cells which suffer most vary with the drug used. The patient is at risk because of anaemia, haemorrhage, and infection, and signs of marrow depression appear earlier when the patient has received previous chemotherapy or radiation, or when the marrow is infiltrated by tumour.

Though some drugs are more toxic than others all produce some degree of bone-marrow depression. The dose should be carefully tailored to the patient, and factors which must be considered in addition to those mentioned already are general condition and weight and age.

Gastro-intestinal Mucosa

Severe diarrhoea can occur due to toxic effects on the bowel mucosa. It is difficult to control and may continue for some time after stopping the drug. A change in bowel habit should be regarded as a danger signal.

Ulceration of the mouth often occurs during the use of methotrexate and 5-fluorouracil. The ulcers are usually painful and may be preceded by erythema, they may be the forerunners of diarrhoea.

These two major toxic effects are not always seen in the same patient. Their severity and time of onset varies with the individual. Signs of methotrexate toxicity can be found after only the first dose, while it may not occur at all in another patient.

Nausea and vomiting are also common. Sometimes this persists for a few days, despite stopping treatment.

Skin and Skin Appendages

All cytotoxic drugs if given in sufficient doses may well cause alopecia. Some of the chief offenders are cyclophosphamide, doxorubicin and daunorubicin, and to a lesser extent bleomycin and vincristine. Usually the loss is not permanent, but patients must be warned and a wig provided as soon as possible.

Nail growth is retarded and occasionally skin rashes can occur. In some patients erythema will return in previously irradiated areas. A patient of mine had radiation to the chest for a carcinoma of the lung. Skin reaction subsided satisfactorily but marked erythema recurred during subsequent cytotoxic therapy.

Specific Organ Effects

Teratogenesis and Fertility

Quite a high proportion of patients who present with malignant disease are already sterile. Cytotoxic drugs have an effect on germinal epithelium and cause secondary changes in endocrine secretions. Whether the changes are permanent depends upon the type of drug used, and, in women, their age. Alkylating drugs are more likely to cause irreversible sterility, although patients under thirty have more chance of retaining fertility. Women may have a premature menopause but this is slightly less likely in younger patients.

Attempts to preserve fertility by banking sperm, or the induction of temporary oligospermia or anovulatory cycles, all prior to chemotherapy, are being made.

Most cyotoxic drugs are teratogenic. If conception takes place during chemotherapy probably abortion occurs, or the child is born with obvious congenital malformation or genetic damage which can be inherited. Therefore, unless it is vital, cytotoxic therapy is avoided in the first trimester and later in pregnancy.

The long term risk of genetic damage in children subsequently born to successfully treated patients is not yet clear. The offspring of acute leukaemia survivors so far appear to be normal, but this may only be due to the type of drugs used. Patients are probably best advised to avoid conception in the first year after treatment is completed. In women there is the additional need to avoid the physical strain of pregnancy and the care of a young child.

C.N.S.

Methotrexate combined with prophylactic radiation has caused some temporary and some long term problems in children, neurological deterioration with fits, decreased reasoning and mathematical ability. This may be avoided in future by limiting the radiation given. The vinca alkaloids may cause peripheral nerve damage with muscle weakness, loss of reflexes, and constipation. Cis-platin may affect hearing.

Heart

Both daunorubicin and doxorubicin affect the heart. This seems to be in proportion to the total dose given. Regular E.C.G. monitoring, and caution if patients already have abnormal cardiac function, are necessary.

Lungs

One drug in particular can cause irreversible lung fibrosis. This is bleomycin and regular monitoring must be carried out. Some of the alkylating agents have also come under suspicion.

Liver

Damage may occur as a side effect of many cytotoxic drugs. Jaundice or abnormal L.F.T.s may be the result. It is difficult to distinguish this from changes due to malignant infiltration of the liver, and a biopsy may be needed to make a correct diagnosis.

Kidneys and Bladder

The drug most likely to cause renal damage is cis-platin. Regular checks of renal function must be made. Adequate hydration or even forced diuresis, will be some protection.

Cyclophosphamide can cause haemorrhagic cystitis.

Immunity

The body possesses the ability to react against foreign protein, it can neutralise this antigen by phagocytosis, white cells taking the protein into their cytoplasm and destroying it, or by an antibody response. An antibody combines with the antigen and neutralises it. This process is a response to infection for instance. The effect can be lasting, after one attack of measles the body is always immune to another attack, or temporary so that one cold does not confer immunity against a new infection. This immune response is responsible for the rejection of skin grafts and other organs from incompatible donors. In these days of transplant surgery the phrase 'rejection reaction' is one with which we are all familiar.

Many cytotoxic drugs have been shown in animals to suppress the immune response. It is probable that in man this causes the liability to infection during chemotherapy. A therapeutic use has been found for this effect, drugs with a low cytotoxic effect are used to control rejection after transplant surgery.

Since it is probable that the body's immune system is capable of mounting a defence against malignant cells, at least initially, there must be some concern that a long term effect of cytotoxic therapy may be the permanent loss of this property. It is also possible that the drugs may induce some malignant change which persists because of the loss of this immunological surveillance.

The higher than normal occurrence of malignancy in transplant and Hodgkin survivors seems to substantiate this concern. It is too early to judge what the level of risk is, but it appears to be linked more with the alkylating agents than other drugs.

Protection against Toxic Effects

Anti-emetics and anxiolytics can be used to reduce the incidence of nausea and vomiting. In an attempt to overcome the effects of bone-marrow depression the return of stored marrow after treatment, or grafts of marrow from a donor, have been tried. Both methods present problems and neither is available for routine clinical use.

In animal work certain chemicals have shown a protective effect against cyto-toxic drugs, but as yet they have not been used in man. There is the risk that not only will tumour and normal cells both be protected, but that due to a greater uptake by the tumour it may be preferentially protected.

In an attempt to prevent the general toxic effects methods have been devised to localise the cytotoxic drug to one area of the body. Two main techniques are, infusion, whereby a catheter is placed in the artery supplying the affected area, and perfusion of an isolated area. Isolation is either achieved by cannulating an artery and vein and circulating the blood through an oxygenating pump at the same time adding the cytotoxic, or by occluding the blood supply to and from the rest of the body while a rapid infusion is given to the treatment area. The technical problems and the morbidity of these procedures have tempered the early enthusiasm. Although pain may be temporarily relieved any regression is rarely maintained, and some leakage into the general system usually occurs producing systemic toxicity.

Folinic acid has the most use as a protective agent. It is one of the metabolites produced in the folic-acid cycle, and can therefore overcome the toxic effects of the folic-acid antagonists such as methotrexate. If this cytotoxic is being used for perfusion folinic acid can prevent systemic symptoms developing, and it will reduce the period during which symptoms persist after the drug's withdrawal when it has been given orally.

In all fields of therapy it is important to remember that drugs can enhance or antagonise the action of other drugs. When cytotoxic chemotherapy is given, other drugs prescribed for completely different reasons may increase the cyto-toxic effect or make a side effect worse. Drugs are bound in varying degrees to proteins in the blood, and those with greater binding power will displace others with a weaker affinity. Aspirin will displace methotrexate thereby increasing the level of active drug, in addition it will potentiate any bleeding tendency. Allopurinol will slow down the fall in the level of available methotrexate, because it inhibits the enzyme responsible for the breakdown of this cytotoxic. Absorption of a cytotoxic may be decreased because anti-emetics have altered the rate at which the stomach empties.

Resistance

Tumour cells may become resistant to the cytotoxic therapy being used, this is particularly a problem when a single drug is used.

Primary Resistance

Bacteria may be resistant from the outset to an antibiotic and a treatment failure will result from its use. Certain staphylococci produce an enzyme, penicillinase, which destroys penicillin, such bacteria are thus naturally resistant. By testing against a range of drugs a laboratory can find the sensitivity pattern of each organism.

Methods have now been devised to culture the 'stem' (primitive) cells of tumours. These cultures can be exposed to various cytotoxics and afterwards the number of tumour colony forming units compared with an untreated culture (control). This should give an indication as to whether the tumour is sensitive to chemotherapy, and if it is, to which drugs.

Adaptation

Earlier in this chapter we learned that sulphonamides block one of the steps in the folic-acid cycle. Over the years many bacteria have become resistant to this group of drugs and they have done this by a metabolic by-pass of this step. It is believed tumour cells can become resistant similarly through a by-pass mechanism.

'Acquired' Resistance

The cells within a tumour continue to undergo mutation. Such mutations are often unstable, but if persistent the cell characteristics may change, and a previously sensitive cell may give rise to daughter cells which are resistant, or resistant to low concentrations of a cytotoxic drug. Within the body there are several factors which can affect the amount of cytotoxic drug reaching the tumour cell, a rapid excretion by the kidney or an equally rapid detoxication by the liver, failure to cross the cell membrane in adequate quantities, or a poor blood supply so that too little drug reaches the site of action.

The emergence of resistance is also aided by the fact that the cells of the tumour may be multiplying at different rates. It will be remembered that in the cell cycle the most vulnerable time is at mitosis. Cells which have a long cycle may well reach this critical point at a time when the cytotoxic concentration is low and less likely to be effective.

Cross Resistance

There are families of antibacterial drugs, the family likeness lies either in the chemical structure or in the similarity in the mode of action. Bacteria which become resistant to one member of a family are usually resistant to all the rest of the drugs of that group. This is cross resistance. To a lesser degree this trait is found in tumours, when one alkylating drug fails response is unlikely to another. On the other hand vincristine and vinblastine do not have such marked cross resistance. Hodgkin's disease which becomes resistant to vinblastine often responds to vincristine.

Phase and Cycle

Some drugs are only effective at one or two points, phases, in the mitotic cycle. Others will attack throughout the cycle. This affects the rate at which cells are killed, in the first case there is a fall and then a plateau is reached, in the second there is a continuous fall. Vincristine is an example of a phase specific drug, alkylating agents fall into the second group.

Some cells are not actively dividing and are in a resting phase, often called Go. They are then insensitive to chemotherapy, as no drug in clinical use at present is active on resting cells. If they remained 'inactive' at least the tumour would have lost some of its growth potential, and if all tumour cells were held permanently in Go then there would be no increase in size. Unfortunately these cells could move back into the active cycle, and it is thought that this may happen when the balance of 'active' to 'inactive' cells is disturbed by cell kill.

Combined Therapy

Having considered each drug in isolation we can now understand the reasoning behind the use of combined therapy. If some cells in a tumour are resistant to one drug from the outset, the simultaneous administration of another with a different mode of action could well attack these resistant cells. Since these cytotoxics are also likely to be absorbed, detoxicated, and excreted at different rates, there is a better chance that a therapeutic concentration will be maintained at the tumour site and resistance be slower to emerge.

When 'culture and sensitivity' becomes a routine procedure the most appropriate drug combination can be predicted, and if resistance develops a switch made to drugs likely to be effective.

The meaning of the word cytotoxic must not be forgotten, nor the fact that all the cells of the body are vulnerable. Combination therapy enables the dose of each drug to be modified, this is often particularly important when toxicity is dependent on the individual or cumulative dose level. It is thought that normal cells recover more quickly from cytotoxic damage than malignant ones. In tissues where not all cells are dividing, the effect will be less as there will be a 'reservoir' of cells capable of carrying on normal function. The bone marrow cells are an example of this 'reservoir' effect. Less than a quarter are in cycle at any one time, but it takes several days for the resting cells to come into active division. Myelo-suppression is a potentially lethal toxic effect of chemotherapy, so regimes are pulsed. High doses are given in a period of less than 24 hours, and then several days rest follow. The next dose is given when resting marrow cells will be in cycle restoring marrow function, but tumour cells will not have made a full recovery.

Sensitisers

Certain drugs 'sensitise' tumours to radiation. It is now known that they also potentiate cytotoxic chemotherapy. Misonizadole and its derivatives are being used.

Principles of Chemotherapy

It would be impossible to specify the uses of individual drugs or the details of various regimes. New drugs are being constantly introduced and incorporated into treatment. It is of more importance to grasp the underlying principles governing their use.

1. Except in maintenance or in treating certain chronic conditions, drugs are used in combination. This lessens the risk of resistance occurring.
2. Combining drugs with different modes of action enables the action of each to be potentiated by the others. Since their toxicities differ, overwhelming toxicity of one type is less likely.
3. Pulsing and combination give attack on cells which are in different phases of the mitosis cycle, while at the same time, allowing normal cells to recover.
4. The signs and symptoms of toxicity must be looked for carefully, particularly these may be masked if steroids are used. They must not be confused with signs and symptoms of the spread of malignancy.
5. Good principles of asepsis must be observed. If necessary reverse barrier nursing or 'special units' may be needed. Discussion of this is reserved for later chapters on leukaemia, Hodgkin's disease, etc.

Handling of Drugs

Naturally there has been some anxiety expressed from time to time as to the effects on personnel who handle and administer these drugs. The situation is constantly under review but there should be no problem if certain rules are followed. In centres where there is a considerable chemotherapy work load, drugs will be prepared centrally. In others preparation should be in an area set aside. Both preparation and administration should be done by nominated personnel who have been trained. Most of the precautions are matters of good nursing technique, they include avoidance of pressure effects causing an aerosol during mixing, drawing up, or expelling air from a syringe, the use of disposable absorbent materials to mop up spills, and the careful handling and disposal of excess drug or patients' excreta. Suitable gloves, long sleeved gown, and face mask should be worn during preparation and administration. If no cabinet is available during preparation a visor or goggles protect the eyes. Splashes into the eye or on to the skin should be washed with plenty of water.

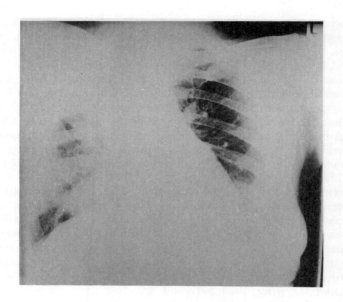

Fig. 4.4a.   Chest X-ray before chemotherapy

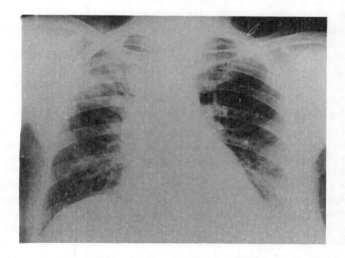

Fig. 4.4b.   Chest X-ray after chemotherapy

Nursing Care

Most local complications following administration occur with injections. Intra-muscular injection is uncomfortable or painful. Large muscle sites will minimise this, and a local anaesthetic may be helpful. If the drug being given causes a platelet fall there is a risk of a haematoma at the injection site.

Inflammation (phlebitis), or thrombosis can occur in veins. Not only is this painful for the patient, it restricts the choice of vein for subsequent injection. The use of an infusion, injection into an infusion running freely, or washing the injection through with saline after injection, all minimise this complication.

Leakage into the local tissues around an intravenous injection site will result in pain and induration. A slowly healing necrotic ulcer may develop. Careful watch should be kept therefore for extravasation into the tissues, particularly when an infusion is being used.

The toxicities of the individual drugs and the general principles of nursing patients receiving this treatment have already been covered in individual sections. Only certain points will be re-emphasised here. Every cytotoxic drug depresses the bone marrow to a certain extent, some more than others. By charting the blood count, it is possible to see the trends and to adjust or stop treatment before a dangerous situation develops. The nurse, either in the out-patient department or in the ward, usually has the responsibility of organising check counts. Laboratories are often busy and may find these repetitive counts a burden, a tactful nurse can be invaluable, particularly if she understands the prime importance of these tests.

Infection is an ever-present threat to these patients. Meticulous care must be taken to send swabs of any discharge, or samples of sputum or faeces for laboratory culture and sensitivity. If the patient is receiving antibiotic therapy his depressed immunity may make it easier for fungal overgrowth to occur. Watch should be kept for this.

The aim of nursing can be summed up as prevention. If the toxicities of the drug in use are known, if the side effects of treatment are expected, a vigilant nurse can do much to prevent them. She is by the nature of her work in con-tact with the patient for longer periods than most other members of the team. She must be the alert sentry who is the first to report suspicious events.

Indications for Chemotherapy

There can be no doubt that this treatment must either be given in hospital or under hospital supervision. Toxic effects are inevitable, and it is important that not only is therapy given where there is ready access to facilities for dealing with these, but that the doctors and staff controlling it should be ex-perienced and so on the alert for early signs of toxicity.

Before deciding on cytotoxic therapy all the implications for the patient and the likely response of the disease must be considered. Chemotherapy is the treatment of choice for chorion carcinoma and for acute leukaemia, and to patients who have disseminated Hodgkin's disease or systemic symptoms cytotoxic drugs often bring dramatic improvement. This still leaves an enormous field, and it must be acknowledged that chemotherapy plays a variable part in the treatment of many other forms of malignant disease. Its usefulness ranges from being an important adjunct to other forms of treatment as in Wilms' tumour, to almost complete failure in solid tumours of the gastro-intestinal tract. Between these extremes there lies a grey area where the decision on its use rests on the experience and judgment of the therapist.

All previous treatment must be carefully considered, radiation or cytotoxics even though used some time before may well mean an early or violent toxic effect. When it is remembered that severe toxicity can occur after only one treatment, even when cytotoxics are being used for the first time, this is less surprising. One of my patients with a lymphoma had had several courses of radiation and chemotherapy. After one injection of vinblastine her blood count fell dramatically, and she exhibited signs of toxicity, mouth ulceration and mental depression.

One of the fiercest debates centres on the timing and use of cytotoxic therapy to treat solid tumours. There are those who advocate its early use. They argue that early in a tumour's life most of the cells will be stem (primitive cells) and so very vulnerable. However when a tumour is detectable by present methods it may already have passed this stage. Many patients may be successfully treated by other means, and to submit them unnecessarily to the toxicity of chemotherapy may be unjustified. Probably nowhere is the debate more fierce than among those who treat breast cancer. It has been suggested that prophylactic cytotoxic therapy should be given to all patients after adequate local therapy. Some of these patients would be 'cured' by local measures, others will develop metastases. If the lymph nodes are not involved there is as yet no known test which will predict to which group a woman belongs, so all must be treated. Metastases appear to be postponed not prevented. The questions therefore to be answered are, should women in the first group be exposed to an unpleasant therapy, and is the lengthening of the disease free interval for the second group sufficient to compensate for the effects of the treatment?

Many are beginning to feel that to ask a patient to endure the unpleasantness of cytotoxic treatment one must be fairly certain of an improvement which will last for a reasonable time. To treat merely in order to do something is easier, to realise the limitations and to refrain, relying on supportive therapy only, is more difficult, but may well be more truly in the best interests of the patient.

Meanwhile efforts must continue to find new drugs which are tumour specific and less toxic. Novel delivery methods, attaching the drug to a carrier so that it is only released at the site of action, are being explored. Carriers may be fragments of D.N.A., lysosomes, and the latest candidate, monoclonal antibodies. Alternatively it might be possible to develop drugs which are cytostatics. They reduce the cell multiplication rate, and some restore the cell's sensitivity to normal growth regulators. They are often natural substances and do not affect normal cells, so there are not the toxic effects of cytotoxic drugs. They are not likely alone to cause complete tumour remission, but if the lessened multiplication rate lowers cell gain below the rate of cell loss (death), growth would be checked, and perhaps shrink to the point where the body's natural defences were once again adequate. In some cases it is just possible that recovery of sensitivity to growth regulators might revert a malignant cell to normal.

Research will continue, and hopefully will result in either some other therapy to replace cytotoxics, or more specific, effective cytotoxic drugs. There is no doubt that while currently cytotoxic chemotherapy is the treatment of choice for several conditions, and is a valuable adjunct in other cases, its use to treat many others is highly debatable. Centres will vary in the policy adopted, but at present there is no accepted regime for this rather large group of tumours, although this may change as a result of research.

In the following chapters discussion of treatment will indicate when chemotherapy is used, and its status as primary or adjunctive treatment. To avoid lists of names and repetitive details of toxicity, a table is given here of drugs in common use. New drugs will be introduced, some probably before this book is in print, but this chapter should enable the nurse to understand the principles governing their use, and also give her some guide to the possible toxicity.

TABLE OF CYTOTOXICS

Nearly all cytotoxics can cause nausea and vomiting.

Drug	Side effects peculiar to a drug	Side effects of the group
Alkylating agents		
BCNU	Pain at injection site Infertility	
CCNU	Infertility	
Methyl CCNU	Infertility	
Busulphan	Infertility, skin pigmentation	
Chlorambucil	Infertility	
Melphalan	Infertility	
Thiotepa	Infertility	
Mustine	Pain at injection site Hair loss	
Cyclophosphamide	Cystitis. Sterility. Hair loss. Sore mouth	Myelosuppression. Second malignancy more commoı
DTIC	Pain at injection site. Pyrexia. Infertility	
Chlorozotocin	Infertility	
Cis-platin	Renal damage. Diarrhoea. Tinnitus, loss of hearing high tones	
Streptozotocin	Pain at injection site	
Procarbazine	Alcohol sensitivity	

Antimetabolites

Methotrexate	Sore mouth. High dosage renal damage	
5-Fluorouracil	Sore mouth. Hair loss	Myelosuppression
Cytosine Arabinoside	Sore mouth	
6-Mercaptopurine		
Hydroxyurea		

Plant origin, natural
or synthetic

Vincristine	Variable myelo-suppression.
Vinblastine	Peripheral neuro-pathy. Hair loss.
Vindesine	Pain at injection site

Etoposide	Myelosuppression.
Teniposide	Hair loss

Antibiotics

Actinomycin D	Pain at injection site. Sore mouth	
Daunorubicin	Hair loss. Cardiac damage if high dose. Pain at injection site	
Doxorubicin		Myelosuppression
Mithramycin	Pyrexia. Pain at injection site	
Mitomycin C	Pain at injection site. Hair loss	
Bleomycin	Pyrexia, skin pigmentation. Hair loss. Lung fibrosis if dose too high	Not myelosuppressive

Enzymes

Asparaginase	Pyrexia, anaphylactic reactions

Drugs which are experimental and not yet fully researched have not been included. Some combination regimes are virtually standard, but as the doses and drugs may be varied, precise details of them have not been given. They are often referred to by the name of the centre or doctor who pioneered them, or by the initial letters of the constituent drugs. So the regime for the treatment of testicular malignant teratomas is named after its originator, Einhorn, while one regime used in the treatment of Hodgkin's disease is called MOPP (Mustine (nitrogen mustard), Oncovin (vincristine), prednisone, procarbazine).

Man is surrounded by hazards,
That he succumbs is not surprising,
What is surprising, is his ability
To survive at all.

5   The Skin

The most frequently occurring malignancies of the skin are rodent ulcers (basal cell) and squamous cell carcinomata. It is interesting that a small percentage of these patients have a malignant growth of another organ. Less common is the melanoma. Carcinoma in situ, Bowen's disease, is usually solitary but left untreated will develop into squamous carcinoma. Occasionally secondary infiltration of the skin may arise from carcinoma of the breast, bronchus, bladder, etc. As the skin is composed of various structures such as sweat and sebaceous glands, blood vessels, lymphatics, nerves, and connective tissue, malignant growth can occur in any of them but this is rare. Benign tumours are warts, corns, and keratoacanthomata. The latter mimic malignant tumours but have a high rate of spontaneous regression. Two conditions which though benign are regarded as pre-malignant, are leukoplakia and senile keratosis.

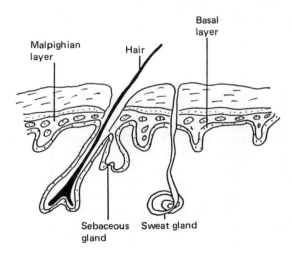

Fig. 5.1   The skin

Rodent Ulcer, Basal Cell Carcinoma

In white races prolonged exposure to sunlight (actinic light) can predispose to basal cell carcinoma, and this explains why it is usually found on exposed parts of the body such as the face. This may be an occupational hazard as with fishermen, sailors, gardeners, or result from living in certain latitudes, it is a common condition among Australians. It is rare for it to arise in races with heavily pigmented skins. Other factors incriminated are long contact with arsenic, this was previously prescribed for skin conditions and was an ingredient in some beauty lotions, and irradiation. A now discontinued practice was the treatment by soft X-rays of ringworm of the scalp in children. This often resulted in middle age in the appearance of multiple rodent ulcers.

The patient is usually male, the sex ratio being M:F 2:1. The disease usually occurs in the sixth decade onwards. However, the modern fashion for prolonged sunbathing may not only result in the tumour arising in unusual sites but also at an earlier age.

Clinical Appearance

The patient complains of a slowly growing lesion of varying appearance, 'a small wart, doctor', 'a little blister'. At this stage it is cystic with fine capillaries running over the surface and can often be transilluminated. This nodular stage is followed by central necrosis producing ulceration. The patient says there is a scab, sometimes irritating, which never heals, and there is occasional discharge or bleeding. There is a variation in size. While growing, small areas may regress spontaneously, so that the appearance is of activity at one edge and healing at another. Thus the typical ulcer is irregular, with a heaped-up beaded edge where there is activity, flattening where healing is occurring, and a centre showing necrosis with bleeding.

Origin and Spread

The precise cell of origin is not certain, but it is thought that these growths arise probably from the basal cells of the hair follicle, so that while the face is most commonly affected any area bearing hair follicles may develop a rodent ulcer. Under the microscope the cells have a typical appearance, densely staining in 'palisades' (clusters), clumps of tumour cells lying separate from the main area and well beyond the clinical edge of the growth. Spread is by local direct infiltration, metastasis to lymph nodes via the blood stream being extremely rare. In special sites such as the inner canthus of the eye, alae nasi, or the ear, because of close proximity, bone or cartilage can be involved, and also any specialised structures such as the lacrimal duct. While spread is generally very slow, invasion is more rapid when other structures are involved and treatment is rendered more difficult.

Squamous Cell Carcinoma

Aetiology

The same factors operate here as in basal cell carcinoma, but in addition should be noted prolonged exposure to hydrocarbons (tar, soot), chronic ulceration as with varicose veins, the previous skin disease leukoplakia, and very rarely malignant change in a sebaceous cyst.

Incidence

This is a disease of the elderly and predominantly males, 4:1 M:F. Cured patients die from other diseases and true incidence is therefore difficult to assess, but some consider this tumour may account for up to 10% of all malignancies.

Clinical Appearance

The patient usually presents with an ulcer as ulceration occurs early. The edge is more pronounced, rolled, everted and nodular, the centre is occupied by scab. Some tumours are very bulky and proliferative. Any part of the body can be involved but it is most common in the exposed sites, face, hands, neck. The growth arises from the prickle-cell layer of the epidermis (malpighian layer), this is where the horny part of the skin, keratin, is formed. Under the microscope small downgrowths of prickle cells containing shiny keratin may be seen, these are known as epithelial pearls. Many pearls are indicative of a well-differentiated tumour, loss of pearls, i.e. keratin, is indicative of a more malignant, rapidly growing, anaplastic carcinoma. Bowen's disease is sometimes a marker of internal carcinoma, particularly bronchus.

Spread

Unlike basal cell carcinomata local infiltration is more rapid, fixation occurring early. Metastases in the lymph nodes are common and blood-stream spread, usually to the lungs, occurs at the last stage of the disease.

Melanoma

The benign form of this tumour is the naevus or common mole. The juvenile melanoma, distinguished by certain histological features, is found in childhood up to the age of puberty and is benign.

The malignant melanoma is uncommon and does not usually occur until the third decade. Exposure to sunlight is a factor in probably 50% of cases, although outdoor workers experiencing chronic exposure are less affected, perhaps acquiring a protective suntan. The very rare disease of xeroderma pigmentosa predisposes to melanoma.

About 0.5% of deaths from malignancy are due to this tumour.

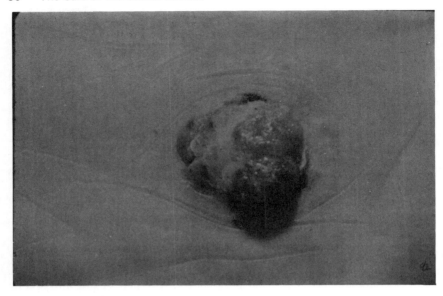

Fig. 5.2.   Melanoma of the sole of the foot

Clinical Appearance

The patient usually consults the doctor because he has noticed a change in a 'mole' which he has had for years. He may complain of bleeding, ulceration, rapid increase in size, the appearance of numerous small pigmented spots, or occasionally of a lump in the regional node site. The previous 'mole' may not always have been raised or pigmented. The common sites are the hands, face, neck, and under the nails of the foot.

In the skin, cells which can convert D.O.P.A. (dihydroxyphenylalanine) to melanin, a dark-brown pigment, are called dopa-positive. The 'naevus cells' from which the malignant melanoma arises are dopa-positive. Under the microscope the cellular appearance of the tumour is variable.

Spread

There is direct infiltration and early lymphatic spread so that nodes are often involved when the patient is first seen. An unusual feature is the ability for spread to occur against the lymphatic flow, retrograde spread. With a lesion on the thigh, glands could be involved in both the knee and the groin. Blood metastases may occur early in the lungs, liver and brain. At autopsy the heavy pigmentation of the lymphatics, nodes, and involved organs is very striking.

Investigations

At the first visit the doctor takes a careful history which will cover aetiological factors, duration and rate of progression, and first symptoms. On examination he will note the appearance, size, fixation, and invasion of local structures, and the presence or absence of regional lymph nodes. To do this the patient must be adequately undressed and the doctor may require a powerful hand lens and torch. As indicated by the history he will ask for a blood test, haemoglobin and white-blood-cell count, X-rays of local bony structures, and chest X-ray.

If melanoma is suspected other specialised examinations are done. These include liver ultrasound or scan, bone scan, and brain scan. In certain situations a CATscan can be helpful.

Histological verification and classification of the tumour is important. A specimen is obtained by biopsy, preferably from the active edge in the case of basal and squamous cell carcinomata. This can be carried out under local anaesthesia in the out-patient department. The biopsy specimen is however very small and should be put at once into the labelled container and sent with the appropriate forms to the laboratory. If there is any suspicion that the lesion is a malignant melanoma, the patient must be admitted for a wide excision-biopsy by an experienced surgeon, since the risk of dissemination by injudicious biopsy is so high. The out-patient excision of moles is a practice to be condemned.

Treatment, Basal and Squamous Cell Carcinoma

Radiation

It is becoming more common for patients to be referred direct to the radio-therapist except when bone or cartilage is involved.

Technique

The area to be treated is marked with a semi-permanent dye, the edge is carried well clear of the palpable tumour to include possible isolated clumps of cells. Lower voltage therapy is used, the exact choice varying with site, extent, and thickness of the lesion. The total dose is spread over 10 to 20 treatments. In specialised circumstances, patients coming long distances as in Australia, one single large dose can be given, but the results are never so satisfactory, particularly from the cosmetic angle. Radioactive moulds and implants, though still employed in some centres, are usually reserved for special sites, lip, dorsum of the hand. The total dose may be modified by special factors, the age and general condition of the patient, the sensitivity of certain areas such as the dorsum of the hand or the lip, or the proximity of other structures, e.g. close relation of the naso-lacrimal duct to the inner canthus of the eye.

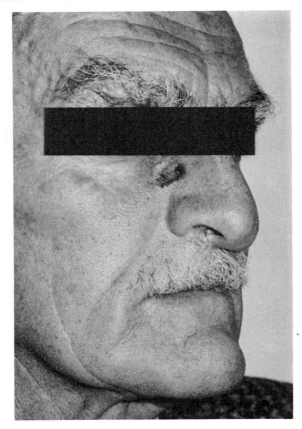

Fig. 5.3.   Rodent ulcer

Special Sites

Eyelids and Inner Canthus

The lens of the eye is very sensitive to irradiation, and when radiating these sites it is usual to insert an eyeshield which prevents X-rays reaching the eye. If a local anaesthetic is used prior to insertion, the patient must wear an eye-pad as the cornea is anaesthetic and the blink reflex lost for some time, so any grit settling in the eye can cause abrasion with possible ulceration. At the inner canthus the skin is very thin and the radiotherapist must bear in mind the close proximity of the punctum and the naso-lacrimal duct.

Alae Nasi

The septum of the nose is composed of cartilage and if it receives too much radiation may later necrose. It is therefore usual to protect it, unless it is involved, by inserting a strip of lead into the nostril.

Nodes

In dealing with squamous carcinoma particular attention must be paid to the lymphatic drainage areas. If nodes are present treatment will be by surgery if mobile, if fixed by radiation. Prophylactic treatment of these areas is no longer practised.

Surgery

Small tumours can be excised and closed with primary sutures. Cryosurgery and diathermy are sometimes used for very small or premalignant lesions. Larger tumours will require skin grafting. When bone and cartilage are involved surgery is the treatment of choice, unless the lesion is too extensive.

Chemotherapy

Very small superficial rodent ulcers can be treated successfully with the cytotoxic 5-FU applied daily in a cream.

In disseminated disease or when the local tumour is very extensive chemotherapy has been used.

Melanoma

Though rare, this is a difficult, but primarily surgical problem. Wide excision with skin grafting is carried out, and at the same time other procedures, such as block dissection, chemotherapy, perfusion, as dictated by the stage of the disease. Where surgery is not possible or incomplete, radical radiotherapy can be employed. While not curative, growth can be arrested in some cases for several years. Where dissemination has occurred radiation is only justifiable to palliate symptoms caused by local foci.

Chemotherapy either as an adjuvant to surgery and radiation, or given after in spaced courses, has assumed some importance. DTIC (dacarbazine) is often used, usually in combination with other cytotoxics such as the vinca alkaloids. Immunotherapy as an adjuvant has also been suggested. This is an attempt to stimulate the patient's own immune defences by using either inactivated tumour cell vaccines, or those unrelated to malignancy such as BCG.

Following some animal work the testing of hyperthermia to kill off the malignant cells has been advocated, but more evaluation is needed.

The diverse treatments used merely reflect the unpredictable, but usually poor results. In addition to better therapy, a predictive test is needed. Some believe that skin reaction to a chemical DNCB may be of some use.

Reaction of the Skin to Radiation during Treatment

This can be divided into stages bearing in mind the structures of the skin, the site, and the dosage related to the period over which it is given. Let us presuppose a four-week period of treatment:

1. No visible reaction, there may be an initial sensation of warmth.
2. A mild reddening (erythema) due to capillary dilation. There may be irritation.
3. The erythema deepens and the skin becomes dry due to loss of secretions from the sebaceous and sweat glands. Loss of hair, epilation, begins.
4. Moist desquamation. Blisters are formed, break, and a raw weeping surface is left. This is painful. Therapy is not pressed beyond this point. If radiation continued ulceration would result and damage to underlying structures.

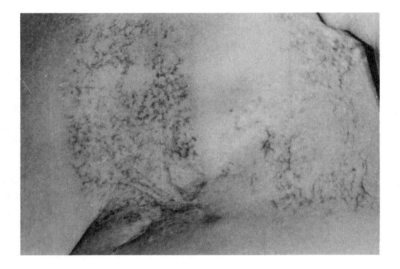

Fig. 5.4.   Late skin reaction, telangectasia of the L. chest wall

Healing takes place rapidly following stages one to three with minimal residual damage, though hair loss may be permanent. Stage four takes longer to heal, and later, leathering of the skin may occur due to atrophy and fibrosis. This is classified, together with the formation of a fine superficial network of capillaries which are incapable of contraction (telangectasia), as the late result of radiation, taking possibly years to develop. In certain cases these late changes can progress to malignancy.

Nursing Care

This can be divided into three parts. In general it must be realised that when dressings are necessary they have to be removed daily for treatment. They should therefore be atraumatic to the skin, any tape containing metallic preparations is avoided since it potentiates the radiation effect. If it has already been used it is usual to allow a few days to elapse before commencing treatment. If infection or discharge is present this requires daily cleansing with a bland antiseptic, and if necessary, the doctor will order a swab for culture and sensitivity, and from the report the necessary antibiotic.

1. Before Treatment

The patient is usually instructed not to wash the area being treated, but tepid sponging may be used if not painful. Any lesion of the scalp will probably entail shaving a wide area so that the skin can be marked easily, and treatment accurately placed. Patients often ask if hair will regrow. The doctor will answer this question, but the nurse should be aware that within the treated area there will most likely be permanent epilation. If there is treatment to the area of the head where spectacles are worn, the patient should if possible do without them, but if they must be worn, the patient should pad those parts of the spectacles which press on the skin.

2. During Treatment

Many ointments and lotions have been used from the outset, and also during treatment, to minimise skin reaction, but they have mostly been abandoned. A baby dusting powder is soothing and alleviates irritation, at this stage a doctor may prescribe an ointment or lotion containing steroid. If moist desquamation occurs the application of 1% gentian violet or similar lotion will provide a cover for the moist surface, this is sometimes applied over small gauze dressings. Antibiotic ointments will also at times be useful.

3. After Treatment

Any scab present will adhere for some time and the patient should be instructed to leave it alone. As healing takes place the scab loosens, becomes smaller, and is finally shed. If it is removed prematurely it merely renews itself until healing is complete. It is important for the patient to realise that the scab, although cosmetically unsightly, is protective. The erythema of the skin is brisk and may take three to four weeks to subside. In areas where there is friction of the surface, such as the neck from clothing, the patient should be advised to wear loose clothing or protect the skin by a silk handkerchief, shaving round the area with an electric razor is usually possible.

Folds of the skin are very liable to maceration and dressings may be required here for some time. If the area is large, it is better for the patient to attend the radiotherapy department for dressings as the nurses are familiar with radiation reaction and healing. Sunlight is another form of radiation. The patients should therefore be advised to avoid excessive exposure to the treated area for the rest of their lives.

Follow-up

Usually the patients are seen within one month of treatment and then at lengthening intervals. This interval will depend upon the pathological nature of the lesion. The patient with a rodent ulcer is usually seen once a year, whilst those with squamous cell lesions will be seen more frequently in view of the possibility of metastatic nodes developing. Follow-up is continued over a period of years to check:

1. Possible skin damage giving rise to necrotic ulcers which usually heal, but may require plastic surgery.
2. Recurrences around the scar requiring excision, with or without skin grafting.
3. Development of fresh lesions.
   An area which requires special attention is the inner canthus where radiation has been given over the naso-lacrimal duct. Watch is kept for the development of, (1) epiphora (overflow of tears), it is indicative of stenosis of the duct, or, (2) eversion of the lid, ectropion. The patient is referred to the ophthalmologist for dilatation and possible surgical correction. If spectacles are worn the bridge pieces may require padding or alteration to avoid trauma to the treated area.

Patients with melanomata are seen more frequently since there is a high tendency to local recurrence, lympathic spread, and distant blood-borne metastases.

Prognosis

Uncomplicated rodent ulcers have a cure rate of over 90%, while for uncomplicated small squamous cell lesions one can expect an 80% survival at five years. Where nodes, bone, or cartilage are involved the prognosis is worsened. Melanoma carries a much less favourable prognosis, five-year survival being in the region of 25%, but dependent upon depth of penetration.

All pass along the highroad,
Both great and small;
But if the road be blocked,
Not even the smallest can pass.

6 The Mouth, Lip, Tongue, Pharynx and Larynx

In this region the anatomy is such that many specialities are involved in both the investigation and treatment of the disease. At some point the services of the surgeon, the neurologist, the ophthalmologist, the dentist, and the radiotherapist may all be required. In addition to general surgery, the specialist skills of the plastic surgeon, or of the ear, nose and throat surgeon may be employed. The patient is best served if all these doctors work in close co-operation.

Occasionally the patient is referred directly to the radiotherapist but more often he comes from one of the other departments. In this latter case the investigations described will mostly have been done already, but for the sake of completeness they have all been included.

Since there are so many similarities in the problems of treating disease in any part of this area, the whole region is dealt with in one chapter. Nursing care follows in the next chapter.

Section I
MOUTH, LIP AND TONGUE

Anatomy

Mouth

This can be divided into two parts, the inner and the outer. The inner is bounded laterally and anteriorly by the teeth and alveoli, above by the palate, hard and soft. Posteriorly it opens into the oropharynx, below it is closed by the floor of the mouth consisting of muscle. I-in the floor are the openings of the sub-mandibular and lingual ducts. Contained within the inner part is the tongue. The outer part consists of the space between the teeth and the alveoli on the

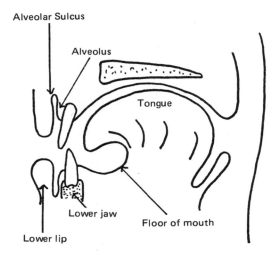

Fig. 6.1.   Tongue and mouth

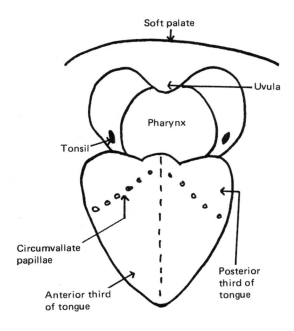

Fig. 6.2.   Tongue, tonsils, and soft palate

inner aspect and the cheek and lips on the outer. The upper part contains the openings of the parotid ducts in the cheek, opposite the second molars. Lymphatic drainage is to the immediately adjacent nodes and then to the cervical and retropharyngeal regional groups.

Tongue

The tongue is muscular with a rich vascular supply and equally rich lymphatic drainage. It is attached in its posterior third by its base to the floor of the mouth. On looking at the dorsum or surface of the tongue, there is a V-shaped line which is formed by large papillae. This demarcates the posterior third of the tongue from the anterior two-thirds, and is an important landmark when considering both lymphatic drainage and prognosis of the disease. The anterior part of the tongue is mobile while the posterior part is tethered.

Lymphatic drainage is eventually to the chain of deep cervical nodes. Immediate drainage may be to adjacent nodes, as from the tip of the tongue to the sub-mental group. An interesting feature is that drainage may not necessarily be confined to the same side, it may cross to the opposite side. Spread of disease therefore may be to both sides of the neck, this is particularly so from lesions of the middle and posterior areas.

Lip

The lips have buccal and outer surfaces and are well supplied with mucous glands. The junction of the red area and the facial skin is the vermiliform border.

Lymphatic Drainage

Nearly one-third of the lymph nodes of the body lie in the neck. As we have already noted when describing the tongue, drainage is first to the nodes in the immediate vicinity, but eventually all lymph passes to the deep cervical nodes. These lie along the line of the carotid artery. The bifurcation of the carotid artery represents a demarcation between upper and lower nodes. As a general rule the anterior parts of this area drain to the lower group, the posterior to the upper. Lesions of the midline and posterior areas can drain to both sides of the neck.

Aetiology

Lip and Tongue

Changes in social habits and disease patterns have been reflected in the incidence figures. The clay pipe smoker with repeated burns and subsequent carcinoma has vanished, but the chain smoker with the wet cigarette stuck to the lip has replaced him. Syphilis is less common and easily treatable, this probably accounts for the fall in the number of cases among men, but the increase in smoking by women may be linked with the rise in female sufferers. Predisposing factors are poor dental care and hygiene, syphilis, excessive alcohol, chronic infection, and long standing iron deficiency anaemia, often associated with achlorhydria. Special factors operate in certain parts of the world, betel nut chewers, fish net menders. Very rarely a possible genetic link may exist, as in Bloom's disease.

Leukoplakia

This is a condition which usually affects the tongue, but can also affect the mouth and lip. In its established state it is described as looking like a coat of white paint. There is fissuring of the underlying tissue. This is a pre-malignant condition in that 32% of cases progress to frank malignancy. The condition becomes more sinister if ulceration supervenes, so a careful watch is kept on patients.

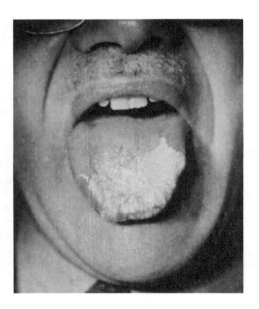

Fig. 6.3.   Leukoplakia of the tongue

Incidence

This is still a disease predominantly of males, occurring from the fifth decade onwards. About 1% of patients are under 30. Tumours of the lip, tongue and pharynx represent about 2% of all malignancies.

Pathology and Spread

Tumours are usually carcinomas of the squamous type. There is a range from well-differentiated keratinising to anaplastic. Spread is by:

1. Direct infiltration, as throughout the tongue.
2. Locally to adjacent structures, from the lip to bone.
3. Lymphatics, to the cervical nodes.
4. Blood borne to distant sites, a late feature of carcinoma of the lip and tongue.
5. Perineural in the case of the tongue.

Sites

The lower lip is involved in about 90% of cases of malignancy of the lip. For the tongue the figures are; lateral border 65%, anterior two-thirds 70%.

Symptomatology

Lip

The patient complains of either a persistent sore which bleeds periodically, or of an enlarging nodule. He may say that before developing this he had noticed a

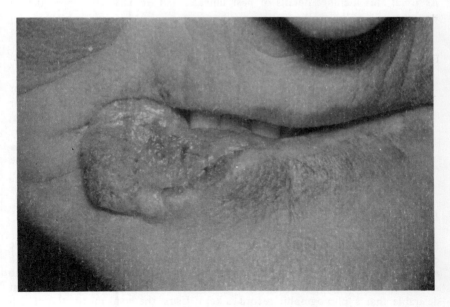

Fig. 6.4.   Squamous carcinoma of the lower lip

whitish patch (leukoplakia). When the lesion is large and fungating, eating will be difficult. The more common site in men is the lower lip, but in the small number of women who develop this disease it can occur with equal frequency in either lip. Despite the fact that it is easily visible, it is astonishing how far patients will allow this to progress before consulting a doctor. At a first visit every radiotherapist has seen the whole lip, both angles of the mouth, and part of the face involved, together with invasion of the mandible, and hard fixed glands in the neck.

Buccal Mucosa

Cheek   The main complaint initially is of discomfort. The patient feels a thickening and often bites this accidentally. Later there is soreness and possibly some bleeding.

Tongue   At first there is a lump or a sore which fails to heal. The lesion in the anterior two-thirds is usually noticed first, carcinoma of the posterior third often escapes notice until a lump in the neck is felt. Depending upon the bulk and degree of infiltration other symptoms may occur, excessive salivation, pain, tethering of the tongue, and occasionally referred pain in the ear.

Hard Palate   Soreness and ulceration are the main complaints.

History

As usual this includes details of past illnesses and of personal habits such as smoking.

Examination

1. General condition. It is obvious that any condition affecting the lip or mouth may mean that the patient has been on an inadequate diet for some time. A search is therefore made for signs of wasting and anaemia, including recording of weight and height.
2 Local condition. In the course of the examination the doctor will examine the inside of the mouth and may require to inspect the pharynx. The examination trolley should accordingly have on it head mirror, lamp, E.N.T. instruments, and a receiver for the patient's dentures.

Lip

After inspection and removal of any crust, palpation is carried out to assess the extent of macroscopic spread. The lesion usually takes the form of an ulcer with rolled, everted, friable edges. Some bleeding or discharge may be visible. The size is measured and a drawing made. As with all accessible disease, it is most desirable that a photographic record is kept. Using the head mirror the mouth is examined. Particular attention is paid to the condition of the teeth and dentures, noting any sharp edges or sepsis. Finally the neck is palpated to discover any evidence of lymphatic spread.

Buccal Mucosa and Hard Palate

Similar inspection and palpation is carried out. If the lesion of the buccal mucosa is extensive, examination may have to be carried out under general anaesthesia. This is because due to infiltration of muscle there is painful spasm (trismus) preventing the mouth opening fully.

Tongue

While the history is being taken the speech can be assessed, this may well be affected by a lesion. The patient is asked to put out the tongue. Its mobility, the extent of protrusion, and any deviation to one side is noted. Inspection then follows noting the appearance of the tongue, whether it is smooth and shiny, has patches of leukoplakia, or an abnormal granular surface. When the condition is very advanced, foetor may be noticeable. As with other lesions of this area, the general state of the whole mouth and also of the teeth is included in the inspection. For adequate examination any dentures are removed, but before doing so, the relation of any sharp edge of tooth or denture to the lesion is noted. Patients referred with suspected carcinoma have occasionally been cured by the removal of a tooth or reshaping the denture.

The doctor will particularly look for the presence of several lesions, since more than one malignancy may occur simultaneously in the tongue and mouth.

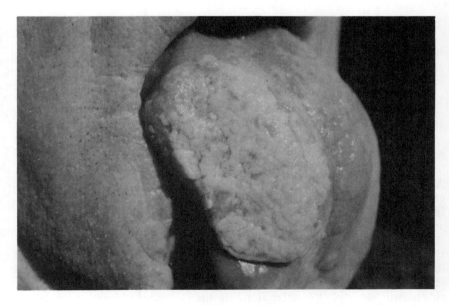

Fig. 6.5.   Carcinoma of the tongue

Attention is now focused on the tumour. Its appearance is variable. It can present, as a nodule with the mucosa unbroken, as an infiltrative thickening, as frank papillary overgrowth (cauliflower in appearance), as fissuring or ulceration. If it is situated in the posterior third, mirror examination is required to visualise it properly. The tongue is then palpated to assess the degree of infiltration.

As will be realised from the description of the anatomy, the lymphatic drainage is such that nodes may be involved on both sides at any point from the base of the skull down to the clavicle. Careful inspection and palpation of the whole of the neck will therefore conclude the examination.

When first seen 40% of patients with anterior lesions have involved nodes, 60% with posterior tumours.

Investigation

Blood Tests

A routine blood count and biochemical profile is made, the latter will include electrolytes, urea and liver function tests. In addition blood is sent for serological testing for syphilis. Although the incidence of this disease is less, it is still a predisposing factor in malignancy and worsens the prognosis. One patient when questioned admitted to having a 'stiff' tongue for years. Her W.R. test was positive and it is likely that she was describing a 'woody' tongue, one of the signs of late syphilis.

X-rays

In addition to the routine chest X-ray, pictures are taken of the jaw, if there is any reason to suspect infiltration or infection, and also if necessary of the teeth. Infection around the teeth will require extraction of the affected teeth before treatment. In the case of an ulcer of the hard palate, as we shall see in a later section, this may originate from malignancy in the nose, nasopharynx, or the antrum. X-rays will be taken of the hard palate and other areas as indicated.

Biopsy

At some point it may be necessary to examine the patient under anaesthesia, at the same time a biopsy will then be taken and any infected teeth extracted. In other cases, such as carcinoma of the lip, biopsy can be done under local anaesthesia. The nurse may ask why, if the lesion on clinical grounds is considered malignant, biopsy is necessary. There are two reasons. If malignant, the information on histology is important, e.g. in the tongue, the degree of differentiation affects the prognosis. Although the pattern of disease has changed, on rare occasions other conditions can mimic malignancy, trauma, tuberculous or syphilitic ulceration. In the last case adequate treatment is important if malignancy is not later to develop. In those rare fortunate cases when the clinician is confident that trauma is the cause, biopsy can be postponed.

The offending tooth or denture is dealt with, and biopsy is only carried out if, in a fortnight's time, there has been no favourable response.

Treatment

Since the lymphatic drainage of the area must be regarded as a whole, treatment of lymph nodes will be dealt with separately at the end of Section II.

The Lip

If the lesion is small and centrally placed, surgical excision can be performed, but radiation is becoming more and more a preferred treatment. It can be carried out in three ways:

1. External radiation.
2. Radioactive needles.
3. Radioactive mould.

External Radiation   The area of irradiation must as always include an adequate margin for safety. This will mean, for example, that for a lesion in the lateral third of the lower lip the lateral extent must include the angle of the mouth and part of the upper lip, while for a lesion in the middle third the whole lip will be treated. Steps are taken to avoid unnecessary irradiation of nearby structures, a protective strip is placed behind the lip and a block used to move the tongue out of the field. These steps can only of course be taken if the size of the lesion permits. Should the bone be involved then megavoltage therapy can be employed, but it is probably better to rely on surgery, due to the sequelae of radionecrosis and pain. Treatment is given daily for about four weeks.

Radioactive Needles   Under a general anaesthetic the tumour is measured and needles of the appropriate size and containing the correct amount of radioactive isotope are implanted. The techniques and principles of implantation will be covered fully in the section on the tongue. The needles remain for a period of six to eight days and can then be removed, provided there is adequate analgesia, without an anaesthetic.

Radioactive Mould   This technique is practised in certain centres. A mould is made which is in the form of a sandwich. A radioactive isotope in an appropriate mounting, is the bread inside and outside the lip, and the lip fits between like the meat. The patient wears the mould each day for a calculated period which is usually several hours. Treatment can last from five to ten days.

Buccal Mucosa

Radiation methods available are, an implant under anaesthetic with radioactive needles, or external megavoltage therapy. If the tumour is radioresistant or bone is involved, surgery will be used. The excision by diathermy of a very small lesion is occasionally undertaken.

Hard Palate

The treatment of choice is irradiation. This can be by:

1. External megavoltage therapy.
2. A radioactive mould usually mounted on a dental prosthesis.
3. The permanent implantation of radioactive seeds (often gold).

If bone is involved, if at all possible, surgical excision followed by plastic reconstruction is the treatment of choice.

Tongue

The commonest of the mouth tumours, its treatment presents a real challenge since speech is part of the personality. Therefore while treatment must be aimed to be curative, it must not be so mutilating that the patient is left with inadequate communication. Fortunately few cases now present at a very advanced stage, and powerful external radiation sources offer an alternative to extensive surgery.

The management will vary according to the site of the tumour and the degree of infiltration. The more posteriorly a lesion is placed, the more it becomes primarily a radiotherapy problem. It should be noted here that although sensitivity increases as the site moves back, the prognosis worsens.

Treatment will now be considered for each primary site.

Tip

The treatment of choice is surgical excision. Functional results are excellent.

Lateral Margin

Surgery   In the anterior two-thirds, surgery is still possible when the lesion is limited to the margin. Hemi-glossectomy is the usual procedure and despite the removal of so much tissue, the cosmetic and functional results are still good. It should be noted that this surgery only involves the anterior mobile portion of the tongue.

Radioactive Implant   Radioactive needles used to be a hollow tube of gold alloy or a platignum iridium mixture containing radium. Now other radioactive sources are used. The principle however is the same. Needles are of standard lengths and strengths.

The aim of an implant is to give a certain area an even dosage of irradiation. If the needles are too close together the dose to one part may be very much higher than the rest. This is called a hot spot. Conversely an area of very low dosage is called a cold spot.

The first step is to measure the maximum area of the tumour and allow a further centimetre beyond it. From standard tables the number, pattern, and strength of needles can be calculated. The original radium tables were devised by two workers in Manchester and named after them, the Parker Pattinson tables. The needles can be implanted in a single layer, two layers, or in a volume implant. The calculations are made in advance so that the necessary number and strength of sources can be prepared and sent to theatre.

After implantation X-rays are taken and the length of time the needles need to remain in place is calculated. Any badly placed needle causing a hot or cold spot must be corrected. Accurate placement of needles in textbook patterns is very difficult.

Until required the needles are kept in a protective container, and if they have to be handled, then this is done using long handled instruments to mini-mise radiation exposure. The needles are secured by stitches, either individually or by one picking up the threads from each needle. If possible a nurse from the ward should witness the procedure.

Wherever the sources move within the hospital there is a check of the number and type. The operation notes will include a diagram of the implant and number and type of sources used. At each change of staff there must be a check that the sources are still in place and the number correct, this is noted in the documen-tation. When sources are removed and returned to the protective store the check must be made, sources returned must tally with those withdrawn.

Posterior Third

Although radical surgery is possible, most clinicians prefer to use external radiation, particularly since many tumours extend on to the epiglottis and in consequence have a worse prognosis. Treatment normally lasts six to eight weeks.

Lymph Nodes

The treatment policy is the same for all sites in this area and will be discussed at the end of the section.

Similarly chemotherapy and radio sensitisers will be discussed.

Combined Regimes

Other methods of radiation such as neutron therapy have been tried, similarly the use of hyperbaric oxygen, none has made any marked impact on results.

Surgery varyingly combined with radiation, chemotherapy, before or after the operation has been attempted. Some successes in particular cases have been reported, but again no marked improvement in results has been seen.

Section II
PHARYNX AND LARYNX

The Pharynx, Anatomy

In order to understand the signs and symptoms of disease here we must first consider the anatomy. The pharynx is a muscular tube lined by epithelium. It can be regarded as a lift shaft with openings at three floor levels, the nose, the mouth, and the larynx. It stretches from the base of the skull above, to the level of the sixth cervical vertebra below. Here it becomes the oesophagus and lies immediately in front of the spinal column. It is in part a common passage for both air and food. For convenience it is divided into three regions.

Nasopharynx

This is bounded above by the base of the skull, behind by the first cervical vertebra and part of the second. In front it opens into the nasal passages. The opening is bounded above by the soft palate and uvula, laterally by the tonsillar pillars, and below by the tongue. Lying in front of the pillars are the tonsils, collections of lymphoid tissue. In the lateral walls of the nasopharynx are the openings of the Eustachian tubes. Due to its proximity to the base of the skull it is close to some of the cranial nerves, particularly the fifth. This nerve contains sensory fibres from the face and some motor fibres. The epithelium of the nasopharynx is mainly ciliated, but with ageing this can become squamous. Lying on the posterior wall are the adenoids, below the mucous membrane there is a rich supply of lymphatic tissue. The lumen of the tube is small.

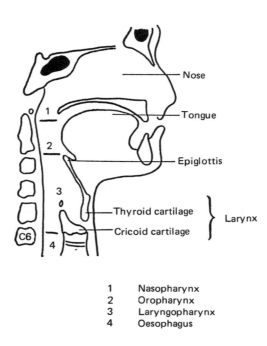

1   Nasopharynx
2   Oropharynx
3   Laryngopharynx
4   Oesophagus

Fig. 6.6.   Sections of the pharynx

Oropharynx

At the level of the soft palate the oropharynx begins, stretching from here down to the tip of the epiglottis. It is bounded behind by part of the second cervical vertebra and the whole of the third and fourth. It opens in front into the mouth cavity. It is lined by stratified squamous epithelium and has a rich lymphatic drainage.

Laryngopharynx

This extends from the tip of the epiglottis to the level of the sixth cervical vertebra where it becomes the oesophagus. It is divided for convenience into the upper and lower parts, the epi- and hypo-pharynx. From the diagram it will be seen that anteriorly lies the epiglottis, the opening of the larynx, and the body of the larynx. Below and lateral to the epiglottis are two fossae, the piriform fossae, these are important sites of carcinoma. Behind, the laryngopharynx is bounded by the fifth and sixth cervical vertebrae. It is lined by stratified squamous epithelium and is closed except during deglutition. As in the rest of the pharynx, the lymphatic drainage is rich.

The nasopharynx conveys air, and the rest of the pharynx, except for the part behind the body of the larynx, both air and food.

Lymphatics

There is a lymphatic plexus lying in close relation to the tube. Further drainage is to the regional nodes, some lying immediately behind the pharynx, others are in the neck, the cervical nodes. These cervical nodes consist of:

1. The tonsillar at the angle of the jaw, the submandibular, and the submental below the chin.
2. A small node close to the mastoid process.
3. The cervical chain lying along the line of the internal jugular vein.

Drainage is from the nodes lying close to the tube to the cervical chain, on to the supraclavicular nodes, and finally discharging into the blood stream through the main lymph ducts.

Aetiology

Nasopharynx

As this is an air passage research workers have studied the role of inhaled substances as carcinogens. There is a high incidence among the Chinese and certain Africans. Factors suggested have been cooking oil fumes, oil lamps, low-grade tobacco, opium and snuff. Since it is equally common in Chinese living in other countries a genetic or racial predisposition must be considered, although it has been reported that in second generation immigrants to the West the incidence falls. In Western peoples smoking and wood dust have also been put forward as carcinogens.

Oropharynx and Laryngopharynx

Here the possible carcinogens are dental sepsis, tobacco and alcohol. There is a close association with long-standing iron deficiency anaemia in women. A very few cases have followed previous irradiation of benign lesions in the neck.

Incidence

Most patients are men in the fifth and sixth decades. There are two exceptions, lymphoid tumours of the tonsil occur in a younger age group, and post cricoid carcinoma is mostly found in younger women.

Pathology and Spread

Carcinoma is of the squamous type. It shows a range from well differentiated to anaplastic. Spread is primarily lymphatic, to the nodes lying behind causing bulging of the posterior wall, and to the nodes on both sides of the neck. Late spread is by the blood stream to the lungs and liver.

In the younger age groups tumours are usually of the lymphoid group. They arise from the tonsil or the lymphatic tissue within the pharyngeal wall. Spread is mainly lymphatic.

In the oropharynx the tumour site is often the tonsil, and in the laryngopharynx malignancy often arises simultaneously in several areas (multicentric origin).

Symptomatology

Nasopharynx

Symptoms may be divided into three groups.

1. Local symptoms due to the presence of growth.
   a. Ulceration giving rise to nasal discharge and bleeding.
   b. Obstruction. The patient complains of being unable to breathe through the nose and of an alteration of voice (nasal speech).
   c. Deafness. This is usually unilateral, but can involve both sides. It is caused by blockage of the Eustachian tube.
2. Symptoms caused by involvement of nearby structures.
   a. Paralysis or loss of sensation. An example is extension to the base of the skull. This will involve cranial nerves, commonly the fifth (trigeminal). There will then be loss of facial sensation on the same side, and in some patients severe pain (trigeminal neuralgia).

3. Symptoms from distant spread.
   a. Lymph nodes. Patients often complain not of local symptoms but of a painless lump in the neck. With such a presentation the pharynx must be carefully examined for a primary. This may be very small, and although sought, is not always found.
   b. Blood stream. If spread has already occurred through the blood stream the symptoms will vary according to the site of the deposits. Lung secondaries will cause dyspnoea and possibly haemoptysis.

Oropharynx

Patients complain of a lump in the throat which cannot be cleared by swallowing or coughing. This progresses to a difficulty in swallowing (dysphagia). There is an increase in the secretion of mucus and this can become blood stained. Presentation with a lump in the neck is found in this group. In some patients the diagnosis is only made after investigation of attacks of recurrent tonsillitis. Late symptoms include pain and hoarseness of the voice.

Laryngopharynx

Symptoms are similar to those listed under the oropharynx. The predominant symptom is dysphagia. Associated with this is a loss of weight due to the inability to swallow an adequate diet. At a late stage there is hoarseness owing to involvement of the larynx or of one of the nerves supplying it.

Examination and Investigation

Examination

A careful history is taken. This will include details of habits (smoking), occupation (furniture industry), past medical conditions (anaemia), and a description of the symptoms. The nurse must have ready a lamp, head mirror, and instruments for examination of the ear, nose, and throat. It is important that the neck is adequately exposed for examination.

1. General. The doctor will look for signs of anaemia (pallor of the mucous membrane), cyanosis, and at the general state of nutrition.
2. Neck. An inspection is made for swelling, deviation of the larynx, abnormal venous engorgement. On palpation the larynx is tested for mobility and a search is made for lymph nodes. If these are enlarged, their mobility, size, and extent are noted.
3. Nose. There is first an inspection for abnormal swelling and signs of haemorrhage/discharge. The patient blocks each side of the nose in turn and sniffs, this assesses patency. With the head mirror and nasal speculum each nares is examined. The doctor is looking for swelling or ulceration.

4. Mouth. In order to get a good light the doctor will use a head mirror. He will assess the general condition of the mouth including the teeth and look for signs of sepsis.

A particular search is made for:

   a. enlargement of ulceration of the tonsils,

   b. swelling or ulceration of the soft palate, this can be caused either by swelling within the palate or by pressure from the nasopharynx above,

   c. any other visible swelling or ulceration, e.g. a mass in the posterior wall of the oropharynx.

Movement of the tongue and soft palate will be noted, this can be affected either directly by the tumour or by involvement of the nerve supply.

Mirror examination is now carried out. The small mirror is used for the post-nasal space and a larger one for inspection of the larynx (laryngoscopy). Any swelling, ulceration, or in the case of the larynx impairment of cord movement, is noted. It is worth remembering that laryngoscopy is sometimes very difficult. Inspection is followed by digital examination, occasionally a swelling is felt when it has not been visible, this is particular true in the nasopharynx.

Investigations

General

As with all patients attending the Radiotherapy Clinic for the first time, a chest X-ray and blood count will be ordered. A swab is taken from any accessible lesion or any septic area.

X-rays

These will vary according to the site of the lesion. Plain X-rays can show soft tissue swellings or erosion of bone. Further specialised X-rays can then be taken in accordance with the findings. These can be:

   a. pictures of localised areas of bone,

   b. a special type to show soft tissue,

   c. tomograms. These latter bring into sharp focus structures at varying pre-determined depths. All these are designed to show the extent of the disease. In addition 'swallow' studies using a contrast medium will add information on the extent of the tumour, the degree of obstruction, and the movement of the muscular tube. CATscans may be helpful.

Theatre

The patient is examined under general anaesthesia. Direct laryngoscopy is performed, or if the lesion is in the post-cricoid area, an oesophagoscopy. This will be necessary as spread may have occurred down the oesophagus. A biopsy will be taken of the lesion, or if no primary has been found, of an enlarged node in the neck. If the airway is threatened tracheostomy may also be performed at this stage.

Treatment

With the full information now available on the extent and nature of the disease, a decision can be made on the method of treatment.

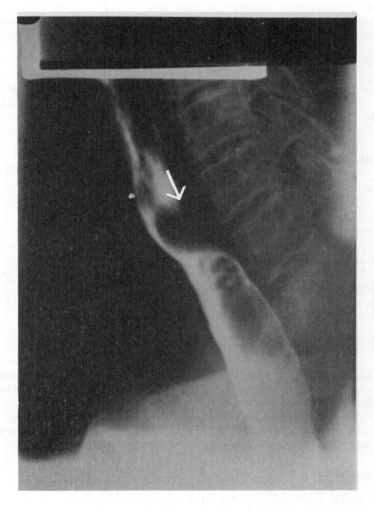

Fig. 6.7.   Barium swallow showing post-cricoid carcinoma

Broad Policy

Dental care   If there is any sepsis so that teeth require extraction, this should be done before irradiation. Sepsis with superimposed radiation predisposes to necrosis of the bone.

Local Condition

As a general rule tumours of the pharynx are treated by irradiation. The exceptions are small tumours of the nasopharynx, and those in the laryngopharynx which the surgeon considers amenable to wide excision and reconstruction procedures. Surgery is also used in some cases of failed irradiation. It should be realised that all these are major procedures which in the lower part of the pharynx may involve removal of the larynx.

Lymph Nodes

Since the principles governing the treatment of lymph nodes in this area are the same wherever the primary site, their consideration will be postponed until the end of this section.

Radiotherapy

Megavoltage therapy is usually employed. Courses of treatment last four to six weeks.

Nasopharynx

The fields cover the full extent of the disease together with a margin. Bearing in mind the anatomy, the upper margin of the field will be the base of the skull or possibly higher. Precautions are taken to exclude vulnerable structures, such as the lens of the eye or the spinal cord. However if the extent of the disease is such that they have to be included, the dose is limited.

Oropharynx

This includes treatment of the tonsil and soft palate. The same techniques are employed, but where electron therapy is available, as from certain betatrons, treatment of unilateral lesions can be so arranged that structures on the other side of the face or neck receive minimal irradiation. This is an advantage when one tonsil is being treated, the mouth and cheek on the other side will be spared avoiding some of the unpleasant sequelae of soreness and dryness.

Laryngopharynx

The main sites of lesions are the extra-laryngeal piriform fossae and the post-cricoid area. Techniques and criteria are similar to those for the rest of the pharynx. For lesions of the post-cricoid area the length of the fields may be relatively greater, since the upper third of the oesophagus may have to be included because of the spread.

Radioactive Sources

In some centres a bougie is loaded with a radioactive source. Under general anaesthesia this is passed down into position in the oesophagus and kept there for a short period. This procedure is repeated at intervals of a few days until the required dose is reached. Occasionally a small radioactive contact source is used to treat lesions of the nasopharynx. Due to the efficiency of the modern megavoltage machines these methods are not in widespread use.

The Larynx, Anatomy

The larynx is the voice box and lies between the levels of the third and sixth cervical vertebrae. It communicates above with the oropharynx and below with the trachea. It consists of the epiglottis and the thyroid and cricoid cartilages, connected together to form a tube by ligaments, membrane, and muscle. The epiglottis which is leaf-shaped is attached to the anterior wall of the upper part of the thyroid cartilage. It acts as a lid closing off the larynx when food is being swallowed. Lying inside the thyroid cartilage are the vocal cords which run from front to back. The true vocal cords are thickenings covered with squamous

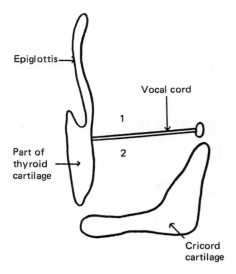

| 1 | Supra-glottic |
| 2 | Sub-glottic |

Fig. 6.8.   Section of the larynx

epithelium. On either side of these closing off the rest of the space, are the false vocal cords. Air passes through the true cords known as the rima glottis, and as the cords are tightened or relaxed during speech the pitch of the voice is altered. The larynx can be viewed in the laryngeal mirror and the cords seen to move. If they move closer together towards the midline, this is adduction, if they move apart, away from the midline, this is abduction. In health the cords move evenly on both sides.

Nerve Supply

Small muscles move the vocal cord and they are supplied by a recurrent laryngeal nerve on either side. If one nerve is involved by disease, the cord on that side will not move, if both are involved, both cords are paralysed. If this occurs when the cords are closed (adducted) this is an emergency and tracheotomy is required. Impairment of cord movement leads to hoarseness of the voice, and, according to its degree, to stridor and airway obstruction. On the left side the recurrent laryngeal nerve runs down in the chest, hooks round the arch of the aorta and runs back up to enter the larynx. A lesion in the thorax, such as enlarged glands, pressing on the nerve will lead to paralysis of the left cord. We shall meet this symptom of hoarseness when considering carcinoma of the bronchus.

Aetiology

Smoking is linked to carcinoma of the larynx, and the risk is increased when associated with heavy alcohol consumption.

Incidence

About 1% of deaths from malignancy are caused by this tumour.

Age and Sex

The patient is usually about 60 and the M:F ratio is about 10:1.

Site

The majority arise from the cords, intrinsic, the rest from the adjacent epiglottis or aryepiglottic tissue, extrinsic.

Pathology and Spread

This is a squamous carcinoma. Figure 6.11 shows the various stages. It usually begins as a swelling of the cord, which later ulcerates, and spreads in most cases forward to the anterior commissure. It can also pass over on to the other cord, upwards known as supraglottic spread, or downwards, subglottic spread. The staging is important since it affects both prognosis and treatment. Prognosis is good when the disease is confined to one cord, but progressively

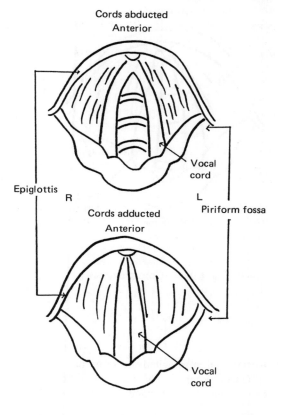

Fig. 6.9.   Cords abducted and adducted

worse as extension increases. The nature and extent of the treatment given will
be determined by the staging. In advanced carcinoma direct extension can occur
into the thyroid cartilage and the pharynx. Lymphatic spread does not often
occur, and when it does it is at a late stage of the disease.

Symptoms

The site of the tumour, its extent, and the nature of its spread will cause symptoms to vary in their order of presentation and in their severity.

Persistent Hoarseness

In lesions of the true cord this is the earliest symptom to occur. It can remain
unchanged for long periods, but as the disease advances it progresses until there
is only a whisper left, or there is complete loss of voice.

Anterior

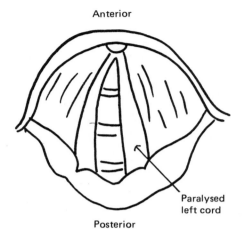

Paralysed
left cord

Posterior

Fig. 6.10.   Cord paralysis

Dyspnoea

This is usually the earliest symptom when the lesion lies below the true cord, but there can be in addition some alteration of the voice and discomfort in the throat. Hoarseness appears when the cord is invaded by upward extension.

Late Symptoms

Pain is a late symptom and indicates infection and involvement of the cartilage. Blood staining of the sputum and foetor can also occur. Very advanced cases will exhibit dysphagia and possibly cyanosis.

Examination

External examination of the neck is carried out and unobtrusively, while this is being done, the condition of the airway is noted, and, whether dyspnoea or stridor is present. Other points to be noted are any enlargement of the larynx, fixation, tenderness, and the presence or absence of nodes. The general condition of the mouth, teeth, and mucosa is noted as before.

Laryngoscopy

In the clinic this is indirect. A large mirror and good light are necessary. The patient requires much reassurance and some will require to suck an anaesthetic

1 Along cord

2 Sub-glottic
   (downward)

3 Supra-glottic
   (upward)

4 Outside the
   larynx

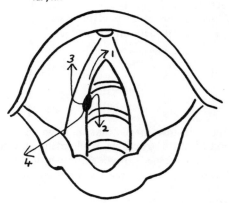

Fig. 6.11.   Spread of carcinoma of the larynx

lozenge or have the pharynx sprayed. The ideal is for the patient to be relaxed, sitting comfortably, and breathing easily.

The doctor will inspect the epiglottis, the true and false cords, the aryepiglottic fold, and the region surrounding the larynx. If a lesion is obvious its appearance and its position on the cord are noted, and an estimate of its size made. The extent and direction of spread is important, whether forward or backward, across to the other cord, and whether up or down. The patient is asked to say 'ee' and the movement of the cord is noted. If there is any airway obstruction it will be accentuated during examination and the cause may be obvious. Obstruction can be due to the size of the tumour, to narrowing by paralysis of the cords, or to restriction of the airway by subglottic tumour. Lesions below the cord can be difficult to visualise and assess in the clinic. Both examination under general anaesthesia and tomograms of the larynx will be required.

Biopsy

Under general anaesthesia direct laryngoscopy can be carried out permitting a fuller examination. At the same time a biopsy is taken. Tracheotomy can be performed at this point if airway obstruction is precipitated by the examination. Of course the patient must be warned beforehand of this possibility.

Investigations

Full blood count and chest X-ray as for all radiotherapy patients is done. In addition an examination of the sputum for tubercle bacilli is made and a serological test for syphilis. These latter two are necessary, as in rare cases both tuberculosis and syphilis can mimic a malignant lesion. Special investigations will include a soft tissue X-ray of the neck, this will show any soft masses distorting the trachea and any destruction of cartilage. Tomograms of the larynx will also reveal any invasion of cartilage and are particularly useful in assessing subglottic spread. If there is any reason to suspect involvement of the pharynx, X-ray 'swallow' studies using contrast medium are made.

Treatment

Radiation

An early lesion of the true cord means that there will be no involvement of the lymphatics or invasion of other structures. While many authorities regard surgery and radiotherapy as of equal value, a growing number now advocate radiotherapy as the treatment of choice, since the results are good, and the voice after treatment is better than after surgery.

Megavoltage radiation is used. The fields are small, 4–6 cm square and accurate positioning essential, both at initial planning and at each treatment. To ensure

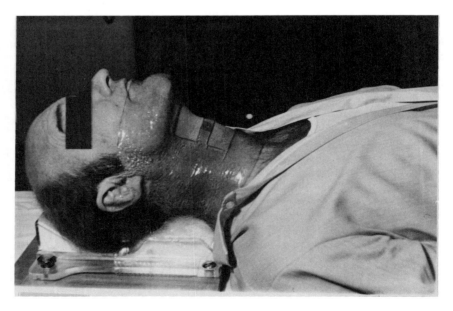

Fig. 6.12.   Carcinoma of the larynx, patient set up for treatment on cobalt machine

this a plastics immobilisation shell may be used, and using lead markers an X-ray check, or a simulator set up carried out. Treatment lasts approximately six weeks.

If the extent of the disease is greater and the decision is still made to treat by radiation, then the fields will of course be larger. Reasons for using radiotherapy in these cases can include the unwillingness of the patient to undergo surgery, or a condition rendering him unfit for operation.

In some centres radioactive needles are still used. This involves removing some of the cartilage and placing the needles palisade fashion in the opening, later removing them. This method is little used now that megavoltage therapy is available.

Surgery

When the lesion is advanced radiation has to be given to a wide area and to a high dosage. If cartilage is involved, the risk of necrosis following radiation is very high since the blood supply is poor. In view of this, if a decision is made to attempt radical treatment, then surgery is the first choice. The operation recommended is usually a total laryngectomy which may be combined with block dissection of the nodes. If primary radiation fails, or if there is a recurrence of tumour, surgery can still be employed.

Rehabilitation

After surgery involving total laryngectomy, the patient can learn to speak with an oesophageal voice. For this he needs the services of a speech therapist to train him. He swallows air and regurgitates, phonating with his lips. The tone is monotonous and the voice easily exhausted. Mechanical resonators can also be fitted, or an external device used.

Chemotherapy

As new and more potent cytotoxics have been introduced, combination drug regimes have been tried to reduce tumour bulk before surgery, combined with radiotherapy, or as palliation. In addition drugs to sensitise the tumour to radiation or chemotherapy have been given. It is impossible to assess results, numbers are so small, but in centres reporting success the combination of methotrexate, bleomycin, and cis-platin has been the most common, although in older patients the toxicity of cis-platin limits its usefulness. The route of administration is intravenous, or a perfusion giving the cytotoxic directly into the artery supplying the area.

Other Methods

The use of hyperbaric oxygen to enhance sensitivity has not, on the whole, fulfilled its early promise. Neutron therapy is still experimental. Sensitisers to enhance therapy are also being used.

Treatment of the Lymph Nodes Draining the Whole Area

The clinician is aware that some of these tumours spread early to the lymph nodes. The extent of the spread may depend upon the site of the lesion.

1. Usually spread is to the nodes on the same side as the primary lesion, but occasionally both sides of the neck can be involved, spread is certainly to both sides from midline tumours.
2. Nodes can be involved although not clinically palpable. This was demonstrated histologically in nodes that were removed prophylactically.

Principles of Treatment

1. No enlarged nodes   When nodes are not enlarged the whole of the cervical chain is not included in the field. Only the regional nodes in close proximity to the tumour are irradiated. Prophylactic irradiation or block dissection is still advocated by some centres. In any case the patient must be seen at regular intervals to check that no enlargement has occurred.

2. Mobile enlarged nodes   If enlargement is due to sepsis, this will subside with antibiotic treatment. Provided that satisfactory control of the primary condition has been achieved, or can be confidently expected, block dissection of involved mobile nodes is universally accepted as the treatment of choice. This would be the policy if enlarged nodes fail to subside after antibiotic treatment. Block dissection means the removal, on the same side of the neck, of all the lymphatic drainage tissue. The usual proviso on the fitness of the patient of course applies.

3. Fixed nodes   Surgery plays no part in treatment, radiation is the treatment of choice. The decision whether it should be given, and if it is given the dose required, will depend upon a careful consideration of the primary and the extent of the metastatic deposits, together with the age of the patient. A small fixed gland would receive a radical dosage, while more extensive deposits throughout the neck would merit only limited treatment.

Section III
FOLLOW-UP AND PROGNOSIS

Follow-up of Patients with Disease in the Whole Area

General Policy

The patient must be seen at regular intervals. The timing of these appointments will vary according to the site of the disease, the histology, policy adopted, and the period which has elapsed since treatment. Since any of these lesions may metastasise quite quickly to lymph nodes, and the nodes then become fixed in a short period thereby becoming inoperable, it is important that a careful frequent watch is kept. A common policy is for patients to be seen monthly for the first year, two monthly for the second year, and at longer intervals, thereafter. The importance attached to follow-up is such that the reason for any patient failing to attend must be vigorously pursued.

If ulceration is present on discharge, then the patient should attend the radiotherapy centre for dressings since the staff understand the nature of the reaction better.

At every follow-up the history and examination will fall into well-defined sections:

1. General condition.
2. The state of the local lesion.
3. The state of other structures.
4. The lymph nodes.

As an example we will look at the points covered during an immediate follow-up appointment. Every patient is weighed and the result entered in the notes. The doctor compares this with the weight on discharge and will learn much, before the patient says anything of how he is managing with his diet. Questions are then asked as to how the patient feels, whether he has had any fresh symptoms, or if he feels there has been any improvement. When the patient is elderly it is rather more fruitful to talk to the relatives. This of course may be so at any age, as some patients are very stoic and minimise their troubles. Specific questions are then asked about diet, pain, dysphagia, sleep and cough. If a tracheostomy is present the patient is questioned as to how this is being managed. When he is being visited at home, by a nurse, her report should be available.

General Condition

On examination any obvious wasting or signs of anaemia are sought. During the earlier conversation the presence of any hoarseness and the strength of the voice can be noted.

Local Condition

The state of the local lesion is next assessed, the doctor is looking for regression of the tumour, repair by normal tissue, and restoration of function. Where inspection is difficult owing to crusting, reliance is placed on palpation alone. The crust is, if necessary, removed but not routinely. A swab is taken of any obviously infected lesion and sent for culture and sensitivity.

Other Structures

Mucosa

The reaction in the mucous membrane and also in the skin settles over a period of approximately a month. At completion the mucosa is covered by a white 'radiation' membrane surrounded by an area of erythema. As the expected appearance is known it is possible to assess whether the reaction is subsiding normally. Eventually the mucosa may become slightly pale and sometimes dry.

Skin

The reaction will vary according to the type of machine used. We may find a deep, fiery red, dry erythema.

Occasionally a moist reaction occurred with the previously used conventional therapy.

Larynx

A mirror inspection is made and the state of the local lesion is assessed, the presence of any fresh lesion noted, and the function of the cords recorded. The airway is tested by asking the patient to breath deeply and listening for stridor.

Cartilage

Any damage to cartilage gives rise to pain which is often out of all proportion to the size of the affected area. The policy adopted is a careful frequent watch with the use of local cortisone preparations. No precipitate action is taken.

Bone

Pain is also the dominant symptom here. Occasionally a swelling is present or even a sinus. An X-ray is taken. The policy will be to treat any infection and wait for a bone sequestrum to separate. In both the last two cases adequate analgesia must be prescribed.

Nerves

For reasons already given earlier in this chapter in the section on anatomy, function of the cranial nerves is assessed. This will include inspection of the fundi and testing of the ocular movements.

Lymph Nodes

The examination as already described is made. Points to be assessed are:

1. In a patient with known nodes, have these progressed?
2. Have any additional nodes appeared?
3. Have nodes appeared for the first time?

According to the findings, policy is formulated by the guidelines already laid down in the section on the treatment of lymph nodes.

Investigations

The routine blood count is performed. If dyspnoea or dysphagia is causing deterioration, appropriate X-rays will be performed. Other investigations may include serological tests if syphilis is being treated, others will be determined by the patient's condition or symptoms.

This description of follow-up includes points not appropriate in every case, since the whole area has been described in this chapter.

Prognosis

There is a range in the prognosis, much will depend on the site of the lesion, the extent, and the presence of metastatic spread. For example a small lesion of the lip with no lymph node involvement should do well, while at the other extreme, the outlook for the patients with carcinoma of the nasopharynx is poor.

Overall Prognosis

Site of Lesion		Five-Year Survival Rate
Lip	Upper	30%
	Lower	50%
Buccal Mucosa		14–17%
Hard Palate		14%
Tongue	Tip	20%
	Lateral	20%
Posterior Third		12%
Pharynx	Naso-	16%
	Oro-	10%
	Laryngo-	5%
Larynx		20%

These figures are only a general guide, those with early disease and no involvement of lymph nodes will do much better. The patient with a stage I carcinoma of the larynx has an 80% chance of surviving five years, and a patient with a small lesion of the tip of the tongue and no involved glands may well survive to a normal age.

We reach outwards seeking in vain for happiness,
Yet all the time
It lies here close at hand in the ward.
For no happiness is greater
Than the happiness we give to others.

7 Nursing Care of the Patients Described in Chapter 6

Before considering the detailed step-by-step care of these patients, we should stop for a moment and consider first the problems of the nurse. Those of us who spend all our time caring for patients with malignant disease, are only reminded when we return from an absence, such as a holiday, of the impact that a ward of these patients makes on the new nurse. She may only recently have left school and has had little experience of life to prepare her. Like all of us she will at first only have eyes for the very ill patients. There is an indefinable sense of withdrawal amongst the patients in contrast with the lively atmosphere of the surgical ward. That is not to say that there is not laughter, but the key is muted. Then she begins to adjust and see that range of conditions, from the early cases with the good prognosis, to those for whom only palliative measures are possible.

Finally she finds her place in the team, and the initial impressions fade as she becomes absorbed in her work. Those in charge of such a ward need to remember their own early experiences, and make this period of adjustment as easy as possible for the new nurse. If she is told that her emotion is natural, but that through her activities she will come to accept, she will be better prepared.

If she understands something of the disease she will realise that the immediate returns are small. The steady improvement and the response to nursing care that she sees in a surgical or acute medical ward, is not repeated in a radio-therapy ward. Those patients who respond do so slowly, others by the very nature of their complaint have a prolonged, sometimes downward, course. All of them require from those treating them a great deal of encouragement. There-fore, despite the nature of the disease we have to convey our own realisation that what we are doing is of benefit. We must steer a course between unqualified, ill-founded optimism and gloomy pessimism, maintaining a steady cheerful atmosphere. The patient responds to a team united in a sincere approach to all these problems.

This chapter is not intended as a detailed description of nursing techniques but rather to emphasise special points arising either from the consequences of treatment or the nature of the disease. Particular fluids or preparations are intended as a guide, each centre will have its own preferred regimes.

The Ward Patient

Some patients with disease of these structures are treated as out-patients, but many are admitted to the ward. We will therefore consider in detail the nursing problems involved for these latter patients.

On Admission

The nurse who admits the patient can learn much which will be helpful later to the doctor. If the relatives come with the patient she can find out what sort of diet he has been taking, whether he has any marked dietary likes and dislikes, whether he is suffering much pain. If it is not possible for the doctor to see the family at this time, then an early appointment must be made for him to do so. When the patient has been transferred from another ward or hospital, these details can be sought from an accompanying attendant, for the transfer letter may need amplification.

Preparation for Treatment

General Condition and Diet

It may be necessary for a period of intensive nursing care to precede treatment. Often the patient is depressed, and may be exhausted by pain, or poor diet, or distressed by discharge from sinuses. Poor nutrition potentiates radiation reaction and delays healing. The dietician is an important member of an oncology team. She needs to learn the patient's likes and dislikes and the nurse who has talked to the relatives can be a great help. A diet must be both attractive and high in calories and protein. It must be easy to take and may even need to be homogenised. Taste if not already lost, is lost or altered during this period, and due to this and the build up of radiation reaction, alterations to the regime will almost certainly be required. As this regime has to be continued at home, attention must be paid to easy preparation and to expense. The nurse complements all this work by continually encouraging the patient. Some may require feeding, a gastrostomy or nasogastric tube is avoided if possible, others though capable of eating will tend to leave food because of the inertia caused by their illness. An adequate fluid intake is also most important, particularly if any vomiting occurs.

If anaemia is present blood transfusion is given, this can be followed by special fluids if the diet has been inadequate, in order to correct the negative nitrogen balance. Any necessary extraction of teeth is carried out at this time also.

The alcoholic and the smoker present special problems. A slow reduction of alcohol intake at first is necessary, but the calories so lost must be replaced in the diet. It may be .impossible to withdraw the alcohol completely. Ideally smoking should stop, but if this would make the patient miserable then a compromise is reached and he is encouraged to cut down. The problem usually solves itself, as towards the end of treatment cigarettes often become distasteful. The exception to this compromise is when the larynx is treated, then smoking must always stop. The ideal must be weighed against the nature of the disease, smoking and alcohol in moderation are unlikely to affect the prognosis at this stage, and to deprive patients may make life less tolerable for them.

Mental Preparation of The Patient

At the planning session in the clinic the doctor will explain to the patient what the treatment involves. If possible the nurse should be present, but even if she is not, she must know what is planned, since she will have to answer questions later from the patient and the relatives. If her knowledge is inadequate she may unwittingly confuse them.

Routine Records

A careful record of weight, fluid intake and output, and the diet calories is kept.

Radiation Reaction

Any infection or discharge makes radiation reaction worse and every attempt must be made to stop maceration of the skin. The reaction in the skin will vary according to the type of radiation employed, and will usually only require active treatment toward the end of the period of treatment. Since the sweat glands and hair follicles are affected the skin becomes dry and loss of hair can occur. When this epilation does occur patients must be warned that it may be permanent.   ·

About the second week the mucosa becomes erythematous, sore, and dry. This reaction reaches a peak seven to ten days after the end of treatment and then gradually subsides. The mucosal condition can cause laryngitis or oesophagitis, and the patient may complain of dysphagia and loss of taste. This latter symptom may continue for up to six months. The cause of the radiation systemic upset is unknown but it may result in nausea, sometimes proceeding to vomiting. These reactions can occur almost at once then die away returning in the second week of treatment. The appropriate remedies are given and the diet maintained, it is here that at this point the nurse must be encouraging and sympathetic but firm. Pain and depression are also treatable. Analgesia must be available when required, this may well be at less than the routine intervals, but if pain is allowed to build up it becomes more difficult to alleviate.

Nursing Care of Special Sites

Skin

Any Elastoplast dressings must be removed and only tapes containing no heavy metals used. The hair should be shampooed before treatment. It is not only a morale booster, but if parts of the scalp are included in the radiation field hair washing may not be possible. The skin usually needs little active treatment except towards the end of radiation. All perfumed preparations, including deodrants, are avoided as they may contain radiation potentiating metals. Although washing and shaving used to be forbidden, gentle sponging with tepid water or shaving with an electric razor are possible and morale boosting, obviously if there is soreness these measures must stop. Clothes must be kept from rubbing, a soft collar or silk handkerchief is useful in preventing chafing. Jewellery should not be worn. In the last week of the course a dusting powder may be needed, occasionally a steroid cream, or aqueous 1% gentian violent for a moist reaction.

Mouth

Oral hygiene is very important. Frequent bland mouth washes are given. Dental floss may be necessary to keep teeth clear of debris. If infection was present when teeth were extracted antibiotic cover may be continued during treatment. When dysphagia occurs aspirin gargles are helpful. Anaesthetic mucilage may be required. A careful watch must be kept to ensure that dysphagia is not due solely to radiation reaction but to supra-added candidal infection.

Lip

If the lesion is being treated with a radioactive source, then this must be carefully checked that it is intact and in position. The nurse should realise that she is very adequately protected. She wears a badge which registers the amount of radiation received, and if she obeys the rules for handling radioactive substances she can come to no harm. A prominent notice will tell her the maximum permitted time she may spend with a patient each day. Armed with this knowledge she will not be afraid. Patients have been made to feel very unhappy and neglected because nurses, through lack of understanding, have hurried their care of the patient and have spent no time talking to them. Since the patient is already isolated because of his treatment and will also undoubtedly be suffering discomfort and pain, human contact is most important to him.

During radiation treatment the lip becomes oedematous and painful. The mucosal reaction is brisk for all types of radiation, the peak being reached seven to ten days after treatment. If external radiation is being given, the daily dose is smaller than usual and the course more prolonged, because of the oedema occurring.

Oral hygiene is practised as described for tongue and mouth, and for a time the diet may have to be entirely liquid.

Tongue

Before the patient goes to the theatre he will have been told what is involved by the doctor. Questions will arise and the patient will turn to the nurse for answers. She must warn him that speech will be difficult and perhaps impossible, but that after the radioactive source is removed the reaction subsides. Speech will return. He must be assured that he will experience no difficulty in breathing. He needs to know that he will have a bell and that he can summon help quickly. Pencil and pad are provided so that he can write down what he wishes to communicate. The pad should be large and the pencil easy to grasp, glasses if needed should be to hand. With all these preparations there will still be a sense of frustration. Writing is not as quick as speech, there must be a pause while others read the message, the quick interchange of conversation is lost. The nurse needs to exercise great patience and let him take his time. The family must have the situation explained to them so that they in turn can help. Above all it must be remembered that the patient though speechless is not deaf, and there must be no discussion of his state as if he were not there.

The radioactive source check must be done carefully. The needles must be checked that they are intact, not loose or partly out of position. It is rare for them to become so loose that they have to be removed, this usually only happens when infection is present.

Oral hygiene is extremely important. Swabbing the mouth would be too painful and mouth rinsing is difficult. Syringing gently is the best method, and dilute hydrogen peroxide keeps the mouth as fresh as possible. The only complication which occurs does so usually within the first 24 hours. There may be some bleeding around the needles and if this escapes it will be syringed away, but if the blood remains within the tongue a haematoma may form. This is painful and alarming to the patient. Every effort is made to avoid premature removal of the needles. Ice is applied locally, and adrenalin swabs may be used. With care the swelling does not usually enlarge further and often subsides. A haematoma of this type may be due to haemorrhage from a small venule. The oedema rarely threatens the airway. The diet is fluid or semi-solid, great care must be taken to ensure the fluid intake is kept up.

If treatment is by external radiation the oral hygiene is maintained by mouth washes and gargles. Treatment is longer and the reaction is slower to develop.

Pharynx

Nasopharynx   There may be discharge and some bleeding. Oral hygiene is maintained as described for the mouth. The problem will be aggravated if the patient is forced to breathe mostly through the mouth. Gentle careful nasal toilet may also be required.

Oropharynx   The problems are the same as already detailed for the mouth.

Post-cricoid area

The emphasis here is on the diet, not only must it be adequate but also suitable. The oedema caused by treatment will add to any obstruction from the growth, and unsuitable food may block the narrowed passage. Sometimes it is necessary to protect the patient from the injudicious gifts of friends and relatives. Though tempting they may cause untold trouble. A tactful word of explanation usually prevents an unwanted complication. Laryngitis as a result of the reaction occurs. Inhalations are helpful and soothing, and a steam kettle at night often makes restful sleep possible.

Larynx

Patients with early disease usually have no complications apart from soreness and radiation reaction. They must not smoke and should keep talking to a minimum. Some find sucking sweets a help. Occasionally an antibiotic is required.

The more advanced cases of the disease often arrive with a tracheostomy. These patients require much more nursing. The tubes must be kept clean, sucked out, and changed when necessary. Some patients who are reasonably fit can learn to suck out their own tubes. Such a variety of tubes is available that no attempt will be made to describe them here. Great efforts must be made to avoid maceration of the skin around the stoma. The risk of developing chest infection is high. The physiotherapist will visit the patient daily, but the nurse will need to encourage him to go on practising the exercises prescribed. Inhalations and steam again are most useful. The lack of communication can be very frustrating. The sympathetic nurse, who gives her patient time to close off the tube and talk, will give his morale a great lift.

Avoiding Tracheotomy

As radiation produces oedema, the patients with bulky tumours or subglottic infiltration are at risk from airway obstruction. Dyspnoea will increase and stridor may appear for the first time or get worse. The need for tracheotomy may be often avoided by careful nursing, inhalations, use of the steam tent, but nevertheless there should always be on the ward an emergency pack.

Cytotoxic Infusion

This is a technique which may be used as the sole means of treatment, as the method of reducing extensive growth and rendering it suitable for radiation, or as a supplement to radiation. Under general anaesthesia the external carotid artery on the appropriate side is cannulated and the tip of the catheter guided to lie within, or close, to the origin of the artery supplying the tumour area. A saline drip is connected. To overcome the arterial pressure the tubing is long, with a Y end at the top. Two bottles are connected to this end and hung high up on the ceiling. The height above the patient gives sufficient pressure to overcome arterial pressure. A trap to exclude air bubbles is included. At certain times of the day the intake is switched from saline to the second bottle containing a measured quantity of a cytotoxic drug. These infusions need careful watching. When changing bottles air bubbles may enter the tubing. A clot can form in the catheter if the drip is allowed to stop and may become detached. Either air or blood clot entering the cerebral circulation can cause infarction of brain tissue. Regular white counts are required, usually daily, as the drug depresses the bone marrow and leucopenia can occur quickly. There is usually a brisk reaction in the tumour area, this can take the form of gross oedema. In certain situations such as the tongue this can cause airway obstruction and a tracheostomy may be needed. The usual systemic reactions also occur. Nursing patients receiving this form of treatment requires the highest skill and vigilance.

On Discharge

The usual reports to the patient's doctor are sent but outside helpers may need to be alerted. If the nurse is to visit she needs to be told the patient's condition and requirements; in some cases the patient will attend the outpatient clinic for daily dressings. An adequate supply of dressings and drugs must be taken out to tide the patient over to the first visit to his own doctor. The medical social worker will have been in close contact with the patient and his family. Where necessary she will arrange financial help, and may also contact local services to arrange home calls and help with the diet. Convalescence can be arranged, but it should be remembered that it is often more beneficial and enjoyable if there is a short rest after completion of treatment before the patient goes away.

The Outpatient

Patients for treatment as outpatients are carefully selected and should have minimal difficulties. Nevertheless the same reactions occur. The nurse or radiographer must assess the patient on each visit and refer to the doctor at the earliest sign of difficulty. All the principles of good nursing apply, and must be conveyed simply but adequately to the family. Often there is an atmosphere of tension because relatives are afraid of doing the wrong thing, and alternate between completely restricting the patient or allowing him to follow exactly his own fancies. When the nurse has established a good relationship with the patient and his family, relatives often in return give information which the patient from fear, diffidence or stoicism, will not volunteer himself.

Throughout treatment the informed patient is more relaxed and will co-operate more fully. The family too must be completely in the picture so that they will be ready to take over on the patient's discharge. The diet must be adequate. Treatment is tiring and the patient must be told that to relax and take things easily is not a sign of weakness but good sense. Depression is often experienced. It has many causes, fear, pain, the disease itself, the inability to eat, the loss of taste and appetite, the sudden cessation of normal activities. Financial problems can be worrying and the medical social worker can be of enormous help here. The nurse can help by being kind, firm, and encouraging. Depression can be improved by drugs and by providing occupation. The occupational therapist is often forgotten, but she can make a valuable contribution to morale. When the date of completion of treatment is known the patient should be told together with the date of expected discharge. All patients, whether in the ward or attending daily, get a great uplift when they know the end of treatment is in sight. This date when given should not be altered unless it is absolutely necessary. Equally the family should know as soon as possible so that they in turn can make any necessary arrangements well in advance.

The ills of Man lay quiet,
Unsuspected in Pandora's box.
So within the body this box can lie,
Its evils hidden and unknown.

8 The Paranasal Sinuses

Anatomy

The paranasal sinuses are air spaces within the skull and the maxillae. Tumours most commonly involve the antrum lying within the maxilla. It is lined with ciliated mucous secretory epithelium, the mucus draining through openings into the nose. Lymphatic drainage is to the retropharyngeal nodes (behind the pharynx).

Only tumours of the maxillary sinus will be discussed, the other sinuses are only rarely involved and then treatment is similar.

Aetiology

There are as yet no firm indications of carcinogenic factors. It is suggested that it is more common in E. Africa and among workers in the furniture industry, in this latter case chronic inhalation of wood dust has been indicted.

Age and Sex

The age groups most commonly affected are the older ones from the fifth decade onwards. The exception to this is the occasional young patient with a sarcoma. Men are slightly more often affected than women, but sarcoma is more common in young women. However the tumour is not common, accounting for about 0.2% of deaths from cancer.

Pathology

An impressive list can be made of the histological types of tumour occurring in this area. Up to 75% of them however are of the squamous carcinoma variety, all degrees of differentiation being found. However, in the case of the wood-worker's tumour, it is unusual, being an adenocarcinoma, arising from the glands in the mucous membrane.

Symptomatology

If the antrum is thought of as a pyramid shaped box with its base lying against the lateral wall of the nose, and its apex (point) in the lateral part of the cheek, the symptomatology is easier to understand.

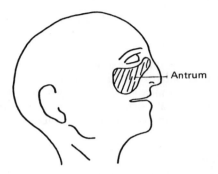

Fig 8.1   The antrum

In the early stages the tumour may cause no symptoms, or only those of sinusitis. Rarely the disease may be discovered when antral infection is being investigated. Growth may originate at any point on the mucosa and spread in any direction, which wall will be involved first is therefore not necessarily related to the site of the tumour on the mucosa. Symptoms which are caused by invasion of one of the antral walls will vary according to which wall is involved. Because of this patients may not always present in the E.N.T. clinic first. If diplopia is the initial symptom referral may be to the neurologist or ophthalmologist.

Symptoms according to the wall involved:

1. *Roof*
   This is the floor of the orbit and the complaint is usually of diplopia and sometimes of proptosis (the eye is pushed forward). The nerve supplying the ocular muscles may be affected giving rise to paralysis. If the fifth nerve is involved there may be pain and loss of sensation over part of the face.
2. *Floor*
   The close relation to the teeth means that toothache is an early symptom followed by swelling and ulceration of the alveolus or of the palate.
3. *Base*
   The drainage of the antrum is affected and secondary infection usually occurs. There is bulging of the lateral wall of the nose with discharge and bleeding. At a later stage ulceration of the palate can also occur.
4. *Apex*
   There is swelling of the cheek, and pain due to involvement of the fifth nerve. Drainage of the lacrimal secretions may be impaired resulting in epiphora (overflow of the tears). When extension of growth in this area

involves the muscles moving the jaw (pterygoids) pain in the jaw occurs, and difficulty in opening the mouth (trismus).

Of all these presentations the most common is that of swelling followed by ulceration in the hard palate, the alveolus, or the junction of hard and soft palates, together with pain.

Examination

From the description of the symptomatology it will be realised that not only will the E.N.T. instruments be required but also the ophthalmoscope. Before proceeding to the special examinations, points to be noted will be, the presence of any deformity or swelling, and signs of discharge or bleeding.

Dentures are removed and the special areas examined.

Nose

Sniffing tests the patency of each nostril in turn, using a special small mirror with curved handle the post nasal space is inspected. The pharynx may need to be sprayed with local anaesthetic.

Eye

The presence of oedema of the conjunctiva, epiphora, or loss of facial sensation is noted. The eye movements are tested and the retina examined. The degree and direction of any proptosis present is assessed.

Mouth

Bulging or ulceration of the palate or alveolus is noted and also the state of the teeth. The antral sinuses are transilluminated, the affected one is often opaque.

Cheek

Swelling or deformity is noted, the infra-orbital area particularly being carefully checked for fullness. Tenderness or loss of sensation is sought.

Investigations

In addition to the routine blood count and chest X-ray, special X-rays are ordered. These include all the paranasal sinuses, the base of the skull, and tomograms if indicated, CATscans may be helpful. As infection is often present, a swab is taken from any discharge and sent to the laboratory for culture and sensitivity of the organisms. It is also advisable to have the vision tested. It is often not possible to spare the eye during treatment, and it may be important to know exactly how good the sight is in each eye.

Biopsy

The final diagnosis rests on the histology. X-rays may be unhelpful or, alternatively may show an opacity with bone destruction pointing to a tumour, which on biopsy proves to be a chronic abcess. The usual approach for biopsy is through the nose or the alveolar sulcus. Occasionally the biopsy is repeated since despite a negative result the clinical picture so strongly represents malignancy.

Treatment

The treatment of choice is radiotherapy but before this takes place there must be consultation with the surgeon and the dentist. The dentist extracts before radiation any teeth likely to cause trouble later. He will also make the dental prosthesis required after fenestration.

Fenestration

The word is derived from the Latin *fenestra*, a window. The surgeon removes part of the palate making an opening into the antrum. The timing of this operation in relation to radiation will vary according to the clinical condition. The purpose of fenestration is to enable inspection of the growth, adequate drainage, and if necessary application of a radioactive source to any residual growth. Initially the cavity is packed, but as soon as possible the patient wears a dental prosthesis. This has an obturator mounted on a dental plate which fits into the artificial opening. Without this aid swallowing is very difficult and speech very altered. Fenestration is usually carried out three to six weeks after completion of treatment, or if there is pressure due to pus, it may be done before the treatment commences.

Radiation

Treatment is given by megavoltage therapy using normally two fields. It is almost impossible to spare the eye on the affected side. Close relationship to the orbit, both below and on the medial side, means that to cover the mucosa adequately the eye must be included in the field. By special shielding devices and techniques the lens is spared as far as possible, particularly if this is the good eye and sight is poor on the other side. By arranging the fields carefully it is possible to spare the other eye from the radiation which comes through from the treatment side. Patients are warned of the risk of lens degeneration (cataract formation), but they are also told that operation is possible should this damage occur. For accurate positioning a plastic shell may be made so that the patient is held still and the beam aligned on the same point daily. Treatment lasts from four to six weeks.

Radioactive Source

For treatment of small areas of residual growth or occasionally of recurrences, a radioactive source is mounted on the prosthesis. The patient wears this for a few hours each day, treatment usually lasts five to six days.

Surgery

If radical clearance is possible this is done, but mutilation may be considerable and require plastic surgery. Usually the surgeon's role is confined to biopsy and fenestration. When radiotherapy fails or there is recurrence, diathermy excision may be carried out.

    When the primary is controlled, palpable, mobile lymph nodes in the neck are removed by block dissection.

Cytotoxic Perfusion

In a few centres the area is perfused with a cytotoxic drug over a period of days. This is usually combined with radiotherapy, and the timing in relation to the course of radiation is variable.

    Results have not been impressive so far.

Complications during Treatment

The skin occasionally becomes sore but the greater reaction occurs in the mucosa. This becomes erythematous, shiny, oedematous, and sometimes filmed. Secretion is reduced and the mouth and pharynx become dry. If there is nasal discharge this adds to the discomfort. The patient will complain of a sore throat, loss of taste; and dysphagia. The eye shares in this mucosal reaction. Epiphora may occur before tear secretion lessens, glands of the eyelids secrete less, and the conjunctiva becomes erythematous and oedematous. The patient has a sore eye and the eyelids may irritate. The hazard is infection which can result in a corneal ulcer leading to loss of vision.

    Nursing must be directed to maintaining a proper diet and food intake. Frequent small drinks and sucking fruit sweets will help to overcome the dryness of the mouth, but oral hygiene is very important and mouth washes must be given regularly. Saline baths are soothing to the eye, a bland cream can alleviate irritation of the lids. At the first sign of infection a swab is taken and the doctor will prescribe the appropriate antibiotic. Atropine may also be used. It is most important that the patient should not rub the eye. Any discharge from the nose or eye must be cleansed away regularly, but this must be done gently to avoid provoking bleeding. Skin care is essentially the same as for any other area. Men will not be able to shave.

    Very occasionally haemorrhage from the growth may occur. This is very alarming to the patient. The nurse should turn the patient on to the sound side, reassure him, and encourage him not to swallow the blood. Because of the site it is usually impossible to apply any external pressure. Often bleeding stops spontaneously, but if it continues the patient is taken to theatre and the cavity packed. Blood transfusion is given if necessary.

When fenestration has been carried out the cavity must be syringed out and the patient taught to insert his prosthesis. At this point a judicious mixture of firmness and kindness is often required by the nurse. As soon as possible the patient learns to carry out the syringing of the cavity himself.

On discharge arrangements may be needed for a visiting nurse to continue dressings for advanced growths, or supervise the oral hygiene of older patients.

When treatment is carried out on an out-patient basis, the nursing procedures must be carefully explained to the patient and his family. It is important also that the nurse or radiographer who sees him daily should watch the condition of the eye, skin, and mouth carefully.

Follow-up

At follow-up there is a general inspection of the face followed by examination of the special areas. The site of the growth is examined through the fenestration. If there is any sign of recurrence a further biopsy is usually taken, it is sometimes difficult to distinguish necrosis from recurrence. Finally the neck is examined for lymph nodes. At intervals routine chest X-rays are taken, and other X-rays as indicated by the clinical findings.

Other Sinuses

These vary mostly in the technique of treatment. To protect the eye when treating the ethmoid sinuses the field is localised to the central area over the nose. Owing to the close proximity to the brain the total dosage is limited by the tolerance of the brain tissue.

Case History

Mr. G. Age 71.
3/12 pain in L. cheek and bleeding from L. nostril. Seen in E.N.T. clinic; apart from slight fullness over L. maxilla no other abnormality.
X-rays. Skull. Changes suggestive of Paget's disease.
Sinuses. Destruction of the outer wall of the L. antrum.

Exploration

Grossly thickened mucosa suggestive of neoplasm.

Histology

Well-differentiated squamous cells? Malignancy. Fenestration performed before radiotherapy. Histology again only suggestive of malignancy.

Treatment

Megavoltage radiation to a maximum tumour dose of 58.5 Gy (5850 rads) in six weeks with cobalt therapy using two fields, a compensator and shell.

During the next 18/12 he was seen at intervals. Crusting and discharge from the antrum was treated with antibiotics and observation was continued. At the end of this period definite evidence of malignancy was obtained on biopsy. While cytotoxic perfusion was being considered the patient developed signs of malignancy in the chest. This was considered to be a second primary, carcinoma of the bronchus. As he was not fit for surgery, but on the other hand had no chest symptoms, radiation was not given. His condition remained reasonable, intermittent infection of the antrum was treated by antibiotics.

Two years after the original diagnosis he developed haematuria. At cystoscopy he was found to have a third primary, carcinoma of the bladder. Ulceration of the cheek and hoarseness of the voice also developed. It was considered un-justifiable to give radiation and he was kept comfortable by the use of antibiotics and antral wash outs.

The patient died three years after his radiation treatment.

Prognosis

This is not a common tumour and so no series of results has large numbers. When adequate surgery is possible 5 year survival figures of 30-45% are quoted, but for all cases 10-30% is the usual rate. Such a prognosis is not good, but hope lay at the bottom of Pandora's box, and to this hope we, and our patients, must cling.

Man's brain enables him to explore the Universe,
Yet it is this very brain
Which defies his efforts at self exploration.

9   The Brain

We are going to discuss tumours of the brain as we would during classroom demonstrations and lectures.

Anatomy and Clinical Signs

This is an extremely complicated subject and we must consider a very simple outline. In clinical practice the divisions we describe will not be nearly so clear-cut, for the symptoms attributable to a lesion of one area must be modified by those due to another.

Anatomy

Grey and White Matter

Within the brain there are nerve cells, neurones, found in the grey matter which forms the surface of the brain, the cortex, and in collections of cells deep within the brain, such as the respiratory centre or the thalamus. From these cells run the nerve fibres, the white matter, which conduct impulses to and from the cells. Between the cells and between the fibres lies the connective tissue of the brain. This is formed of 'packing cells' known as glial cells.

Cerebrospinal Space and Fluid

Within the brain are communicating spaces, ventricles, containing cerebrospinal fluid. They are the lateral (paired), third (single) and fourth (single). The space continues down as the spinal central canal. Clear cerebrospinal fluid is secreted by the choroid plexus, circulates in the ventricular system, central canal, and subarachnoid space. It is absorbed back into the blood stream through venous channels.

Coverings of the Brain

The brain is covered by three membranous layers, meninges, varying in texture. The very thin pia mater covers the convoluted surface of the brain, and between it and the next layer, the arachnoid, is the subarachnoid space. The tough third layer, dura, is attached to the skull's inner surface and also projects between parts of the brain, the falx cerebri between the cerebral hemispheres, the tentorium cerebelli between the cerebral hemispheres and cerebellum forming the roof of the posterior fossa. Brain is designated either supra- (above) or sub- (below) tentorial. The great venous sinuses run within the dura mater.

Cranial Nerves

Within the brain there are collections of nerve cells known as nuclei. Connecting certain of these nuclei with definite structures, face, tongue etc. are the nerve fibres known as the cranial nerves. They are twelve in number, paired, and are either motor, sensory, or mixed.

Areas of the Brain

For convenience the brain is divided into three parts for descriptive purposes.

Forebrain,   supratentorial. The cerebral hemispheres and connecting corpus callosum.

Mid brain,   short, connecting cerebral hemispheres with hind brain and spinal cord. All fibres to and from the cortex are here contained in a small space.

Hind brain,   sub (infra) tentorial. Pons, medulla oblongata, cerebellum, all lying in the posterior fossa. Motor and sensory tracts cross to the other side. Vital centres controlling heart and respiration lie in the floor of the fourth ventricle.

Symptoms and Special Areas of the Brain

From the evidence gained from stimulating the exposed brain, from excising parts of it, and from identifying the areas affected by disease, it has been possible to map out the function of some areas.

The Frontal Lobe

Anteriorly a so-called silent area, a lesion here may only cause personality changes. The motor area lies in front of the fissure of Rolando, the body being represented upside down. Stimulation causes movement on the opposite side of the body. A lesion may irritate causing Jacksonian epilepsy, or if an area is destroyed, weakness and later paralysis of the represented part.

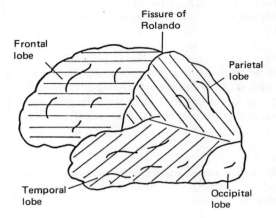

Fig. 9.1.   Lobes of the brain

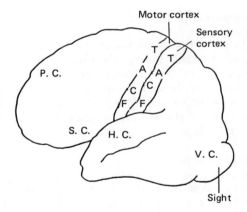

T =   Toes
A =   Abdomen
C =   Chest
F =   Face

P. C. =   Personality Centre
S. C. =   Speech Centre
H. C.=   Hearing Centre
V. C. =   Visual Centre

Fig. 9.2.   Localisation of the cortex

Parietal Lobe

The sensory cortex lies behind the fissure of Rolando, the body again represented upside down. Discrete lesions will cause alteration or loss of sensation.

Temporal Lobe

Lying below the Sylvian fissure it has a close association with the hearing and speech centres, and with the optic tract passing from the retina to the occipital cortex. Lesions may cause visual or auditory hallucinations, partial loss of the field of view, or speech disturbance such as inability to name known objects.

Occipital Lobe

This lies posteriorly. It is a small but important area and concerns sight.

Dominant Hemisphere

Most patients are right or left handed. This means that the cerebral hemisphere on the opposite side is dominant. A lesion in the speech centre of this hemisphere will cause profound disturbance of the speech.

Mid-brain and Internal Capsule

Fibres connect the motor cells of the cortex with the appropriate motor neurone in the spinal cord. They pass through the narrow area of the internal capsule, the equally narrow area of the mid-brain, cross in the medulla oblongata, and run down the spinal cord. Incoming sensory fibres pursue a similar course to the sensory cortex. While lesions of the cortex may cause localised symptoms, even a very small lesion of the internal capsule or mid-brain affects many fibres and so a much larger body area, even to causing a hemiplegia.

Pons, Medulla, and Cerebellum

Many of the cranial nerve nuclei lie within the pons and medulla. Muscle tone and co-ordination are controlled by the cerebellar hemisphere on the same side. Cerebellar lesions cause inco-ordination on the same side, fumbling, failure to carry out fine movements, ataxia of the lower limbs giving an abnormal gait. In the other areas signs may be focal due to involvement of cranial nuclei, e.g. wasting of the tongue on the same side as an involved cranial XII, widespread because of motor or sensory fibres being affected, or life threatening due to pressure on vital centres.

Pituitary

Better knowledge of the relationship between the pituitary and the hypothalamus means that whereas regulation of the levels of hormones secreted by the pituitary was believed to occur in the gland, it is now known that the hypothalamus

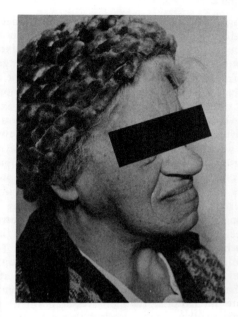

Fig 9.3   Acromegaly. Enlargement of the jaw, coarse textured skin

regulates their release by means of releasing and inhibiting factors or hormones, e.g. hypothalamic thryotrophin releasing hormone stimulates the release of thyroid stimulating hormone from the pituitary.

Lying in a saddle shaped fossa in the sphenoid bone, the sella turcica, the gland is close to the crossing of the optic fibres, optic chiasma, its enlargement can therefore interfere with vision. Many substances secreted by the anterior part affect other organs or functions, e.g. growth, lactation, thyroid, adrenal glands, ovaries, testes. One of the most interesting discoveries has been that endorphin secretion occurs here. These are opioid like substances 'natural analgesics', their action can be blocked by opioid antagonists, and their existence may explain the analgesic effect of placebos in some people, formerly believed to be psychological.

Excess of diminished secretion of pituitary chemicals may cause widespread effects, e.g. acromegaly, amenorrhoea.

The posterior part of the gland stores anti-diuretic hormone (A.D.H.) which controls excretion of water by the distal tubules of the kidney. Any fall in A.D.H. results in the patient passing abnormally large quantities of urine and always being thirsty, a condition known as 'diabetes insipidus'.

Clinical Histories

Now let us look at some histories, and meet some patients who have had cerebral tumours and been referred to us from neurological centres. Our first patient is a married lady aged 50. As you will see the head has been shaved and she has the horseshoe shaped scar of a R. temporo-parietal craniotomy. She is alert but you will notice that she is holding her left arm in a flexed position. If we asked her to pick up her spectacles she fumbled because her grip was weak. For years she suffered from Jacksonian epileptic fits involving the left hand and arm and occasionally the left side of the face. They became more frequent, more severe, and on two occasions she lost consciousness. Earlier examinations at the neurological centre could detect no anatomical abnormality and she was maintained on anti-convulsants. Six weeks before surgery she developed headaches, nausea, and slight weakness of the left arm. This time X-ray studies showed a space occupying lesion of the area immediately in front of the right fissure of Rolando. From this history alone it is possible to visualise a slowly growing lesion involving the motor cortex. Since it is only the upper limb involved it must be a very localised lesion. At first there was irritation leading to excitability of the cortex provoking fits, and later as the lesion spread, pressure on the motor areas produced weakness of the arm. As the right side of the cortex controls the left side of the body, the damage must be on the right. The late symptoms of headache and vomiting were due to the expanding lesion causing a rise of pressure within the skull. When I used the ophthalmoscope after her operation it was easy to see that the papilloedema noted before the operation had resolved. The optic discs were flat and pink, the blood vessels normal, whereas before, the discs would have been swollen and the vessels engorged due to pressure obstructing the venous return. Failure to relieve the pressure would have resulted in optic atrophy and possibly permanent damage to the vision.

You will remember that in the film we saw yesterday a young lady in her twenties told us her story. She began with a sudden focal fit which progressed to unconsciousness. The other lady had her problems before the introduction of CATscanning, but even with the aid of this powerful technique, it was impossible to say definitely there was tumour present in the second patient. Biopsy would probably have been negative and there was a small but definite risk that she would have been made worse. So she too was placed on anti-convulsants, but within a year she developed signs of progression, severe headache, and the second set of investigations were positive. If we compare, particularly the CATscans, we can see the difference. The first lady's X-rays, particularly the right carotid arteriogram, show a space occupying lesion pushing the right anterior cerebral artery across to the left, the ventriculogram shows a right lateral ventricle which is narrowed compared with the left.

This lady holds a responsible position, a head teacher, and she obviously agrees when I say that she was quite well until about six weeks ago. Then she developed headaches and had a fit with loss of consciousness about six weeks ago. A sudden event like that obviously worries both the patient and family very much. Just before she goes I'll put my fingers in the palm of her right hand, notice how she grasps them involuntarily, the grip tightens as I pull away.

Although she is obviously very intelligent I prefer to keep the general discussion to this stage when she has left us. It is all too easy for a patient to pick up some generalisation, apply it to herself, and become very alarmed.

We are always stressing the value of a careful history, and that patient's family told us that before her fit she had been getting forgetful and was not her usual self. Based on the history a provisional diagnosis was made of a lesion in the frontal lobe. In this so-called silent area a tumour can be present for years and cause little disturbance. The radioactive isotope scans showed dense uptake in the area. The evidence was so conclusive that no X-ray studies were done, it was quite possible to pinpoint the lesion and to diagnose a meningioma with confidence. This is a benign tumour and usually post-operative radiation is not given, but here the surgeon is not entirely happy with the clearance and has sent the patient for treatment.

Our next patient has a Cushingoid appearance. He is overweight, mainly the trunk with enlargement of the breasts. There is a loss of pubic and axillary hair. He is 60 and attributed his weight increase to his age. He found he could not see things out to the sides (peripheral vision) and went to an optician who very wisely advised him to see his doctor. On questioning he admitted to feeling the cold badly. His appearance is due to over production of cortisone.

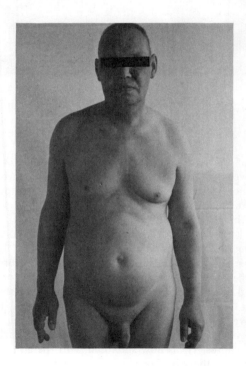

Fig. 9.4.   Pituitary hypoplasia

Next we have a very happy family group, parents and four boys. The father first went to his doctor because he too had eye problems and also loss of libido. Since he was not long married this was a severe problem. I can remember a young woman who also had visual problems, and it was then found when she

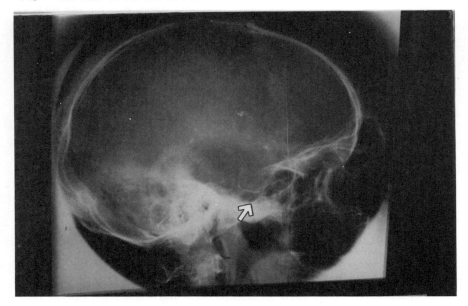

Fig. 9.5.   X-ray of the skull showing enlarged pituitary fossa

saw a doctor that she had experienced an early menopause at the age of 24.

The link between all three patients is the visual disturbance and obvious hormone imbalance. All three have had adenomas of the pituitary gland. Although benign due to their position they can cause quite severe problems by pressure. Within the gland they expand and cause atrophy of the secretory cells, and when they rise above the sella turcica they press on to the inner fibres of the optic tract causing loss of vision at the sides.

In all three patients biochemical tests established the hormone disturbance, X-rays showed the characteristic enlargement of the sella turcica. The fields of view were mapped out and the extent of the visual loss assessed.

The two men have had surgery followed by radiation, the young woman only radiation. We can give hormone supplements, but this was only partially successful in the young man's case. As you can see he did achieve a family, but he kept having relapses. He is now stabilised with the addition of a new drug, bromocriptine, to his therapy. We now know that the pituitary is controlled by the hypothalamus and adenoma formation is probably in response to an excess drive. This young man's tumour secreted prolactin and bromocryptine reduces this. Combined with thyroxine and testosterone supplements it has restored normal sexual function.

In the next few years there is good reason to believe that drugs capable of controlling the hypothalamic hormones will enable pituitary adenomas to be treated medically.

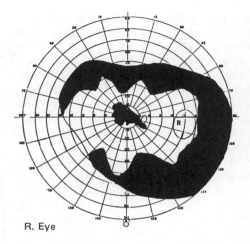

R. Eye

Fig. 9.6a.   Pituitary tumour, loss of field of view before radiation

So far with the exception of the young lady in the film, all our patients have had benign tumours. She has a glioma, a malignant tumour. After surgical removal of as much tumour as possible, she was given radiotherapy, and is currently receiving cyclical courses of chemotherapy. On the whole the outlook for many gliomas is not good, and this regime is an attempt to improve the prognosis. She has tolerated all her treatment well, but it is too early to predict either her future course, or whether this combination treatment will improve survival times for this type of tumour.

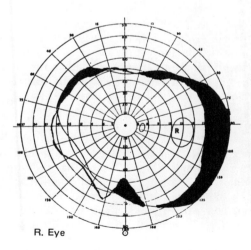

R. Eye

Fig. 9.6b.   After radiation, showing marked improvement

Our last patient is having treatment and we can go to the children's ward and see him there. He is three and passed his milestones normally. Then his mother noticed he was dropping his toys and was not walking so well. This progressed to a loss of balance, he became irritable, fretful, and complained his head hurt. He went off his food and started to vomit. By this time he was quite unable to walk and his mother noted a squint in the left eye. He is still unsteady, walking with his feet wide apart, and the squint, though less marked, is still present. You can see he has had treatment to his head, there is loss of hair and the skin is red. If we look under his pyjama coat we can see the treatment marks for the field to the whole spine.

His packet of X-rays is a fat one. The plain X-ray of the skull shows widening, 'springing' of the suture lines, the bones at this age are not yet firmly united, and the skull has a 'beaten copper appearance'. Both are signs of persistent and prolonged raised intracranial pressure. All the other investigations pointed to a diagnosis of a tumour in the posterior fossa obstructing the fourth ventricle. At operation this was confirmed, histology showing it to be a medulloblastoma. This type of tumour, and also the ependymoma, tends to seed along the cerebrospinal fluid pathway, so it is necessary to give radiation to the brain and the spinal cord. A very careful watch has to be kept on the white cell count as the spine is being irradiated. He is not going to receive chemotherapy.

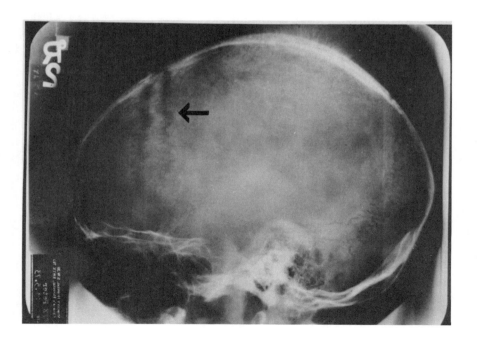

Fig. 9.7a.   Skull X-ray, springing of the sutures

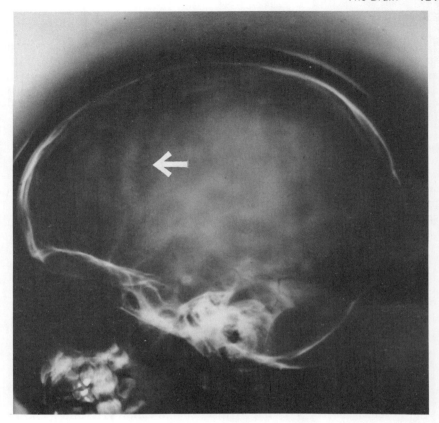

Fig. 9.7b.   Skull X-ray, copper beaten appearance

History

If you have been looking at the notes you will have seen that a full history is taken from both patients and relatives. Very often this will give a pointer to the site and nature of the tumour. A long history will suggest a slowly-growing tumour. Obesity, amenorrhoea, or loss of libido, indicates a hormonal dysfunction related to the pituitary, while loss of balance will direct our attention to the cerebellum. Headache and vomiting are signs of raised intracranial pressure and give no clue to the site. On the other hand the history of a fit and its details (part of the body involved, preceding aura, loss of consciousness, incontinence, duration, frequency) may all yield clues. If a nurse observes a fit in the ward, these are the details she needs to note for the doctor's information.

Examination

The clinical examination establishes the level of consciousness and the mental state of the patient. This gives a base line and subsequently it will be possible to assess progress or deterioration. If the patient cannot be roused and is unable to swallow he will present an entirely different problem from the patient who has only a slight paralysis. The cranial and peripheral nervous systems are examined fully and a clear note made of the patient's gait.

We must look at the investigations performed on these patients and at the pathology of the tumours. The findings from the history and the examination will fall into two groups, generalised and focal. During our last discussion we concentrated on the focal, let us now turn our attention to the generalised signs and symptoms. The skull is a closed box, and any extra tissue within it will cause pressure on the brain and its vessels giving rise to a condition of raised intra-cranial pressure.

Symptoms

Raised Pressure

1. Headache, this varies in site, but characteristically in the early stages it is worse in the morning improving during the day, and aggravated by coughing or sneezing.
2. Nausea and later vomiting, the latter is sometimes projectile in nature and must not be confused in children with vomiting due to alimentary tract causes.
3. Papilloedema, always an important sign but not always present.

General

Varying mental symptoms, epilepsy, mental deterioration, slight personality changes.

Focal

1. Failing vision, double vision, loss of part of visual field.
2. Deafness, dysphasia.
3. Ataxia, weakness.

Other signs may be found, but not in every case, they are alterations in the pulse rate and the respiratory rhythm. A generalised convulsion may precede loss of consciousness, and pressure may alter pituitary hormone secretion. So it can be seen that signs of intracranial pressure do not localise the lesion necessarily.

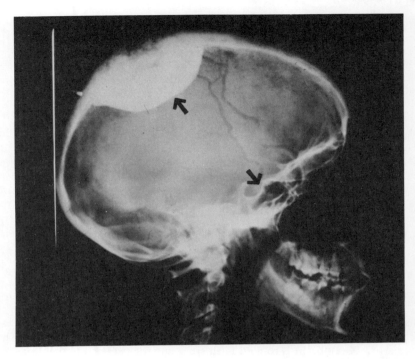

Fig. 9.8.   Skull X-ray. Calcification in a meningeal sarcoma (upper arrow).
Note the normal pituitary fossa

Investigations

Faced with a patient with a suspected tumour the doctor wishes if possible to
answer three questions. 'Where is it?' 'What is it?' and 'How is it to be treated?'.
To supplement the clinical findings in answer to the question 'Where is it?'
investigations are carried out. We have already mentioned some of them, now we
can list them and the information which can possibly be gained from them.

X-rays

1. Plain pictures of the skull. This is a simple procedure.
   Infants: 'springing of the sutures and 'copper beaten' appearance due to
   raised intracranial pressure.
   Adults:
   a. erosion or thickening of bone due to prolonged pressure or irritation,
   b. expansion of the sella turcica with/without erosion of bone, by a
      pituitary tumour, or following raised intracranial pressure,
   c. specks of calcium lying within certain tumours,
   d. shift of the calcified pineal to one side, it normally lies in the midline.

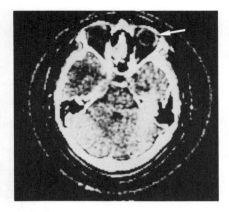

Fig. 9.9a.   CATscan at the level of the orbit. Note outline of the eye

Computerised Axial Tomography (CATscan)

This specialised form of X-ray, with and without radio-opaque contrast, has become the most important single examination in diagnosing brain tumours. The very narrow X-ray beam is rotated in an arc round the patient and the degree of X-ray absorption by the brain tissues recorded. The enormous number of measurements can only be handled by a computer which produces pictures in any desired plane. New developments have produced CT directed biopsy and even enabled pictures to be taken during operation.

Angiography

This has not been superseded by the advent of CATscans but now follows these and skull X-ray. Opaque contrast material is injected under general or local anaesthetic into the carotid/vertebral artery. The angiogram may show shift of vessels by a mass, abnormal circulation characteristic of certain tumours, e.g. angioma, and helps the surgeon in planning surgical approaches.

Ventriculogram

This is now less used since the information can be obtained from CATscans. The ventricles are outlined either by a direct approach through a burr hole and the injection of air or other contrast materials, or by air introduced at lumbar puncture. It may be useful for tumours in particular areas, e.g. pituitary, brainstem, third ventricle.

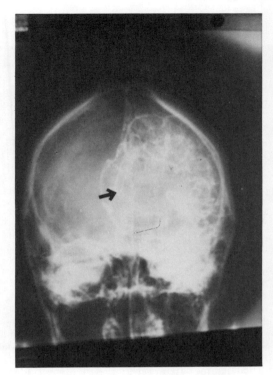

Fig. 9.9b.   L. carotid arteriogram. Displacement of L. anterior cerebral
artery across the midline by left-sided tumour

Isotope Scan

Again this is less used since the advent of CATscans. Following the venous
injection of a small quantity of radioactive material which concentrates in the
brain tumour, a detector moves over the skull in a set pattern. The scan is
mainly used for precise localisation or for information on the likely type and
vascularity of a tumour.

Electro-encephalogram

The tiny pulses of electricity generated by active cells are detected, magnified,
and recorded. Again less used since CATscans have superseded this examination,
it may give localisation clues but the information is non-specific.

New Examinations

Two methods as yet experimental, may in future become more widely used.
The first, positron emission tomography (PET) looks at the way in which a

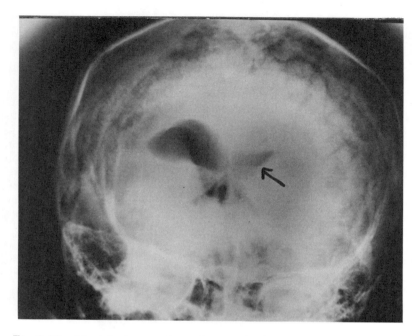

Fig. 9.10.   Ventriculogram. Lateral ventricle partially occluded by tumour

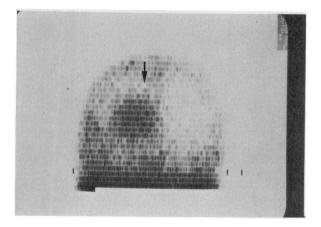

Fig. 9.11.   Brain scan, arrow indicates concentration of radio-isotope in
the tumour

substance, radioactively labelled, is transported and metabolised in the brain. Nuclear magnetic resonance (NMR) applies a magnetic stress and utilises the resultant changes in the magnetic fields of the chemical constituents of the brain tissue to produce pictures. This method has the advantage, like CAT scanning, of being non-invasive.

Other Examinations

Lumbar Puncture   Occasionally it may be necessary to examine the cerebrospinal fluid either biochemically or cytologically; if carcinoma invades the meninges malignant cells may be shed into the CSF. Puncture is at the level of L3, 4 where the needle will enter the subarachnoid space but avoid the cord which ends at L1.2. The examination is more likely to be made if a spinal tumour is suspected, then radio-opaque medium will be injected to produce a myelogram. Lumbar puncture can be dangerous if the intracranial pressure is raised, since a drop in pressure may cause descent of the medulla into the foramen magnum, 'coning', and pressure on the vital centres. If unrelieved by immediate surgery this causes death.

Blood Tests   A rise in ESR may be associated with cerebral metastases. Abnormal levels of prolactin, growth hormone, thyroid hormone and cortisol may be found if a pituitary microadenoma is present.

Pathology

The nervous system is formed from the embryonic ectoderm. The embryonic cells of the central nervous system differentiate into two types of mature cell, the nerve cell, and the glial, or 'packing' cell, the connective tissue of the brain.
Primary brain tumours account for about 2% of deaths from malignant disease.

Gliomas. Astrocytomas

The commonest brain tumours arise from the glial cells and are known as gliomas. Tumours arising from nerve cells are very rare within the central nervous system. There are three types of glial cells and hence three types of glioma, the most common being the astrocytoma arising from the astrocyte. They are graded from I to IV, I being the most benign, IV the most malignant, this is based on the history and knowledge of the clinical behaviour of these tumours. It is important to look at sections from different areas of the same tumour, as some may have more malignant tissue. In adults, in whom the majority of these tumours occur, the usual site is the cerebral hemisphere. More rare in children they then appear in the cerebellum.

Other Gliomas

These are rare and are the oligodendroglioma and the ependymoma. The latter arises from cells lining the cerebrospinal spaces and gives rise to symptoms of C.S.F. obstruction.

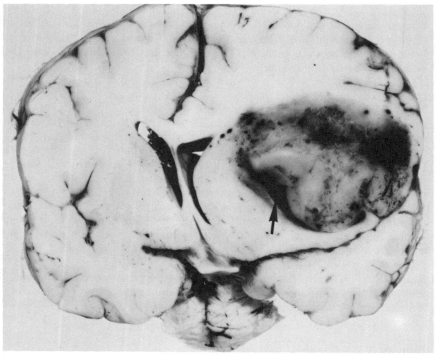

Fig. 9.12   Astrocytoma. Patient had a one year history of headache

Medulloblastoma

This is a tumour of childhood. It has been diagnosed in a child of one day old.
It arises from the roof of the fourth ventricle and the midline of the cerebellum.
Histological identification of these various brain tumours is always difficult.
The presence of carrot shaped cells in 'rosettes', is regarded as strong evidence
of a medulloblastoma.

Meningiomas

These tumours arise outside the brain substance from the meninges. They can
occur anywhere but are more common in certain sites, close to the venous
sinuses, along the spinal cord. They can be rounded, 'golf ball', or lie like a
sheet over the bone. This latter type does occasionally invade bone producing
a reaction which shows on X-ray as a patch of denser bone (hyperostosis).
They are slow growing, damage is done by pressure, and they are usually classified
as benign. A very small number do invade the brain and behave in a more malignant
way. Seen under the microscope the cells are arranged in whorls. Meningiomas
account for about 15% of primary brain tumours.

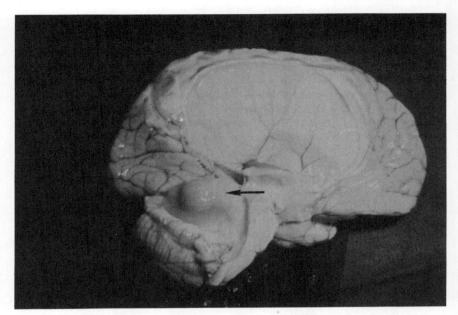

Fig. 9.13.   Medulloblastoma. Tumour obstructing the fourth ventricle
causing hydrocephalus and gross distension of the lateral ventricle

Pituitary Adenomas

Previously these were classified on the basis of staining, and were called chromophil or chromophobe. Now they are known as macroadenomas and are subdivided into functioning, e.g. prolactinoma (secretes prolactin), and the rare nonfunctioning. Microadenomas are usually non-functioning but may occasionally secrete prolactin. It is believed that tumours may be caused by hypothalamic overactivity raising the level of releasing hormones. They are benign, causing symptoms, locally by pressure, or systemically by increased, or decreased, hormone production.

Other Tumours

More rare are the other tumours, pinealoma, craniopharyngioma, and the vascular tumours.

Spread

Central nervous system tumours spread directly. This causes symptoms of raised intracranial pressure and also atrophy of adjacent tissue. The gliomas are usually infiltrative to a greater or lesser degree. Pituitary tumours and meningiomas are

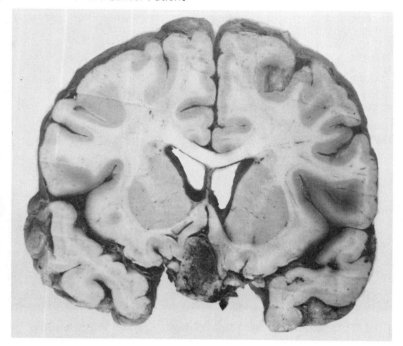

Fig. 9.14.   Pituitary chromophobe adenoma splaying apart the orbital
surfaces of the frontal lobes

usually well demarcated, a small percentage of meningiomas may invade the
skull or brain.

Ependymomas and medulloblastomas seed along the C.S.F. pathways.

Metastasis outside the central nervous system does not usually occur unless
there has been surgery. In a few children with medulloblastoma, metastases
have occurred in lymph nodes and bone.

Metastases

Spread of primary cerebral tumours outside the central nervous system is very
rare, but spread to the brain from tumours of other parts of the body is quite
common.

We can now consider the patient with an established diagnosis of a brain
tumour. The site has been mapped, and in some cases, for example the ladies
with meningiomas, its nature has been predicted. We must now answer the
third question, 'How do we treat it?'

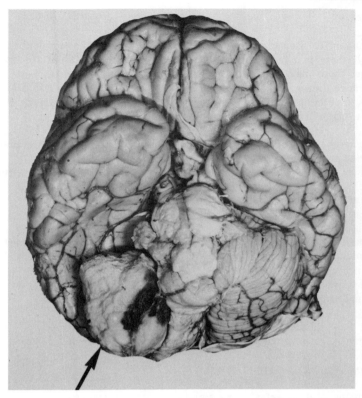

Fig. 9.15   Meningioma, base of the brain. Encapsulated tumour eroding the
cerebellum

Treatment

Surgery

If operable the first treatment of choice is surgery. This will vary from total
excision to biopsy only. In some areas even biopsy is impossible as the lesion
is deep seated and inaccessible. If the surgeon is unable to remove the tumour
completely, he aims by removing as much as possible to reduce the pressure on
surrounding tissues. This often relieves symptoms and gives the radiotherapist
more time. Other operations are done to overcome obstruction to the cerebrospinal fluid pathway, such as the insertion of a by-pass tube, from the
ventricle to the great veins of the chest, with a Spitz–Holter valve. The biopsy
is valuable because it establishes the pathology and thereby gives an indication
as to the advisability of radiotherapy, the response if radiation is used, and
the prognosis. Even when decompression has not been possible, the introduction
and use of the steroid dexamethasone by reducing oedema has also given time
to the therapist.

Radiotherapy

On admission to the radiotherapy ward a full neurological assessment is made. Although there is a record in the neurological centre's notes of the state on discharge, there may have been a change, and it is important to have noted, for reference during the patient's treatment, the exact state on admission. The patient's first contact in the ward is with the nurse, there is much she can observe which will help the doctor. These observations are:

1. General condition, basic physical signs, pulse, respiration, blood pressure, urine analysis.
2. Level of consciousness, mental state, e.g. alert and co-operative, type of personality, reaction to surroundings, speech, intelligibility.
3. State of sphincters and skin.
4. Gait. Paralysis, if present how much of the body involved.

When patients are unaccompanied the nurse should seek to make an early appointment for relatives to see the doctor, for as we have already said their information can be very valuable.

Since some patients may be semi-conscious or deteriorate later a careful note is made of the level of consciousness defined as:

Coma   — failure to respond to any stimulus.
Semicoma — response to painful stimuli — ranging from small to large organised movements.
Confusion — mild, moderate, severe.

In passing it is as well that we should not let our preoccupation with brain tumours cause us to forget that the causes of unconsciousness are many. The unconscious patient in Casualty may have suffered a brain haemorrhage, or a simple test on the urine may reveal a diabetic.

Chemotherapy

Cytotoxics have been given either after surgery and/or radiotherapy, or alone when there is recurrence, to treat malignant gliomas. The results are not a great advance, and further research is needed. The use of substances such as misonizadole, to sensitise the tumours to either radiation or chemotherapy, may be one hopeful development.

Bromocriptine is not a cytotoxic, but it specifically acts on functioning pituitary tumours. It lowers the secretion of prolactin or growth hormone, and may reduce the size of the tumour.

Immunotherapy

Foreign proteins cause the body to mount an immune response, part of which is the production of antibodies to the protein. It had been hoped that specific antibodies to brain tumours could be used. Research results have varied. One speculation is that if such antibodies could be produced then perhaps they could be combined with a cytotoxic, the resultant molecule targetting on to the tumour but remaining inactive until combining with the tumour cell proteins.

Nursing

General

For convenience we may class patients as conscious or unconscious, and discuss some of the special points which arise.

The conscious active patient such as any who has had a pituitary macro-adenoma removed, requires little active nursing. He is usually up and about all day, will probably go home at weekends, and in fact the main problem is usually boredom. A.D.H. in an injectable/snuff form, pitressin, may have to be given to these patients as they cannot regulate their urinary water loss. They require a high fluid intake, this usually adjusts in a matter of weeks. Obviously such a patient requires to be on a fluid balance chart. At the other extreme we have a quadriplegic patient who though conscious is helpless but can swallow. This patient requires careful attention to pressure points, to feeding and diet, and the care of the sphincters. Between these two extremes we shall find a range of states, the hemiplegic, the monoplegic patient, and the nursing will vary accordingly. The active but confused patient presents a challenge to the nurse's vigilance, she needs to see that he is fed properly, that he does not burn himself with a cigarette or set his bed on fire, and that he does not wander away.

Preparation for Radiation

The techniques of planning and treatment involve careful consultation between doctor and physicist. The decision as to the location and extent of the area to be treated depends upon the extent of surgery, results of investigations, histology. It must include the full extent of the tumour and a margin beyond, in practice this often means that virtually the whole brain receives radiation, though the dose will be less in some parts.

It is usual to shave the treatment area so that skin markings can be made. As much hair as possible is kept as patients are naturally sensitive about their appearance. A mild shampoo is desirable, this removes flaking skin and dandruff. It may not be possible to do this later during treatment.

Normally more than one treatment field is required to give an adequate tumour dose. The fields are marked on the skin. To ensure that the applicators are aligned correctly every day the patient may wear a plastic head shell. This is made for each patient by a technician, some with seatings for the applicator face. The patient is immobilised, setting up is easier, and treatment accurately reproduced day by day.

Pituitary tumours are treated slightly differently in that the fields are much smaller. They are centred on the pituitary fossa. When the tumour is a medullo-blastoma prophylactic radiation is given to the spinal cord. This is because spread is known to occur down the central canal.

Treatment

The aim of the therapist is to deliver an adequate dose to the tumour area avoiding excessive dosage to normal structures. Some tissues, such as the lens of the eye, may require special protection, and for these it is usual to use shielding. The length of treatment will vary from four to six weeks, and will last a few minutes a day, five days a week. Conventional X-rays, cobalt, or electrons, can be used for treatment, and technique will vary with each.

Nursing during Treatment

During the planning session the doctor will explain to the patient what is involved in the treatment. A nurse may be present during this time. Patients are often unable to grasp all the details and will ask questions of the nurse later. She should therefore make herself familiar with the department, the machines, and the minor problems which arise during treatment. One of the most frequent questions concerns the hair, and we will include this under the description of reactions.

Reactions

At first treatment produces slight swelling of the brain tissues and there may be some rise in intracranial pressure. Dexamethasone cover may therefore be given. Our previous description will alert the nurse as to the signs for which she must watch, slight headache or drowsiness, nausea or any decrease in the level of consciousness, occasionally an epileptic fit may occur. Sometimes the pressure will manifest itself as a bulging of the bone flap. When these signs are reported the doctor will decide whether to rest the patient, slow the rate of treatment, or give drugs such as dexamethasone or Lasix to reduce the oedema. If there is a Spitz–Holter valve in position this must be checked that it is still working.

Skin

Skin reaction, when it occurs, is usually apparent by the end of the second week and the same general measures apply as already described. The external auditory meatus if included in the field becomes dry and the patient complains of irritation. Hydrocortisone cream is very useful in soothing this. The reaction usually stays dry, any moist desquamation, if it occurs, is slight and appears towards the end of treatment.

Eyes

Where the eye is included in the field as in treating gliomas of the optic nerve, the eyelids and conjunctiva become oedematous and irritate. Eye baths are necessary, usually saline, and if any infected discharge occurs a swab is taken for culture and sensitivity and the appropriate antibiotic prescribed. Some patients find tinted glasses helpful.

Hair

When hair loss occurs it is complete within the field. Regrowth can commence at about six months later but epilation may be permanent. To tide patients over this period a wig may be ordered and the fitting is usually done in the hospital.

Auxiliary Treatment

The medical social worker is invaluable. She can cope with problems that often seem mountainous to the patient, and by liaison with the general practitioner and the community services ensure that the patient continues to receive supporting care and treatment after discharge, for example a home help, financial assistance, or a visitor to enable a relative to get out for short periods. From this it is obvious that a ward round, at which all these workers are present with the nurse and doctor, will ensure that the whole team understands both the patient's needs and the individual contribution each can make to his care.

Discharge

On discharge a full assessment of progress is made for future reference. Return to normal life will be graded according to the patient's condition. After a short rest some patients are able to return to full employment, others need longer convalescence and may require retraining, sometimes in special centres. Yet other patients will return to their referring hospital since they are not fit to go home. It is important that patients take an adequate supply of any necessary drugs to cover the period before the medical discharge letter reaches the general practitioner. Skin care follows the normal rules, but it is always worth repeating the warning about friction of clothes and exposure to sunlight.

The patient may ask about driving. He should be referred to the doctor in charge who will advise him not to drive until he is given medical clearance. It is often a matter of years before this is given, particularly if there is a history of epilepsy.

Follow-up

The patient is usually seen at regular intervals by the neurological centre. Radiotherapy centres vary in their policy, but usually the first appointment is three months, and thereafter at six to twelve month intervals. At these appointments a full neurological examination is made to assess recovery. Patients on hormone supplements may need adjustments of the dosage. If there are signs of deterioration there will be referral back for an early appointment at the neurological centre. Retreatment with radiation can be carried out, but it must be very limited, and only done in special circumstances. Chemotherapy may also be used. However it may be judged better to rely on dexamethasone with little or no adjunctive treatment.

Prognosis

This will vary with the histology and the site of the tumour. The best results are seen in the pituitary macro-adenomas, figures of 80–90% five-year survival are given. Most meningiomas, in the region of 70%, will do well. For the rest there is a scale of from 50% five-year survival Astrocytoma grade I, to a few weeks or months for Astrocytoma grade IV. Although the prognosis for children with medulloblastoma is generally considered poor, a 3 years survival of 15%, figures of five years 40–50% survival have been cited.

However these are only guides, the occasional long survival of a patient with a highly malignant tumour will surprise and please both the relatives and the therapist. It is for this reason that a prognosis should only be given to relatives by an experienced doctor, and also since response can be so unpredictable, that treatment, even in patients with a bad prognosis, is justified, particularly since worthwhile palliation of symptoms may be achieved.

Swift, silent, unbidden,
The message passes to and fro.
Break the chain,
The message is lost, and all purpose too.

10   The Spinal Cord

In this chapter we complete our survey of disease in the central nervous system by considering the spinal cord. We must include the spinal nerves; these contain motor fibres which run out from the cord to the muscles, and sensory fibres which run into the cord and convey impulses from the sensory nerve endings.

Anatomy

The spinal cord extends from the medulla oblongata (hind brain) at the level of the foramen magnum down to the level of the disc between lumbar vertebrae 1 and 2. Thirty one pairs of nerves leave the spinal cord and through the intervertebral foraminae. Each contains both motor and sensory fibres serving certain muscles and well defined areas of skin (dermatomes). Pain or numbness (anaesthesia) of an area can indicate damage to a nerve or to the level of the cord from which it arises. During embryonic development the vertebrae grow faster than the cord, the segment of cord and its nerve often therefore lies at a higher level than the dermatome. Cervical nerves run out almost straight sideways, but the last sacral nerve S5 leaves the cord in the lumbar region, and then runs down beside the cord before leaving at a much lower level. This difference between cord level at which the nerve originates, and vertebral level at which it leaves the column is important clinically. If we are considering symptoms in the dermatome supplied by a spinal nerve, say L4, we have to look at the peripheral nerve, at the L4 vertebra, at the nerve within the column, and at the segment of cord from which it is derived. At any of these points the nerve can be involved giving rise to symptoms. It is now possible to see why, if disease in the bone is suspected, the X-ray must include not only the vertebra at which the nerve leaves, but also all those up to the level of the cord from which that nerve arises.

Structure of the Cord

The cord is composed of grey matter, nerve cells, and white matter. This white matter consists of nerve fibres which are collected into tracts. These tracts run

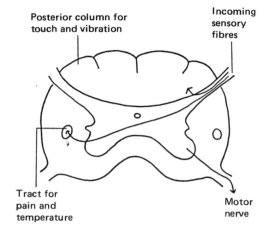

Posterior column for
touch and vibration

Incoming
sensory
fibres

Tract for
pain and
temperature

Motor
nerve

Fig. 10.1.   Spinal cord

to and from definite areas of the brain and are specialised. For instance the
posterior tracts, the posterior columns, run up to centres in the brain and
convey sensations of vibration, light touch, position and joint sense; the pyramidal tracts run down from the cortex and convey impulses to the motor cells
in the grey matter. This grey matter, which in cross section is shaped like the
letter H, surrounds the central canal and is composed of motor and sensory
cells, the motor cells lie anteriorly and are called the anterior horn cells. The
canal contains cerebrospinal fluid and communicates above with the ventricular
system of the brain. It is lined by ependymal cells as in the ventricles.

Coverings of the Spinal Cord

The spinal cord has the same three coverings as the brain; pia mater, arachnoid
mater, and dura mater. Between the arachnoid mater lining the dura mater, and
the pia mater lining the cord, there is the subarachnoid space containing cerebrospinal fluid. This fluid bathes the surface of the cord just as it bathes the
surface of the brain.

Lumbar Puncture

In performing a lumbar puncture use is made of the fact that the dura mater
ends at a lower level than the cord. The needle enters at the disc level L3-4,
it then lies in the subarachnoid space but below the cord, thereby avoiding
injury to the cord.

Arterial Supply

The anterior and posterior spinal arteries arise from the vertebral artery within the skull and run down the length of the cord. The segmental arteries also supply small branches to the cord.

Vertebral Column

The vertebral column is composed of 33 vertebrae. A vertebra is basically a ring surrounding the vertebral canal containing the spinal cord. On this ring are various thickenings and projections.

Anteriorly the ring is thickened to form the body of the vertebra. Posteriorly the bony spine projects backwards. The bone forming the rest of the ring is called the neural arch. Notches on the anterior part of the neural arch form with similar notches on its neighbouring vertebrae, the intervertebral foraminae. It is through these openings that the spinal nerves leave the vertebral column.

Nervous System Considered as a Whole

The whole nervous system, central (brain and spinal cord) and peripheral (nerves and nerve endings) forms a delicate system of checks and balances. Sensory impulses are constantly passing into the central system and motor impulses passing out to the peripheral. This relay of information can occur at many levels. A tendon jerk such as the knee jerk, is activated by a reflex arc passing solely through the spinal cord and never reaching the conscious level in the brain. A sensory impulse from the muscle passes into the spinal cord, acts upon the anterior motor horn cell, and a motor impulse passes to the muscles moving the knee. It is therefore possible for involuntary movement to take place independent of the consciousness or will. The motor cell can also be affected by

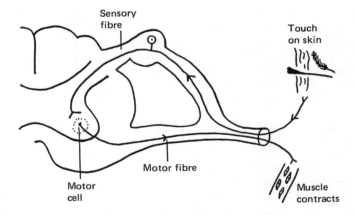

Fig. 10.2.   Reflex arc

impulses passing down in the pyramidal (motor) tract from the motor cortex in the brain causing voluntary movement. In addition the muscles of the body are in a state of 'tone'. This represents a balance between contraction and relaxation and can be appreciated by moving passively a normal limb. This balance is reached because of impulses passing from centres in the brain down other spinal (extrapyramidal) tracts and acting on the motor cell. Sensory impulses pass into the cord and reach various centres of the brain, these may be the cerebellum, the thalamus (nucleus deep in the cerebral hemisphere), or the conscious level in the sensory cortex.

A man walking normally represents the final outcome of the interplay of many impulses either accelerating or slowing action, and this action is further constantly modified by sensory impulses passing into the system. With such complicated mechanisms it is only possible in this book to state certain broad principles, these would on closer study be qualified in many ways.

Basic Principles

1. Interruption of the reflex arc results in loss of tone, the muscles are completely relaxed (flaccid).
2. If the motor cell or nerve is damaged the muscles are paralysed, tone is flaccid, the tendon jerk is lost.
3. Interruption of the tracts conveying impulses to the motor cell from the brain results in:
   a. paralysis of a voluntary movement,
   b. increase in tone – there is more contraction than relaxation – the muscle is spastic,
   c. exaggerated tendon jerks due to loss of the impulses from the brain modifying the reflex arc.
4. Interruption of the sensory tracts results in loss of sensation in the dermatomes supplied by the segments below the lesion.
5. Complete transection of the cord gives a picture of paralysis of voluntary movement of all structures supplied by nerves originating below the level of the damage, and anaesthesia of those areas passing sensory impulses into the cord below the same level. Tone is spastic and tendon jerks below the level of damage are exaggerated. Partial damage to the cord, pressure or destruction by tumour within the cord, will cause a variable clinical picture according to the nerve cells and tracts involved.

The Bladder

The muscles of the bladder are smooth (involuntary) and innervated by the sympathetic and parasympathetic systems. Micturition takes place when the sphincter muscle relaxes. This is an involuntary process accomplished through a reflex arc, but it can be over-ridden by impulses from the brain giving voluntary control. In the paraplegic the arc is interrupted and opening of the sphincter is lost causing retention. When the bladder is full over flow occurs, dribbling incontinence. A lesion of the cord above the L2 segment, or damage below this to the nerves supplying the bladder, will interfere with control of micturition.

Pathology

In discussing the pathology of tumours in this region we have to consider (1) the cord, (2) the space between it and the vertebra, and (3) the vertebra itself. Because of this the range of histology is much wider than in the brain.

(1) Within the cord itself the same histological types of tumour occur as in the brain. They are called intramedullary because of their position.

(2) In the space between the cord and the bone, tumours can arise from the coverings of the cord, meningiomas, and more rarely tumours arising from other structures can occur, such as neurofibroma.

(3) Malignant deposits in the skull rarely cause symptoms by pressure on the brain, but disease in a vertebra on the contrary usually gives rise to symptoms of cord compression. The vertebral column is weight bearing. The weakness of the bone produced by disease causes the vertebra under pressure to become deformed and press on the cord. When the body of the vertebra is affected it can collapse giving a wedge shaped appearance on X-ray. Primary bone tumours are rare but secondary deposits are more common. There are five sites of carcinoma from which spread to bone can be expected, breast, bronchus, kidney, prostate, thyroid, of these the first two are the most commonly found in the spine, indeed they may be the first indication of the primary disease. Rare tumours are the neuroblastomas occurring in children. They arise from sympathetic nerve tissue. Also found, even more rarely, are chordomas which grow from embryonic remnants in the spinal column.

Aetiology

No aetiological factors have so far been discovered.

Age and Sex

In children the most usual tumour is the medulloblastoma seeding down from the cerebellum. Patients are usually under the age of five. A neuroblastoma may lie partly in the vertebral canal and partly outside the column forming a dumbbell tumour. These are more rare than the medulloblastoma. In adults, tumour can occur at any age, although secondary bone deposits are more common in the older age groups. In young adults tumours are usually those arising within the cord or from its coverings. Occasionally they are formed by deposits similar to those found elsewhere in the lymphomas, or in children they may be leukaemic deposits.

Symptomatology

With such a complicated subject any attempt to give all the possible symptoms and presentations would involve far too long a section. Instead we can look at the case notes of three patients with symptoms of spinal cord compression due to spinal tumours. Each case represents one of the sites discussed in the section on pathology.

Tumour Within the Cord (Intramedullary)

Mrs. T. At the age of 57 she noticed that she had numbness in her left hand and that she burnt the hand without realising it. Three years later she developed weakness and numbness in the right hand and found she was unable to write properly. The condition in the hand gradually deteriorated. At the age of 62 she was admitted to a neurological centre. When she was examined, the positive findings were:
Excessive sweating of the palms.
Wasting of some of the small muscles in the right hand.
Gross loss of control of movement, ataxia of the right hand with the eyes closed.
Light touch and pin prick impaired over the hands.
Joint sense absent in the fingers of both hands, and impaired in the right and left big toes.
Vibration absent in the arms and the part of the body below the level of L5.
Temperature sense absent in both hands.
We can deduce that the posterior columns (light touch, pin prick, vibration and joint sense) are affected. The tract close to the canal serving temperature is also involved. The site of the signs and symptoms indicate a lesion in the cervical cord. This was confirmed by the myelogram which showed an expansion of the cord extending from C5 to T1. A laminectomy, removal of part of the vertebra, was performed and the swelling needled for biopsy. The histology showed an astrocytoma grade I. She received radiotherapy. Ten years later her physical signs were unchanged but there was no evidence of recurrence.

Tumour Outside the Cord (Extramedullary)

Mrs. R. At the age of 35, two years before her hospital admission, she had experienced pain in the right shoulder and difficulty in raising the arm when she was dressing. Because of the pain she thought she had rheumatism. The weakness progressed until 18 months later she was unable to raise the arm at all. On admission to hospital, she was found to have wasting and weakness of the muscles in the arm supplied by the right cervical fifth and sixth nerves. At this time she developed a slight hesitancy of micturition. Careful testing showed impaired vibration and joint position sense in the right arm. A myelogram showed a complete block at the level of C6. A laminectomy was performed and a fleshy mass arising from the covering of the cord was partially removed. The histology proved the tumour to be a meningioma.

The physical findings made an accurate prediction of the site of the tumour possible. The localisation of pain and weakness pointed to involvement of a spinal nerve and gave the level, and the sensory changes indicated pressure on the posterior tract. A myelogram showing a block rather than an expansion of the cord indicated a diagnosis of a lesion outside the cord rather than of one within it.

She received radiotherapy. Three years later, apart from weakness in the right arm she was well and had no signs of recurrence.

Tumour Within the Bone

A woman of 52 had received radiation following a mastectomy seven years previously. Menopause had occurred at the age of 42. She was on six-monthly follow-up, and when seen four months previously had been well with no evidence of recurrence. X-rays were clear. She was admitted as an emergency with pain in the back, weakness of the legs, and urinary retention. X-rays showed collapse of thoracic vertebrae 5, 9 and 11. The neurosurgeons considered the disease was too extensive to justify laminectomy. She was placed on androgen injections and radiation to the spine begun. Intensive physiotherapy was given. Initially she improved, movement in the legs was stronger and pain was less. At the end of the third week she became very dyspnoeic. Chest X-ray revealed lymphatic infiltration of the lungs. She died a week later.

Summary

Lesions within the cord give a variety of signs depending entirely on the tracts and nerve cells involved. There will always be some interruption of tracts running down to lower levels of the cord giving signs of sensory and/or motor loss. Usually sensory impairment is found in dermatomes corresponding closely to the level of the lesion. This is called the sensory level and is sought very carefully during examination.

Those tumours which arise between the cord and the bone give very precise motor and sensory symptoms corresponding to the spinal nerves involved, and at the same time symptoms in part of the body supplied by lower levels of the cord. This latter is again due to pressure on the tracts in the cord and will vary according to which are involved. Often it is the posterior tracts, carrying the sensations of light touch, position and joint sense, and vibration sense, which are first involved.

The symptoms caused by disease in the body of the vertebra and its subsequent collapse are, at first sight, a little more difficult to understand. The body of the vertebra lies in front of the cord, yet often the first symptoms are either girdle pain, due to involvement of both spinal nerves at a specific level, or those due to pressure on the posterior tracts. At this point it is as well to remember that pressure on a nerve produces first irritability, signalled by pain and exaggerated sensory symptoms (hyperaesthesia), followed often by decrease of symptoms due to adaptation of the nerve, and finally anaesthesia caused by the interruption of conduction of nerve impulses due to complete occlusion. To return to the picture of a collapsed vertebral body, the collapse distorts the bony ring and causes abnormal angling of the spine and slight forward movement of the vertebra. These changes cause pressure on both spinal nerves and the spinal tracts, usually the posterior. When collapse is slow the signs gradually increase, but if it is sudden often the first warning is severe pain or slight hesitancy of micturition. This latter symptom shows dangerous pressure on the cord involving all tracts to the lower levels. If unrelieved, retention of urine develops and permanent paraplegia.

Investigations

Most of these patients are referred to the radiotherapist from neurological centres, but the full investigations required are described, for during the follow-up of patients, symptoms of cord compression may appear necessitating immediate investigation.

The history is always extremely important. In retrospect minor symptoms can be seen to be part of the clinical picture, and from their timing may give a clue to the nature, the site, and the pathology. The slowly growing more benign tumours, often lying in the vertebral canal, give a long history, while a more rapid progression may indicate a lesion within the cord.

The neurological examination is exhausting to the patient, requiring great concentration particularly during sensory testing. If he is very ill or unco-operative the examination may not always be completed in one session, but the doctor usually tries to establish a sensory level and a basic neurological state, this serves as a comparison should the patient's condition deteriorate.

Based on the clinical finding the special investigations will follow. A full blood count including a differential white count is always done. In a young adult, and particularly in a child, signs of spinal cord compression may occasionally be the presentation of a leukaemia or lymphoid disease. Straight X-rays of the chest and the spine are taken, for pressure due to mechanical injury such as a prolapsed disc must be excluded. If disease of the bone is suspected tomograms may be necessary. In the case of an angioma a selective arteriogram is performed to show the abnormal vessels.

If a CATscan is possible this may be helpful.

Myelogram

When lumbar puncture is carried out it is often convenient to inject contrast medium at the same time and proceed to myelogram. Puncture at other sites (cisternal puncture) is done under X-ray control. A spinal tumour giving rise to a block often gives characteristic findings both on lumbar puncture and myelogram. The pressure is often low, the rise and fall on coughing or compressing the jugular vein is slow, and on laboratory examination the protein content is high. The X-ray pictures may also be diagnostic, a spinal tumour expanding the cord only allows a thin trickle of contrast medium to pass, the so called 'candle grease' appearance, while a block may show as a complete cut off often with a rounded edge.

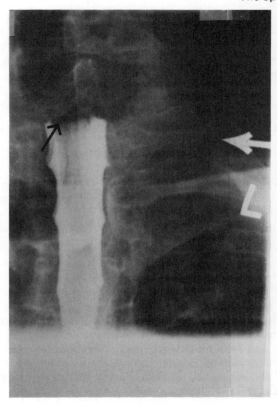

Fig. 10.3. Myelogram. Note failure of contrast medium to pass up beyond
arrow due to a tumour

Further Investigations

These will depend entirely on the suspected pathology. If a diagnosis is made
of a metastatic deposit with unknown primary, or of a primary bone tumour,
then investigations will be directed to establishing the histology. A full skeletal
survey is carried out, and then the full list of special tests, Bence Jones protein
and plasma proteins for myeloma; for secondaries, tests of thyroid function,
kidney, and prostate, and mammography for the breast. It may be that diagnosis
can only be firmly established at operation when biopsy is taken.

Bladder Investigations

The patient with an indwelling catheter must have a full survey of the urinary
tract including C.S.U., blood urea, electrolytes, and if necessary, I.V.P.

Treatment

The aim is first to relieve pressure and if possible eradicate the tumour. Since the aims of treatment vary slightly with the nature of the pathology, primary and secondary tumours are considered separately.

Primary Tumours

Surgery

If at all possible the tumour is excised as completely as possible. In order to gain access part of the bony ring of the vertebra is excised, laminectomy. This in itself will relieve pressure and prevent further damage. Often, coupled with needle biopsy this is all the surgeon can do, for excision, particularly of intramedullary tumours, can make the neurological deficit worse.

Radiotherapy

This can follow surgery or be the only treatment if surgery is not possible. The aim is to treat the full extent of the tumour plus a margin to allow for microscopic spread. Treatment can be given by conventional X-rays, by supervoltage, or by electrons, and lasts four to six weeks. Very careful steps are taken to centre treatment accurately. Special devices are used to ensure day to day reproduction of the placing of the field. Closely related structures such as the kidney are shielded from radiation.

Dosage   The spinal cord can only tolerate a certain dosage of radiation in a given time. The longer the length of cord, the less the total dosage that can be given. Radiation damage to the cord results in damage to the blood vessels supplying it. The tissues supplied suffer ischaemia and both white and grey matter can later undergo necrosis. In the case of the former it is not certain whether damage to the blood vessels is necessarily the cause of this, or whether necrosis occurs independently. The condition is known as transverse myelitis and is equivalent to a traumatic section of the cord. The result is a loss of function in all structures supplied by the cord below the damaged area, this usually means a development of paraplegia.

In addition there is a further limitation to dosage by the effect of radiation on the bones of the vertebral column. These make up one of the blood forming areas of the body and are therefore very vulnerable to X-rays. Depression of the bone marrow first shows itself in a fall in the white blood cell count. It is usual therefore to have a twice weekly count, and in some cases it may have to be done every other day. Treatment is sometimes interrupted to allow the count to recover, but occasionally recovery does not take place and the planned dose cannot be reached. This usually only happens when the whole spine is treated as for a medulloblastoma.

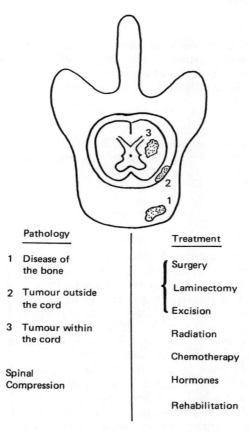

Pathology

1 Disease of
   the bone

2 Tumour outside
   the cord

3 Tumour within
   the cord

Spinal
Compression

Treatment

⎧ Surgery
⎨ Laminectomy
⎩ Excision

Radiation

Chemotherapy

Hormones

Rehabilitation

Fig. 10. 4

Secondary Tumours

Radiotherapy is usually the treatment of choice and gives good relief of pain.
The weakness in the spine is helped by a supporting corset. In some cases, after
a period of months there is some recalcification of bone.

Radiation takes time and if cord compression occurs suddenly, or there are
signs of bladder disturbance, hesitancy or occasionally frequency, then emergency
laminectomy can be carried out. Even if retention has already occurred, provided that operation is done within 24 hours, many patients recover bladder
function. Although the prognosis is poor and a survival of only a few months
expected, no patient should ever be allowed to develop into a catheter cripple
if it can be avoided. The physical discomfort, the risk of infection, and the
psychological shock can make these last few months an intolerable burden.

Hormone Therapy

In addition to radiation and laminectomy, certain forms of cancer may be amenable to hormone treatment, either by surgical or medical ablation. The two common tumours which can be treated in this way are the breast and the prostate. More will be said about this in the appropriate chapters.

Chemotherapy

If the metastasis is part of generalised disease considered responsive to cytotoxics then chemotherapy may be the treatment of choice, with or without radiation.

Nursing Care

The attitude to treating spinal tumours, whether primary or secondary, has altered. The aim now is to institute vigorous measures designed to restore as much function as possible. The severely disabled patient is no longer regarded as being permanently in this state, but as undergoing active rehabilitation.

Most patients will be in hospital for treatment, but where they are visiting daily the nurse must ensure that the full details of nursing care are understood by both the patient and the relatives, and that any rehabilitation physiotherapy is being faithfully carried out. In addition, the nurse and radiographers who see the patient daily must be alert for any signs of deterioration, and should learn to ask about bladder function, muscle weakness, and paraesthesiae, for many patients will not volunteer such information.

Much that was said in the chapter on brain tumours applies equally to the nursing of patients with spinal tumours. Some patients will be up and about with little or no disability, while at the other extreme will be the paraplegic patient with an indwelling catheter. Very rarely with a high cervical tumour the patient may in addition require a respirator and have a tracheostomy. Nursing of the paraplegic patient is time consuming and represents a challenge. The patient is at risk from pressure sores, infection, and development of flexure contractures. If the tumour is metastatic causing collapse of the vertebra, to add to his difficulties the patient may turn but must not sit up. To maintain his morale and self-respect in these conditions needs all the understanding of the nurse. Almost his first need is to be assured of speedy help. A method of summoning help must be provided and assurance given that it works. Where a ripple bed is not available, particular care must be taken to turn the patient frequently and to use padded rings to relieve pressure points. A rucked sheet may easily be the start of skin damage. In the older patient the vitality of the skin is less and damage occurs more readily.

Analgesia must be adequate and must be given regularly. When the patient has to be moved for treatment, an intramuscular injection of analgesic may be needed before this is done. The Stryker frame avoids moving him unnecessarily. For those who have not seen one, it is a form of stretcher which holds the patient firm between rubber mattresses and canvas slings so that he can be turned over in one piece.

Where there are anaesthetic areas particular care must be taken to avoid burns or other trauma. Patients who smoke can easily burn themselves or set the bedding alight. A casual knock can set up an area of bruising which may be difficult to heal.

The care of the sphincters is important both to the health and comfort. Great attention must be paid to asepsis when emptying bladder drainage bags and watch kept for signs of infection. Patients with indwelling catheters are very liable to urinary infection, and once established it can be very difficult to eradicate. It is usual to attempt to re-educate the bladder by clipping off drainage for increasing lengths of time, and then when changing the catheter letting the patient try to micturate normally. Incontinence of faeces may also occur but more often constipation is the problem.

If a nurse will try the experiment of lying flat and attempting to eat and drink, she will speedily appreciate a patient's difficulties. Most will require help, and some will actually need to be fed. All will tend to drink too little and therefore fluid balance charts must be kept and drinking encouraged.

Physiotherapist and Occupational Therapist

The team work necessary in caring for all patients is very much in evidence here. The physiotherapist and occupational therapist have much to offer.

The physiotherapist can make light splints to prevent flexure contractures developing, and can devise exercises, both active and passive, to preserve muscle tone and encourage and strengthen residual activity. When mobilisation is possible she will provide walking frames and gradually teach the patient to manage small flights of steps. For some, calipers are required, and the orthopaedic surgeon and fitter will be needed to advise. While the patient is being mobilised and is sitting out, a special chair to provide adequate support is useful, and if he can be wheeled to the bathroom and toilet his morale will receive a tremendous boost.

The occupational therapist can provide occupation for both mind and body. Mere repetition of exercises is boring, but making a rug or painting a picture exercises weak muscles and provides interest. The truly supine patient can be helped greatly by a special bed table which can act as a book rest, by the provision of mirrors, and by devices for turning pages easily. The daily newspaper can be very troublesome to hold, and the simple device of large elastic bands to hold it on the book rest may make all the difference to a patient's enjoyment.

Medical Social Worker

During this period of treatment the medical social worker is able to assess the needs of the patient and family, and liaise with the community services. This may range from simple convalescence to financial support, and a rearrangement of the home or even rehousing. Where a patient is in an upper flat with no lift, with patience and persistence, rehousing can often be arranged, or in a house assistance to make a bedroom downstairs can be given. In other cases she may arrange the preliminaries to a course of retraining at a government rehabilitation centre.

When a fully disabled patient returns home the nursing burden on the family is great. The medical social worker through her contacts can often trigger the provision of sitters and helpers so that the family can get a much needed respite. Arrangements to provide any special apparatus needed and community nursing must also be made.

Deterioration

The nurse must always be on the alert for signs of deterioration in a patient who has not had surgery. Any unusual paraesthesiae, difficulties of micturition, or weakness should be reported. It cannot be emphasised too strongly that sudden spinal cord compression is as much of an emergency as appendicitis, and that prompt surgery can often prevent the patient becoming paraplegic.

Relatives

The doctor is responsible for the explanations to the family of a patient's condition, but often the nurse is called upon to repeat and clarify what has been said. In turn she can often learn much that is useful to the doctor and the rest of the team. When rehabilitation is taking place, she can explain to the relatives what the object of therapy is, and persuade them not to wait on the patient hand and foot but allow him to make his own efforts. This last advice is often most needed in the case of mothers of young children. She can demonstrate nursing procedures to the relatives when necessary, and finally on discharge see that the necessary drugs and special appliances are sent out with him.

Prognosis

It is extremely difficult to give any meaningful figures since the pathology is so varied. At one end of the range, only 1-2% of children with medulloblastomas survive 10 years, while at the other extreme a patient with a spinal meningioma may have a normal life span. In the case of metastatic deposits the progress of the disease elsewhere determines the prognosis.

Follow-up

The intervals between the follow-up visits are dictated by the nature of the underlying disease. If it is metastatic the first appointment is usually a month later and thereafter at longer intervals. Most other patients will be seen first

at three to six months, and thereafter six monthly. At each visit a full neurological examination is made.

The final word must be that all these patients must be regarded as in a phase
of rehabilitation. Every effort must be made to avoid them spending long
periods on terminal care. Their physical situation is already difficult. If some
activity can be preserved for them, then they can retain self respect and avoid
the frustration of feeling completely dependent on others.

The mind has its exits and its entrances.
When the portals are closed,
The exit gate stands open but unused,
The mind turns inwards,
Frustrated, upon itself.

11   The Eye and the Ear

THE EYE

Anatomy

In shape the eye is two overlapping globes, the smaller filled with aqueous humour is the anterior segment containing cornea, iris, ciliary body, lens. The internal layer of the larger posterior segment is the retina (receptors of the retinal nerves), external to this is the choroid. The macula, the sensitive spot, lies on the eye's central axis. The retinal nerves leave the eye at the optic disc. They form the optic tract, eventually reaching the occipital cortex. Retina and optic disc are part of the brain, swelling of the disc is one of the first signs of raised intercranial pressure. Blood supply, through branches of the ophthalmic artery and vein, is rich, except to the cornea.

The eyelids are formed by skin externally, conjunctiva internally, with the cartilaginous tarsal plate between. The margins carry eyelashes, and openings of sebaceous and mucous glands. Lids protect the anterior chamber, shutting out light when closed. Blinking occurs involuntarily several times a minute, and also in response to a foreign body or threatened blow. The lacrimal gland, lying laterally beneath the upper lid, secretes tears. The blink sweeps them across to the inner canthus, cleansing and lubricating. Tears drain by two punctae into the naso-lacrimal ducts which open into the nose.

Cranial nerves supply six muscles moving the eye. Paralysis of one or more muscles causes faulty movement and inco-ordination of the eyes. This results in diplopia (double vision).

The orbit, the bony socket of the eye, is formed by seven bones. Posteriorly and medially lies the brain, antrum medially and below, nose medially. Lymphatic tissue and fat lie between the eye and bone.

In order to follow a logical sequence we shall begin with the lids and discuss tumours in each part of the eye separately.

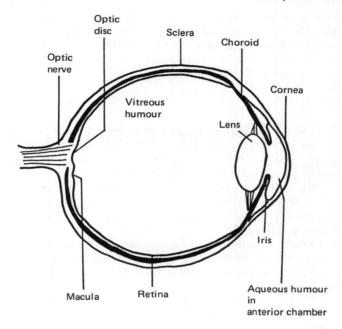

Fig. 11.1.   The eye

Eyelids

The commonest tumour being skin carcinoma, aetiology is probably the same as for other skin areas, but little is known. The site is usually the lower lid. Patients are in the fifth decade onwards, more men than women being affected.

Pathology and Spread

Basal cell and squamous cell tumours occur, the former being more common. Spread is direct for both, but additionally for the squamous type lymphatic and blood borne in the later stages. Extensive tumours can involve tarsal plate, lacrimal duct, conjunctiva, deeper eye structure, and the orbit. More rarely pre-cancerous melanosis, melanoma may occur, and very rarely involvement by generalised Hodgkin's disease, non-Hodgkin's lymphoma, or leukaemia. Gland tumours can also occur.

Symptomatology

The patient complains of a small nodule which has ulcerated and failed to heal. The edge is rolled, everted, and irregular. There is intermittent discharge and occasionally a little bleeding. Extensive tumours can interfere with the tear drainage, with the vision, and can cause pain, for they are often infected and may involve cartilage or bone. More rarely, the story is of a mole which has begun to grow or bleed.

Examination

During the taking of the history, an attempt is made to enlist any aetiological factors. Examination includes measurement of the lesion, a diagrammatic sketch, and photography if possible. Patency of the puncta is assessed, and the presence of any ectropion (turning out of the eyelid) or entropion (turning in of the lid). By palpation the infiltration of the tumour is estimated and also the presence of any fixation. When examining the upper eyelid it is necessary to evert it in order to inspect the conjunctival surface. Finally the nodes around the ear and in the neck must be palpated.

The eye is examined with the ophthalmoscope. In the uncomplicated lesion the doctor notes any opacities present in the lens. Where there is invasion of the eye he examines the whole retina carefully, if this is possible, searching for signs of tumour.

Investigations

Routine tests include blood count, swab of any discharge for bacteriology and sensitivity, and chest X-ray. The latter is also useful as a check for other conditions. A biopsy is taken to establish histology, but not of a suspected melanoma, this is accomplished by wide excision. If the tumour is extensive, orbital and skull X-rays are checks for bone infiltration or destruction.

Radiation Effects on the Lids and Eye

Before treatment is described, it will be convenient to consider first both immediate and late radiation effects in the eye and lids.

Lids

Immediate skin effects are as elsewhere in the body. Late changes include pallor, telangiectasia, and possibly fibrosis causing tarsal plate or lid deformity. Healing of lesions with fibrosis may cause lids turned in (entropion), causing conjunctival and corneal irritation, or outwards (ectropion), with soreness and disturbed tear drainage (epiphora = overflow). Eyelid epilation is usually permanent.

Lacrimal Duct

As it is closely related to the inner canthus, stenosis, caused by fibrosis, may lead to epiphora as a late effect.

Glands

Both lid and lacrimal glands are affected. Lid irritation is usually present. Tears initially increase, then share in the general decrease of secretions. Resultant dryness and soreness may persist leaving the eye liable to infection.

Conjunctiva

The erythema threshold is lower than for skin. Initial change is congestion followed by oedema (chemosis) with a liability to infection.

Cornea

This is an avascular structure and is very resistant to radiation. If keratitis and ulceration occur this is usually a result of trauma and infection, and not of radiation. If not treated adequately, corneal ulceration with the resultant loss of vision follows.

Lens

This is the most vulnerable structure of the eye. Radiation can cause cataract formation. Unlike the senile variety it develops rapidly, and fortunately therefore remedial operation is possible much earlier. A single dose of 200 rads (2 Gy), a very small dose, can cause lens damage, and certainly doses lower than those required to treat lesions of the lid can induce cataract formation. These lens opacities appear from eighteen months to seven years after radiation.

Retina and Optic Tract

These are very resistant to radiation. Any damage which does occur usually does so following overdosage.

Treatment

Either surgery, radiotherapy, or radioactive plaques can be employed. The choice will depend upon the site, extent, histology of the lesion, and the age of the patient.

Radiation

Basal cell and squamous cell carcinomata   Low voltage conventional external therapy is used for all except extensive lesions involving the bones and the eye, the penetration required is very small and therefore megavoltage is not used. In some centres, plaques containing radioactive isotopes emitting radiation travelling a very short distance (β emitters) are employed. Higher voltage conventional X-rays, megavoltage irradiation, or electron therapy are used for the extensive tumour which involves the eye. The area to be treated includes an adequate margin of healthy tissue, and treatment will last from two to six weeks depending upon the type of lesion and the radiation employed. Except for patients with major lesions, or the elderly, treatment is given on an outpatient basis.

Protection

In treating the lids, protection of the vulnerable structures in the eyelids and in the eye is vital. Lead of the necessary thickness is used. The eyelashes and the other lid are protected by a lead strip or by a lead cut-out, and by using an applicator which is well shielded. The eye is protected by inserting a lead eye shield coated with plastic to absorb secondary irradiation under the eyelids. This must be done with scrupulous attention to asepsis and the avoidance of trauma.

Insertion of eye shield   The patient is positioned lying down comfortably. The head is stabilised with sand bags. The procedure to be followed is explained carefully to the patient.

The tray contains the eye shield selected for the patient by the doctor, it lies in antiseptic solution, sterile gauze swabs, disposable sachets of sterile liquid paraffin and of a local anaesthetic, a small quantity of sterile water or saline, disposable forceps, and sterile scissors. The whole tray is covered. It is extremely important that nothing else should ever be put on the tray so that the possibility of irritant solutions being used in the eye by mistake is avoided. If disposable sachets are not available, sterile oil and anaesthetic must be obtained, and frequently checked bacteriologically.

The nurse or radiographer washes her hands thoroughly. The doctor inspects the eye to see that no inflammation or infection is present. The nurse then uncovers the tray, snips off the end of the anaesthetic sachet, after having this checked, and inserts the drops in the conjunctival sac. To do this, she should stand at the patient's head and bring the sachet in from the side, explaining all the time what she is doing and warning the patient that he will blink and possibly feel a slight smarting. The upper lid is retracted slightly and the lower lid is gently pulled down to form a well. The drops are inserted at the lateral fornix so that the natural action of the lids and tears sweeps the anaesthetic across the cornea. The patient then waits 10 to 20 minutes for the drops to take effect. Meanwhile, using disposable forceps the nurse takes the eye shield out of the antiseptic and places it in sterile water or saline. The doctor washes his hands. The nurse now instils oil, after checking, in the conjunctival sac, this blurs the patient's vision. After drying the eye shield on a sterile swab the doctor may ask for a few drops of oil to be put in the concave surface of the shield. He runs his finger over the surface to make sure that there is no roughness to traumatise the cornea. Standing in the same position as the nurse he asks the patient to look up. The upper lid is gently retracted and the shield carefully slipped into position, the lower lid quickly pulled down and allowed to slip back up over the shield which floats in position on a thick layer of oil. With proper care no damage to the cornea should result. After treatment the lower lid is gently pulled down, slight pressure on the shield causes it to slip out. Since the eye is anaesthetised

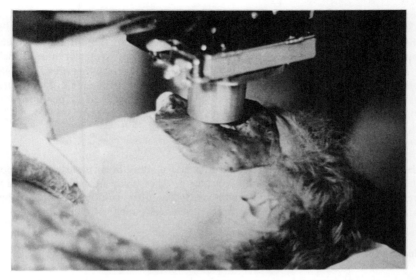

Fig. 11.2.   Lead shield in position over the eye with applicator

and the corneal reflex lost, the patient is given an eye pad and instructed to wear this for at least an hour. He must also be constantly reassured about his sight, but warned that he will lose his eyelashes in the treatment area.

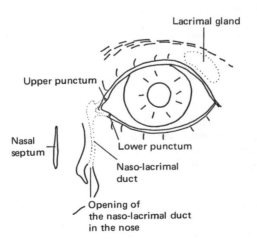

Fig. 11.3.   Lacrimal gland and nasolacrimal duct

Lead Shield

The other lid is protected by a strip of lead moulded to the correct curve and kept in place by Sellotape. If the lesion is larger and more irregular, a lead shield is prepared. A plaster cast is taken of the eye and surrounding area. The lead shield is moulded over this and a window for the treatment area cut out. After insertion of the eye shield, the face shield is then secured in position with sellotape.

Inner Canthus

The close proximity to the lacrimal duct has already been mentioned. If possible the duct is avoided and the applicator directed away from the other eye to prevent radiation reaching it. If radiation to the duct cannot be avoided, then careful watch is kept during follow-up for the development of epiphora.

Nursing Care

Care during treatment is directed to the skin, the conjunctiva, and the cornea. Watch must be kept for signs of infection. The conjunctiva after installation of anaesthetic may be reddened, but this should have settled by the next appointment. If it persists, infection should be suspected and a swab for culture and sensitivity taken. The doctor may decide to rest the eye from treatment, or alternatively prescribe eye-drops keeping a very careful watch. If infection is proved, treatment is stopped until this subsides. Radiation conjunctivitis and oedema may occasionally be severe enough to require hydrocortisone eye-drops. Oedema of the lid, unless with electron therapy, does not usually require treatment to be halted. Any extensive ulcerative lesion will require careful cleansing and dressing. Irritation of the eyelids usually responds to a bland ointment. If a lesion of the cornea is suspected, the patient is referred immediately to an ophthalmologist and treatment stopped. The development of a corneal ulcer is an avoidable complication.

Surgery

This involves plastic reconstruction and skin grafting. It is the treatment of choice for major extensive lesions, for melanoma, and in some centres is also the first choice for the smaller lesions. The recurrence of any lesion after radiotherapy is also treated surgically.

Radioactive Isotopes

Plaques containing β emitters can be used as the primary treatment. Although penetration is only a few millimetres, full eye protection should still be given. In the elderly patient who is not fit for surgery, the recurrences are sometimes

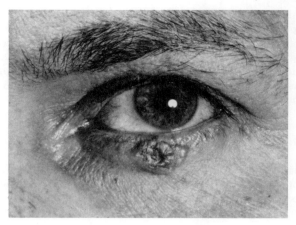

Fig. 11.4.   Lesion of the lower lid before surgery

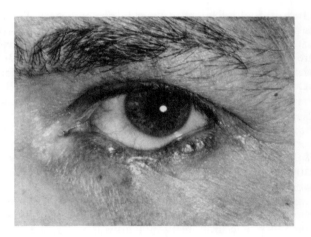

Fig. 11.5.   Lesion of the lower lid after surgery

treated by the implantation of radon seeds. The risk of cataract formation is high and therefore this method should only be employed when the natural life expectation is short.

Follow-up

After radiation, the patient is seen again in one to four weeks depending on the severity of the reaction. Patients with extensive lesions requiring dressings are best treated in the department, where nurses are familiar with the radiation reaction. Within six weeks, the reaction settles and in eight weeks healing is usually complete. The intervals between follow-up will then depend upon the histology of the lesion. At each visit the local condition is inspected, and where appropriate an examination is made of the lens and of the nodes in the neck. A careful watch is kept for signs of the late complications of radiation, deformity of the lids and epiphora. Since the eye has been fully protected cataract formation will not occur.

Nodes

When lymphatic metastases develop the same policy is adopted as described in Chapter 6, block dissection or irradiation. This is true for all parts of the eye and so this section will not be repeated in this half of the chapter.

Prognosis

Much depends on the histology, but for a small basal cell or squamous cell carcinoma, treatment either by radiation or surgery is successful in 90% of cases. For larger lesions, the prognosis is rather better for basal cell than for squamous cell lesions, but once bone is involved the prognosis progressively worsens. Adequate treatment is essential, for even a small lesion which fails to respond, can, through extension, involve the eye, eventually requiring major surgery including enucleation.

The Eye

Tumours of the eye itself are rare. Their treatment involves two considerations, the preservation of life, and the preservation of the sight. Since they are so rare, it is customary to refer the patient to a radiotherapist familiar with these tumours and skilled in their treatment. It must be obvious that there must be close cooperation between the therapist and the ophthalmic surgeon. Both primary and secondary tumours can occur. Primary tumours will be described first.

Conjunctiva, Cornea and Iris

Tumour can arise in any of these structures but it is rare.

Cornea and Conjunctiva

Intradermal carcinomata and squamous carcinomata can occur. They are rare and usually affect the elderly. Treatment is by radiation.

Melanoma

This can affect all three structures and can occur either as a diffuse or circumscribed lesion. Treatment is by excision followed by the application of β emitter plaques. Surgery gives good results in early cases and in tumours of the iris, but the results are poor where the disease is diffuse. For the latter, radical surgery is the treatment of choice. Metastases are the commonest cause of death. They may occur in the central nervous system, or in the rest of the body, most commonly the lung.

Choroid Body

The lesion here is usually a melanoma. Again it may occur as a circumscribed tumour or as a diffuse lesion. Spread is similar to that described in the preceding paragraph. The patient complains of loss of part of the field of view (field defect), and deterioration of vision due to tumour. Retinal detachment can occur and also glaucoma (this is blockage of drainage from the anterior chamber raising the pressure and sometimes causing pain). Inflammation may also be present. Treatment is by surgery if possible, followed by megavoltage radiotherapy.

Follow-up

Since spread can occur to distant parts of the body as well as to the nodes, chest X-rays and palpation of the nodes should be routine examinations.

Prognosis

This is very variable and ranges from two to twenty-odd years. It is not unknown for a patient to present with a large liver, obvious systemic signs of metastatic disease, but with no indication of the primary. The alert doctor who notices the glass eye will have a very strong clue and suspect previous removal of the eye for melanoma many years ago.

Retinoblastoma

A very rare childhood tumour arising spontaneously in about 1 in 34,000 live births, but there is a strong familial tendency. Of children born to previously affected parents, 50–70% develop the disease, while only about 4% of the second children of non-affected parents have the tumour. About 75% of patients present before the age of three, only 8% in the over sixes. Bilateral tumours, differing in the degree of development, are found in 20–30% of patients.

Pathology and Spread

The tumour arises in embryonic retinal cells. Histologically areas of necrosis and calcification are seen. Cells, with numerous mitoses, may be arranged in rosettes. Spread is within the eye, backwards to the optic nerve, meninges and brain, and outwards through the eye to bone and occasionally lymph nodes. Blood borne metastases occur usually in the bone but occasionally in the lungs.

Symptoms

Presentation is often late with complaints of squint, inflammation, or 'ox eye' (prominent eye). Tumour may already extend to the anterior surface. Vision is affected if retinal detachment or glaucoma is present. Parents may notice 'cat's eye' (reflections in the eye).

Examination

Viewed through the ophthalmoscope the tumour is usually cream cheese coloured, hemispherical, flocculent in texture, with thin walled vessels. On X-ray calcification is seen. Chest X-ray is routine, and skeletal survey if there is complaint of bone pain.

Treatment

Although the retina is radio-resistant, the tumour is very radio-sensitive.

1. If more than half the retina is destroyed but the other eye unaffected, full excision is the treatment of choice, with as much uninvolved optic nerve as possible. If histologically the nerve is not clear, post-operative radiation is given.
2. If one third or less of the retina is involved, radioactive discs are sewn into place and left for one week. Prospects of both tumour destruction and some useful vision are reasonable. Prior megavoltage radiation may occasionally be used to shrink large tumours.
3. External radiation alone is less successful for primary tumours, but is useful for recurrence, metastases, or to treat the other eye after enucleation of one (bilateral disease).
4. Some centres have used a combination of radiation and intra-arterial cytotoxics in advanced cases.

Follow-up

Careful watch is kept both on the primary site and the other eye. As tumours do not disappear, but only become whiter and denser, examination under anaesthesia may be required. Chest X-ray is routine. Other young children in the family are screened regularly.

Prognosis

If the lesion is small, posterior, with no nerve involvement, the prognosis is good, but worsens with increased size or invasion. When death occurs it is usually within one year of treatment, but is rare after a disease free period of 4 years.

The Orbit

Tumours may arise in orbital structures lying between the eye and the bone, lymphatics, lacrimal glands. Sarcomas and vascular tumours have been described, and Hodgkin's disease, lymphomas, childhood leukaemia can also involve the orbit. A common symptom is diplopia caused by proptosis. Treatment depends upon histology. The rare sarcomas receive surgery and radiation, or radiation alone. Results are poor. Lacrimal gland tumours are usually ectopic salivary tissue, highly malignant, and treated by surgery and radiation with eye protection if possible.

Adult lymphomas confined to the orbit respond to surgery and radiation, otherwise lymphomas and leukaemic deposits are treated as part of the generalised disease. In children a metastasis from an adrenal neuroblastoma is quite often found.

Secondary Tumours

Metastases from other primary sites may occur in the eye, the commonest is from the breast, but lung, kidney and stomach secondaries are known. Retinal detachment causes complaints of field defect or deteriorating vision. Radiation is given to relieve symptoms, and, in the case of the breast, hormone or cytotoxic therapy if appropriate.

Extraorbital Disease

Reference to the anatomy explains how invasion from extraorbital tumours can cause proptosis and diplopia. Primary sites include brain and meninges, more rarely optic nerve, nasopharynx, paranasal sinuses. Treatment depends on the primary site. Secondary recurrences are irradiated.

THE EAR

Anatomy

The ear is divided into three portions, the external consisting of the pinna and external auditory meatus, the middle, and the inner (internal) ear. We can imagine we are walking inwards from the pinna to the inner ear.

External Ear

This is formed by the pinna, cartilage covered by skin, and external meatus. This is an S-shaped tube, the lateral third of the walls being cartilage, the rest temporal bone. It is lined by skin with fine hairs, and glands secreting 'wax' (thick sebum) which has some antibacterial action. Sound is funnelled to the middle ear, some animals can move the pinna towards sound (pricking).

Middle Ear

This begins at the tympanic membrane (junction of external meatus and middle ear) and ends at the small window in the bone closing off the inner ear. Lying within the petrous (hard) part of the temporal bone it is related above to the brain, below to the jugular vein, and behind to the mastoid air cells. The ossicles, a chain of three small bones, connect the tympanic membrane with the inner ear window. The facial nerve runs in a bony canal above the inner ear window.

Inner Ear

It is a bony labyrinth consisting of two parts, the cochlea containing the organ of Corti (organ of hearing) and in front three fluid filled semi-cricular canals. These lie closest to the centre of the head and serve balance. The eighth cranial nerve supplies both parts of the inner ear. Lymphatic drainage is initially to pre- and post-auricular nodes, then to the cervical chain.

Hearing

Sound sets the tympanic membrane vibrating. The ossicles conduct the movements to the inner ear window, setting up vibrations in the cochlea resulting in nerve impulses. These are conveyed to the brain's auditory centre. Deafness is of two types, conduction (interruption of ossicle vibration), and nerve, vibrations reach the cochlea but no nerve impulses are set up. Sound can travel through

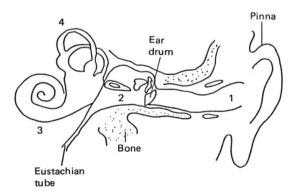

1 External ear

2 Middle ear

3 Organ of Corti

4 Semi-circular canals

Fig. 11.6.   The ear

bone to the cochlea, e.g. tuning fork on the forehead. So hearing aids can help conduction, but not nerve deafness.

Lymphatics

Drainage is to the immediate nodes, pre- and post-auricular, and thence to the cervical nodes.

Tumours

Aetiology

Certain predisposing factors are known. The same factors affecting the skin elsewhere influence the pinna. Chronic otitis media may precede a middle ear tumour. An offensive waxy discharge may be associated with a cholesteatoma, not a true tumour but squamous epithelium overgrowth superimposed on chronic infection. Rarely a glomus jugulare tumour may arise in the specialised chemoreceptor cells of the jugular bulb.

Age and Sex

The glomus tumour is three times more common in women, otherwise there is no sex bias. Carcinoma of the pinna arises in older age groups, the rare middle ear tumour in patients over fifty.

Pathology and Spread

External Ear

The histology of pinna tumours is usually squamous, occasionally basal cell. Middle ear tumours may present in the external meatus. Spread is direct, also lymphatic to auricular and upper cervical nodes.

Middle Ear

Again histology is usually squamous cell, probably due to metaplasia of the normal cells as a result of prolonged irritation or infection. Spread is usually direct, but occasionally lymphatic along Eustachian tube tissue to the pharyngeal nodes, or outwards to the cervical group.

Glomus Jugulare

Histologically cells resemble those in the adrenal medulla but stain differently. Spread is by direct invasion.

Symptomatology

Signs and symptoms of pinna tumours are as for skin elsewhere. Due to the close adherence of skin to cartilage pain is an early symptom, often out of all proportion to tumour size.

Usually external meatus tumours arise in the middle ear, but a true tumour can spread inwards. Symptoms are deafness, discharge, pain and occasionally facial stiffness on the affected side. The latter is due to involvement of the facial nerve as it crosses the middle ear wall, resulting in paralysis of varying degree.

Glomus jugulare tumours lie close to cranial nerves at the base of the skull, and can cause various paralyses including facial. Invasion of the middle ear causes deafness, tinnitus (ringing in the ear), giddiness (vertigo) and in the late stages bleeding and pain.

Examination

The pinna is examined in the usual way for skin tumours. Particular attention is paid to assessing fixation to the underlying cartilage. Palpation of the cervical and auricular nodes is never omitted. Patients with tumours of the external meatus and middle ear are usually referred to the E.N.T. clinic. Examination includes inspection with the auroscope, points noted are the condition of the drum and the present or absence of a normal wall around it. Lymph nodes are palpated. Tests of hearing include the Weber and Rinne, these are carried out with a tuning fork. All the cranial nerves are examined. Positional vertigo is also investigated. The patient is asked to sit up and down several times and then when lying the head is turned sharply to one side, the length and duration of giddiness is noted and any nystagmus. Cold and warm water can also be placed in the meatus and vertigo noted. These tests assess the function of the eighth nerve and occasionally give clues to the pathology.

Patients with a glomus jugulare tumour will be referred either to the E.N.T. clinic or to the neurologist according to symptoms. The examination does not differ from that of a patient with a middle-ear growth.

Investigations

In addition to the full blood count and chest X-ray, skull X-rays, with tomograms of localised areas if necessary, are taken. Knowledge of the extent of bone destruction is important in planning treatment. If required, audiometry assesses the type and degree of deafness. CATscans can be helpful.

Swab of a discharge is taken for culture and sensitivity, and occasionally for cytology. Histological confirmation is obtained from biopsy or operation material. An exception is the glomus jugulare tumour, biopsy can cause torrential haemorrhage.

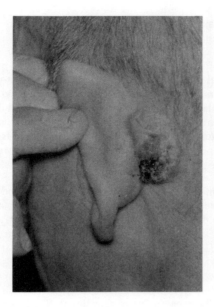

Fig. 11.7.   Treatment of the pinna by radiation (before)

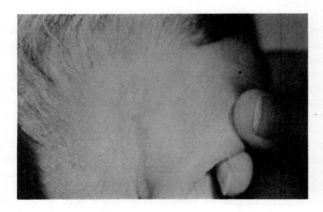

Fig. 11.8.   Treatment of the pinna by radiation (after)

Treatment

External Ear — Pinna

Radiation

Low-voltage external beam irradiation can be used. Although the histology is usually of the squamous cell type, the dose is limited by the close relation of the skin to the cartilage. Treatment usually lasts 10 to 14 days. In some centres radioactive applicators are used, either on one surface, or where the lesion extends on to the back of the pinna a sandwich technique is employed.

Surgery

Large lesions or tumours involving much cartilage can be treated by excision. Almost half the pinna can be removed and a good cosmetic result still achieved. If the whole pinna is removed, the patient subsequently wears a prosthesis. Surgery is employed if radiotherapy fails or there is a recurrence.

External Meatus

These tumours can be treated by conventional X-rays or occasionally by the use of radioactive applicators. The tumour is rare.

Middle-ear Tumours

Treatment is usually by a combination of surgery and radiation, but the latter can be used alone. After excision of the tumour a course of radiation lasting four to six weeks is given. Megavoltage or high energy electron therapy is used. A brief revision of the anatomy section reminds us that the middle ear lies in the petrous temporal bone, so, even if there is no evidence of bone invasion, irradiation must include the whole of the bone and extend virtually to the midline of the head. At the same time, the plan must spare brain tissue, either by using more than one field or by using high energy electrons. Because of the risk of haemorrhage glomus jugulare tumours are often treated solely by radiation.

To ensure accuracy in positioning the fields each day a plastic shell is constructed. It immobilises the patient and enables the treatment position to be reproduced daily.

Localised recurrences can be treated with applicators carrying radioactive sources. In some centres perfusion with cytotoxic drugs has been employed.

Lymph Nodes

The policy which we have already discussed at length in Chapter 6 is followed.

Nursing

Pinna

The same measures are taken as for the treatment of any skin cancer. Heavily infected or necrotic lesions will need daily cleansing and dressings, also possibly the use of topical antibiotics. When cartilage is involved pain can be quite severe, adequate analgesia is required. Following treatment during which daily dressings have been required, it is often advisable if possible, for the patient to attend the department.

Middle Ear

Here, despite the fact that a large cavity is often present, nursing problems are few. Until a new epithelium has grown over the raw surfaces crusting will occur. This requires periodic gentle cleansing and removal. Watch must be kept for any signs of infection. The patient can attend the department or be visited at home.

Follow-up

Since most of these tumours are squamous cell carcinomas, follow-up needs to be at frequent intervals initially, lengthening out as time passes. The first visit will be at one to two weeks depending on the reaction. At each visit the local lesion is assessed and the lymph node areas palpated. Patients who have had external lesions treated must be warned about undue exposure to sunlight, this precaution is virtually a life-long one. The tolerance of the cartilage to a further dose of radiation, although of a different type, is very low and necrosis easily occurs. One patient took a day's sea trip in the summer, subsequently developed cartilage necrosis, and was left with a small neat hole through the pinna. This damaged cartilage is not only painful but liable to infection. An expectant policy is adopted. The site is kept clean and free of infection. Hydrocortisone cream may be helpful. If epithelium fails to grow back local excision is carried out with plastic repair.

Any patient who has had involvement of lymph nodes or whose condition seems to be deteriorating should have a chest X-ray. This should be repeated at intervals. Although blood borne spread is late, it does occur.

Prognosis

Patients with external-ear tumours and no lymphatic involvement do well. At five years, 90% will have survived. The outlook is worse if nodes are involved and fixed. Tumours of the middle ear have carried a gloomy prognosis. A three-year survival rate of 26% is quoted from some centres. Although more powerful radiation has slightly improved the chances, substantial improvement can only follow if diagnosis can be made much earlier. The glomus jugulare tumour carries a rather better prognosis.

Patients who have progressive disease die from the effect of lymphatic spread, extension into the brain, or haemorrhage.

Life is a dance,
The body moves slow or fast,
Swaying to an unseen orchestra,
Its tempo set by a silent master.

12   The Thyroid

The main action of the thyroid is to secrete hormones, thyroxine and tri-iodo-thyronine which speed up body metabolism. They do this by increasing the usage of oxygen necessary to metabolic processes. It is as if the body fires are stoked up and burn more brightly and rapidly. The hormones are synthesised by the gland from iodine circulating in the blood, this iodine is derived from food. The

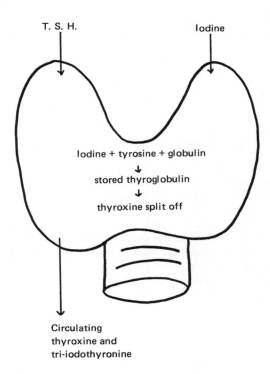

Fig. 12.1.   Formation of thyroxine

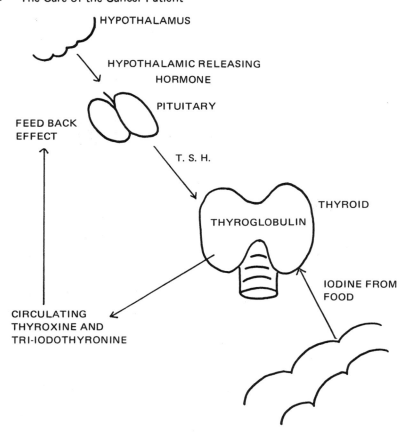

Fig 12.2   Regulation of thyroid activity

thyroid acts as an iodine trap. The synthesised hormone is bound to a protein and stored as colloid in the vesicles of the gland.

When the thyroid hormones are required they are split off from the protein and secreted into the blood. This process is regulated by hormones from the hypothalamus and anterior pituitary, and is a response to the circulating levels of thyroid hormones. If these are low, hormone production rises and vice versa, an example of a feed-back control. Other centres in the brain can affect this control, for instance emotional stress can occasionally trigger off a rise in circulating hormone levels.

Anatomy

The thyroid gland is found in the front of the neck and is wrapped around the trachea which lies behind it. It is shaped like a bow-tie and consists of two lobes joined by a narrow isthmus. Occasionally a small lobe, the pyramidal lobe, projects upwards from this isthmus. The main lobes stretch from the side of the thyroid cartilage down to the sixth ring of the trachea, and the isthmus overlies the second to fourth rings. Running close to the gland on either side are the recurrent and superior laryngeal nerves. During any operation on the thyroid they must be sought and carefully preserved or the patient will develop hoarseness and possibly stridor. The parathyroid glands lying on the deep surface of the thyroid must also be carefully guarded during operation.

During swallowing the gland moves upwards together with the larynx, and the examining fingers should be able to get below the lobes. Failure to do so indicates a retrosternal extension of the gland or fixation to surrounding tissues.

As would be expected in an endocrine gland the blood supply and drainage are very rich. Arteries are derived from the external carotid and the sub-clavian arteries. Lymphatic drainage is to the cervical glands.

Thyrotoxicosis

A short description of overactivity of the thyroid gland, thyrotoxicosis, is given as this condition can be treated by the radiotherapist. Increased thyroxine production results in the patient complaining of symptoms which can be divided into groups.

1. Metabolic effects – increased feeling of heat with sweating, loss of weight with a voracious appetite. 'I eat like a horse, Doctor, but I still lose weight'.
2. Cardiovascular effects – palpitations, a rapid pulse, sometimes irregular. Occasionally cardiac failure occurs.
3. Neurological effects – changes of mood are exaggerated. The patient is irritable and weepy. The hands show a fine tremor of the fingers.
4. Eye signs – the eyes are staring and wide open. Thyroxine acts on the lid muscles causing retraction. Protrusion of the eyes, exophthalmos, is not due to excess thyroxine but probably to the action of another pituitary secretion.

Investigations

The object of all investigation is to test the various steps in the control of the synthesis of thyroxine. Radioactive isotopes can be used to monitor the concentration of iodine in the gland or the uptake of thyroxine into the red cells. The levels in the blood of cholesterol (only useful in myxoedema) or iodine can be determined, and now also various hormone levels. The rate of metabolism as measured by the consumption of oxygen at rest (B.M.R.) is an older test but can still be used.

Since the gland takes up iodine so readily, it is important to avoid, prior to these tests, the administration of iodine containing substances, particularly radio contrast media.

Testing is carried out to confirm the diagnosis of thyrotoxicosis, myxoedema, or to determine whether tumour tissue is hormonally active and secreting thyroxine.

Antibodies

Occasionally proteins of body tissues which are not normally in contact with the blood are released into the blood stream. The body treats this protein as foreign, not self, and antibodies to it are formed. These antibodies then attack the body tissue which contains this protein. Such a disease is called auto-immune. The serum levels of such antibody can be determined. This process can occur in the thyroid and is called auto-immune disease of the thyroid or Hashimoto's disease.

Since iodine is taken up so readily by the thyroid, radioactive iodine can be used not only in minute quantities to measure the activity of the gland, but in slightly higher amounts to depress its activity, or in still higher quantities to destroy certain tumours and their metastases.

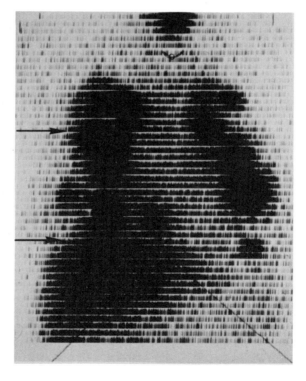

Fig. 12.3.   Radioactive iodine scan. Dense concentration in lung metastases

Originally the unit dose of radioactivity was the curie, further divided into one-thousandth part, milli-curie, or one-millionth part, microcurie. The name was chosen to honour Marie Curie, the discoverer of radium. In the SI system the unit is called a becquerel.

Treatment of Thyrotoxicosis by Radioactive Iodine

The aim of treatment is to depress thyroid activity not to induce myxoedema. The iodine concentrates in the gland giving off radiation and reducing activity. Only certain patients are considered suitable. Although follow up studies have not so far demonstrated a risk of induced malignancy, nevertheless patients under 40 are not usually treated in this way, both because of the long latency of carcinoma, and a possible risk of genetic mutation in the germ cells.

Other contraindications are pregnancy, the iodine can pass to the foetal thyroid and affect it, a large goitre, a possibility of associated carcinoma, poor follow-up, the presence of uraemia or bone-marrow depression.

Nursing and Administration of the Dose

Since a nurse may look after not only the patient with malignant disease receiving ablation therapy, but also the outpatient attending for tracer studies, and the thyrotoxic patient receiving a therapeutic dose, a description is given of the procedure for administering the radioactive isotope, the precautions to be taken subsequently, and the reaction to ablative doses.

Administering the Dose

It is best that the patient is given the dose in the radiotherapy department. In this way the chance of the wrong person receiving the iodine is minimised. The name is checked against the notes and the previous decision to give isotope therapy is verified. The nurse should do this and the doctor will do a repeat check. Radioactive iodine is given in the morning with the patient fasting. The liquid isotope is dispensed so that it will have the correct amount of activity at the time when it is given. The bottle is labelled with the patient's name, placed in a lead container which is also labelled with her name, and the lid closed. The lead pot is placed on a tray covered with absorbent paper. Also on the tray are disposable gloves, straws, a squeeze bottle of distilled water, paper wipes, a plastic bag, and a receiver for dentures. The whole procedure is carried out without removing anything from the tray to avoid contaminating the area with radioactivity. The patient is asked to remove her dentures if worn. The doctor puts on gloves, checks the name, the label on the pot and the one on the bottle. The bottle is kept in the pot all the time. A straw is then put in the bottle and the patient is asked to drink the iodine, the doctor steadying the pot. To ensure that all the dose is taken water is added and the patient drinks this too. After using a tissue wipe on the lips she should put this in the plastic bag. The doctor puts the straw in the bag, recaps the bottle, closes the lid, and taking care not to contaminate his hands peels off the gloves and puts them in the bag.

Occasionally a patient feels sick but vomiting very rarely occurs. Since the vomit would contain radioactive material patients are kept for an hour in the department, as the staff would know how to cope with any radioactive spill. Afterwards a cup of tea and a light lunch can be taken.

Precautions

After a tracer or therapeutic dose there are no after effects and the patients present no nursing problems. They are warned to take particular care to wash the hands when preparing food and also when using the toilet.

The patient who receives an ablation dose presents a different problem. There will certainly be after effects and there is also the problem of radioactivity in the excreta. Normally these patients are in a cubicle in hospital. Any vomit the first day and the excreta over the next few days must be monitored for activity. If it is low enough disposal can be in the usual way, but if it is too high storage in safe containers must continue until disposal is safe.

Reactions

After an ablation dose a patient will suffer from radiation sickness within 24 hours, anti-emetics are helpful. Inflammation of the gland can occur, thyroiditis. The symptoms are a sore throat and dysphagia, and there will be local swelling and tenderness. If this reaction is very severe prednisone or A.C.T.H. injections will lessen it. A similar inflammation of the salivary glands is a rare occurrence. Bony secondaries become more painful, this is due to temporary oedema causing local pressure. If the deposits are in the spine careful watch must be kept for signs of cord compression. Menstrual rhythm is disturbed occasionally amounting to amenorrhoea. A slight temporary fall in the platelets and lymphocytes is noticed. Long-term effects may be pulmonary fibrosis if the metastatic deposits were in the lungs, or following large doses myeloid leukaemia can occur.

Follow-up of Thyrotoxic Patients

Patients with thyrotoxicosis are usually seen after six weeks and a clinical assessment is made. Thereafter follow-up is made either by the physician or the therapist. A careful watch is kept for recurrence of over activity, this can be treated with further radioactive iodine, and also for signs of myxoedema, this necessitates replacement therapy. Before treatment of either condition studies of thyroid function are made.

Tumours of the Gland

Malignant tumours are uncommon, less than 1% of deaths caused by malignancy are due to them. The age range of the patients is wider than usual and one type, papillary, can occur in childhood. The histological cell type of tumours is closely related to age, and at all ages females predominate, being 3:1, F:M. In a man a solitary thyroid nodule is always regarded with suspicion, for although rare, the chance of malignancy is very high.

Although still uncommon, malignant tumours occur slightly more frequently in some areas where goitre is common, such as parts of Switzerland and Columbia.

Aetiology

Very rarely a benign adenoma of the gland may undergo malignant change. The only known carcinogenic factor is irradiation to the neck in childhood. Malignancy has occurred following X-ray therapy of benign skin conditions, radiation of the thymus, and most rarely of all following successful treatment to the spine for a medulloblastoma.

Medullary carcinoma may be familial. Non-Hodgkin's lymphoma may possibly arise when there is Hashimoto's disease present.

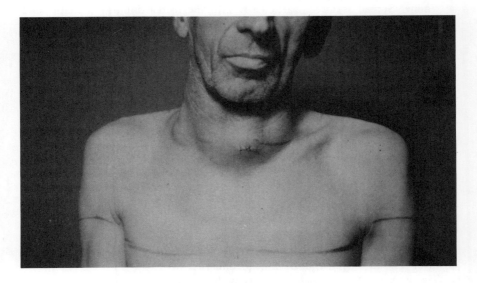

Fig. 12.4.   Carcinoma of the thyroid

Pathology

There are four types of growth.

1. *Papillary*
   The tumour is often a small nodule with microscopic papillae. The cells are frequently well differentiated and of a low-grade malignancy. It metastasises in half the cases to lymph nodes in the neck. When the metastasis is the

first overt presentation it used to be called 'the lateral aberrant thyroid' in the mistaken belief that this was a primary originating in aberrant thyroid tissue. Patients with this tumour are young.

2. *Follicular*

This is usually a tumour of middle years. Most of them resemble normal tissue with very slight evidence of invasion. Less commonly in older patients the type is obviously invasive. Spread is direct particularly in the more invasive type, to lymph nodes, or blood borne to lungs and bone.

3. *Anaplastic*

The cells are poorly differentiated although some areas may have a more normal appearance. Lymphatic and blood borne spread is common. The tumour is rarely found below the age of 60. About 10–15% of thyroid carcinomas are of this type.

4. *Medullary*

Certain cells, C cells in the thyroid, secrete calcitonin. Malignancy can arise in these cells and the tumours then secrete calcitonin and possibly other substances. Histologically polygonal cells containing amyloid are found. About 5% of thyroid carcinomas are of this type. Patients are usually over 40, but a familial type, often associated with other endocrine tumours, occurs in the young. Spread is direct particularly into the mediastinum, lymphatic, and particularly in fatal cases blood borne.

Lymphoma

A non-Hodgkin's lymphoma can occur. Previously some of these may have been classified as anaplastic carcinoma. Patients are usually elderly.

Secondary Deposits

Although uncommon deposits blood borne from other primary sites may be found.

Symptomatology

The story told by patients varies according to the type of tumour. The complaints will be related to the degree of local infiltration, to the lymph nodes involved, and to the presence of bone secondaries.

The young patient usually presents with a story of a slowly growing lump either in the thyroid or in the side of the neck. There is usually no pain although occasionally there may be a complaint of discomfort on swallowing. Occasionally malignancy is only discovered as a result of the microscopical examination of a routine operation specimen.

Over half of the middle-aged patients with a follicular carcinoma have metastases when first seen, and their symptoms may be those of the secondary deposit rather than of the primary growth. A middle-aged woman who was referred to my centre had first been seen complaining of back pain. On X-ray she was found to have a collapsed lumbar vertebra. The physician asked an orthopaedic surgeon to do a drill biopsy. Histology of the specimen showed this to be a secondary deposit from a follicular thyroid carcinoma.

It is those patients who have invasive carcinomas, more commonly the older age group, who most often have symptoms due to local infiltration and pressure. The tumour is usually bulky, hard, and fixed. Invasion of the long thin muscles of the neck, the strap muscles, gives pain. The veins may be engorged due to obstruction, and one-third of them have paralysis of a vocal cord giving rise to hoarseness. This hoarseness is due to involvement of the recurrent laryngeal nerve. The close anatomical relationship to the trachea and the oesophagus means that complaints of dyspnoea, stridor, and dysphagia are often encountered, stridor may be severe enough to call for a tracheostomy. At least half of these patients will have metastases, either local or distant, which may or may not give rise to symptoms.

Examination

The doctor during examination will aim at deciding whether the growth is within the thyroid or not and whether there are symptoms of toxicity or myxoedema. First to be assessed is the general appearance of the patient, any eye symptoms, the type of movement, the condition of the hair and skin, and the emotional state. The pulse is taken, its rate and character noted, and on stretching out the hands the presence of any finger tremor sought. The legs are examined for signs of pretibial oedema. Movements of the eyes are tested and lid retraction is specifically sought. During this time it is easy to notice without alerting the patient any dyspnoea, stridor, or hoarseness. Examination of the gland now follows.

Examination of the Gland

The size and texture of the gland are noted and also its general shape. The doctor always stands behind the seated patient to palpate the gland. He tests the mobility of the thyroid and asks the patient to swallow, the gland should move with deglutition and the examining fingers should be able to palpate below its lower limits. Any pain or tenderness is noted. The lymph nodes are then palpated, the presence of enlargement, its nature, and any fixation assessed. Using the head mirror and the laryngoscope the vocal cords are examined. Finally the chest is examined and the abdomen palpated for any sign of liver enlargement.

During the history taking any treatment which is being given, including self medication, is noted. Many compounds, among them the contraceptive pill, interfere with radioactive iodine studies of thyroid function.

Investigations

After the routine blood test and chest X-ray, investigations will be dictated by the clinical findings. A soft-tissue X-ray of the thoracic inlet may show deviation of the trachea or a retrosternal soft-tissue mass. A barium swallow is often performed to assess pressure on the oesophagus or its invasion by growth. If there is suspicion of invasion and extension into the trachea tomograms may be requested, and if necessary, an examination made under anaesthesia with direct laryngoscopy and bronchoscopy. Any skeletal pain is an indication for a skeletal X-ray scan. Studies of thyroid function are carried out, these will include antibody estimation as Hashimoto's disease can, on rare occasions, mimic carcinoma. Radioactive iodine studies are performed in carefully selected cases, usually the young patient in whom the diagnosis is uncertain. Finally malignancy is either clinically obvious as in the advanced cases, or is confirmed at operation or biopsy.

Treatment

The principles are simple. The gland can be removed, depressed, or destroyed. We can examine each method in turn and its application. The choice will be governed by the state of the tumour, its histological type, and the age of the patient.

Surgery. Removal

This is the treatment of choice for the young patient with a papillary tumour. The extent of the operation will vary from a hemi-thyroidectomy together with any enlarged nodes, to a total thyroidectomy with or without block dissection. Symptoms due to the removal of the parathyroids with the thyroid are usually only temporary. If the operation is less than total a careful watch is kept and the function of the remaining tissue is depressed by giving thyroxine.

Thyroxine keeps the level high enough for normal body function, but depresses the supply of hypothalamic and pituitary regulating hormones. When metastases are functional they can be treated with radioactive iodine.

The middle-aged patient who is in good condition and who has a follicular tumour is treated initially by total thyroidectomy with removal of any involved glands. Radioactive iodine is only given six to eight weeks after operation, the rationale for this is given later.

Hormone replacement will be necessary.

Medullary tumour is treated by total thyroidectomy with removal of lymph nodes if necessary. Hormone replacement must be given.

The indication for surgery in lymphoma is the same as for anaplastic carcinoma, cytotoxic therapy has also been used. Hormone replacement is given as necessary.

An anaplastic tumour is not as a rule suitable for surgery. Generally the only operation carried out is biopsy, preferably by needle aspiration. Where pressure symptoms are severe tracheotomy may be required, with some local surgery.

After surgery a patient is allowed to become myxoedematous. If there is any functional residual tissue or metastases these will become avid for iodine. This may be enhanced by supplementing the normal T.S.H. or depressing release of T.S.H. Six to eight weeks after surgery a tracer dose of radioactive iodine is given and a whole body scan carried out. Functioning tissue can then be ablated

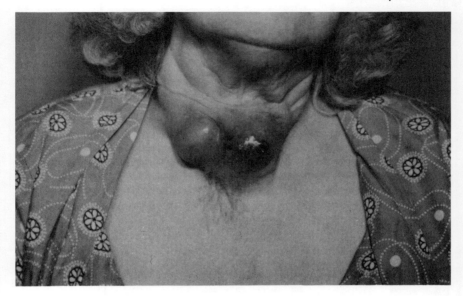

Fig. 12.5.   Thyroid carcinoma recurrence

by a larger dose of radioactive iodine. The procedure can be repeated several times.

Radiotherapy

Primary radiation of the thyroid is difficult as the tissue is fairly radioresistant and therefore high doses are required. Treatment is given to the anaplastic tumour which is often radiosensitive, to the inoperable papillary tumour, and to metastatic deposits. Irradiation may also be given after surgery or for recurrences which occur later. If primary treatment is being given either conventional X-ray or megavoltage radiation can be used. In both cases multiple fields are angled to treat the gland and the cervical lymph nodes avoiding high dosage to the spine. If necessary mediastinal nodes in the chest can be treated. A course of therapy lasts four to six weeks. Metastases are given a small dose of radiation when they are causing symptoms or there is danger of a pathological fracture. Recurrent nodules in the neck often regress on high energy electron therapy, the betatron can be used very satisfactorily.

Place of Radioactive Iodine in Treatment

Treatment by this isotope may be the primary choice in the aged. It can also be used when surgery is impossible or refused, and is the treatment of choice for functioning metastases.

As already mentioned if regular isotope scanning is required replacement hormone therapy must be stopped for the necessary time before the follow up visit.

Hormones

Thyroxine is used to replace the normal secretion of the gland but it can also be used to suppress the activity of metastatic deposits. Patients with multiple pulmonary metastases have survived for long periods on suppressive therapy. It is now usual to give a different form, tri-iodothyronine, T.I.T. This can be continued much closer to the date of the scan than other agents. This suppressive therapy is most often successful in the papillary type of growth, in about half of the follicular type, while with anaplastic tumours there is usually failure.

Chemotherapy

A trial has been made in some centres of the use of cytotoxic drugs, so far the results have not been encouraging.

Lymph Nodes

It will be obvious from the preceding paragraphs that if not fixed involved nodes are removed at the time of thyroidectomy, or subsequently if they later become the site of metastases. Fixed nodes are irradiated or treated with radioactive iodine according to histology.

Nursing Care

The patient who has received an ablation dose to the thyroid is started on replacement therapy 24 hours later. This can be thyroxine or T.I.T. It is continued for life and only interrupted for periodic scanning and if necessary further radioactive iodine treatment. It is important that patients are taught that they must remember to take their tablets faithfully.

If radiation is being given to the gland or to the neck the same reactions will occur as in the patient who has a lesion of the pharynx. The same attention to hygiene, to diet, and to analgesia is required. When the tumour is very advanced, the patient may have a tracheostomy. The special care to prevent maceration of the skin and infection of the lungs has already been described. We have already discussed the care of a patient with a collapsed vertebra and the special routines necessary for a paraplegic. If a pathological fracture elsewhere is present or feared, unless fixation has been carried out, a plaster cast or splint is required. Within the limits set by the orthopaedic surgeon the physiotherapist will work first to preserve muscle tone and later to promote active rehabilitation. It is not surprising that so many branches of medicine are called on in treating this disease if the site and the nature of the spread is borne in mind.

Tumours

Follow-up

The usual routine is followed, the patient's history is taken, particular attention being paid to symptoms of myxoedema, local recurrence, or metastatic deposits in bone or soft tissues. During the examination thyroid function is assessed and also the local condition, with laryngoscopy if necessary. The lymph nodes are palpated. Blood tests, chest X-ray, and any other X-rays indicated by the history are ordered.

Examination of the lymph nodes can never be omitted even after several years, the following history illustrates this.

Mr. – was first seen at the age of 50. He complained of a lump in the left side of the neck which had been increasing in size over a period of eight weeks. On examination he had no toxic symptoms, X-rays of the chest and thoracic inlet were normal. A left hemi-thyroidectomy was carried out. Histology showed the tumour not to be a non-toxic adenoma as expected but a poorly-differentiated adenocarcinoma. He received post-operative radiation to the left side of the neck. Four years later he was well, and owing to difficulty in getting him to attend he was placed on postal follow-up. Ten years after the original operation, he was sent up by his private doctor. He complained of a lump in the left side of the neck, this had not increased in size. On examination he had a hard nodule. This was excised and proved to be a secondary from the original growth. As he had done so well previously a waiting policy was adopted and he was closely followed at regular intervals. Eighteen months later a further nodule was found. Block dissection of the left cervical nodes was carried out, histology of the involved node was identical to the two earlier specimens. It is now a year since this operation and he remains well.

Prognosis

The outcome is very dependent on the histology of the tumour, the stage of the disease, and presence or absence of metastases. At 10 years 80% of patients with papillary tumours are alive and well, older patients do less well. Slightly invasive follicular tumours do very well, but in the invasive type survival at 5 years is only 50%, and only 25% at ten years. Patients with medullary carcinoma have a 50% survival at 10 years after surgery. It has been suggested that survival of patients with metastases treated with radioactive ^{131}I is dependent upon site, lung only, doing better than skeletal. For lymphomas overall survival figures of 45% at 5 years have been given, but many survive only a few months. Survival for anaplastic carcinoma patients is extremely poor, those with metastases die within six to twelve months usually.

Parathyroids

Although the function of these glands is quite different, they are so intimately related to the thyroid that they are described here. Four in number they are pea-sized, yellow, and lie two on each side on the posterior surface of the thyroid. The hormone secreted, parathormone, regulates the calcium metabolism of the body. A carcinoma of the gland is extremely rare. It is usually associated with over-activity of the gland. The effects of over-activity are manifested either by calcification in abnormal sites, or more rarely by rarefaction of the bone and replacement with fibrous tissue. Malignant tumours are slow growing but may eventually metastasise. Treatment of choice is surgery, radiation can be used for recurrences but is not usually successful.

It is not always ignorance of the disease that kills,
Rather it is Man's ignorance of himself.
For while the wisdom of a few may be understood by the many,
The folly of the many is understood only by the few.

13   The Lung, Bronchi and Pleura

Ninety per cent incurable, ninety per cent
preventable

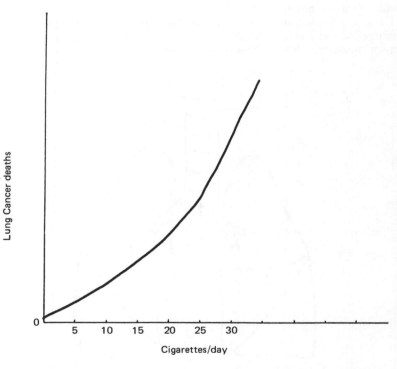

Fig. 13.1.   Relation of lung cancer deaths to cigarette smoking
(after Doll and Hill (1956). *Brit Med. J..*) 1071–1081)

Anatomy and Physiology

Trachea

The lower respiratory tract consists of the air passages and lungs. The main passage, the trachea, runs from the level of the lower cricoid cartilage, down into the chest (thorax) and ends behind the sternum at the level of thoracic vertebrae four to five. Here it divides into two main bronchi, right and left, this division is called the carina. Stiffened with U-shaped rings of cartilage, open ends pointing backwards, it is lined with a ciliated epithelium well supplied with mucus secreting cells. The cilia beat keeping a lubricating flow of mucus moving and sweeping upwards any foreign matter.

Lungs and Bronchi

The point at which a main bronchus enters the lung is called the hilum. The bronchus subdivides until finally the small bronchioles end in a cluster of air sacs called alveoli. These have a lining a single cell thick, and are in close contact with the pulmonary capillaries. Across this very thin membrane gaseous exchange takes place, oxygen out into blood, and carbon dioxide into the alveolus from the blood.

Lungs are divided into lobes, the right has three, the left two. Each lobe has a number of segments. Each lobe has a well defined blood supply enabling the surgeon to remove a lobe (lobectomy) or a whole lung (pneumonectomy).

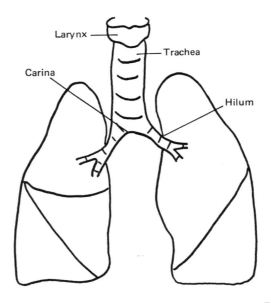

Fig. 13.2.   Trachea, carina and hilum

Pleura

The pleura, a thin sheet of tissue, covers the lungs. It is formed of two layers which are continuous at the hilum. Normally these two layers though they are not attached to each other lie close together, but they can be separated by air, pneumothorax, by blood, haemothorax, or by a pleural effusion (fluid).

The Mediastinum

The mediastinum, a fibrous structure, runs from back to front of the thorax, separates the lungs, and among other important structures contains the heart and the main vessels. The lungs which are conical in shape have a depression of their mediastinal surfaces to accommodate the heart.

Surface Markings

The apex of the lung reaches above the first rib, while the base rests upon the diaphragm. This means that at the back the lungs reach a lower level than at the front. Naturally the level varies with respiration.

Diaphragm

The thorax is separated from the abdomen by the diaphragm, which is attached at its margins to the ribs and the ligaments lying in front of the vertebrae. It is pierced by the oesophagus, aorta, inferior vena cava, lymphatic ducts, and nerve trunks. On contraction the diaphragm flattens enlarging the thoracic cavity.

Rib Cage

The walls of the thorax are formed by the ribs and the intercostal muscles connecting them.

Nerve Supply

Segmental nerves from the thoracic spinal cord supply the intercostal muscles. Right and left phrenic nerves, originating in the cervical cord, run down into the mediastinum to reach the diaphragm. If one nerve is involved by disease in this course there is paralysis of one half of the diaphragm. On X-ray screening this half does not move down on inspiration, but is forced up by the pressure of the abdominal contents, paradoxical movements.

One nerve which does not supply the lungs nor the muscles, but which enters the thorax, is the left recurrent laryngeal nerve. It is important because it runs down, hooks round the arch of the aorta, and then returns to the larynx supplying the left vocal cord. Enlarged nodes can press on the thoracic part of the nerve causing cord paralysis. Hoarseness can be a sign of thoracic disease.

The lungs themselves are supplied by branches of the tenth cranial nerve (the vagus) and by the sympathetic nervous system. The centre for these branches lies in the hind part of the brain, the medulla, and is called the respiratory centre.

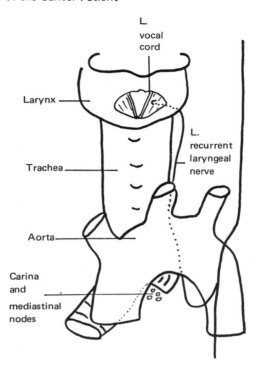

Fig. 13.3.   Relation of L. recurrent laryngeal nerve and mediastinum

Respiration

Mechanical

During inspiration the diaphragm contracts and flattens, the intercostal muscles lift and tilt the ribs. This increases the space within the thoracic cavity, the pressure is lower than that of the external air, so air is drawn into the lungs, inspiration. Muscle relaxation reduces the space, the pressure of the abdominal contents on the relaxed diaphragm contributes to the reduction, air is forced out, expiration. The diaphragm is the main muscle of respiration. If it is paralysed, inspiration is effected only by the intercostal muscles, and breathing is weak and shallow.

Nervous Control

The rate and depth of breathing is controlled by impulses from the respiratory centre. This in turn receives stimuli from the rest of the brain so that emotion can affect it. Stimuli are also received from the lungs and blood. Nerve endings in the lungs register the stretching of the alveoli, impulses reach the centre, and return impulses cut short the inspiratory process. At points in certain of the main arteries there are cells which respond to the carbon dioxide content of the blood. If this reaches too high a level the respiratory centre sends out impulses which quicken and deepen respiration. This is the basis of Cheyne–Stokes breathing. Patients who have had long standing respiratory disease may have become accustomed to a high blood concentration of carbon dioxide. To such patients an oxygen tent may be dangerous, as they breathe oxygen the carbon dioxide level is lowered, stimulus to the respiratoty centre is lost, and respiration depressed.

Gaseous Exchange

De-oxygenated blood from the right side of the heart reaches the lungs in the pulmonary arteries which divide until the capillary system is reached. Here carbon dioxide diffuses from the blood into the air spaces, oxygen passing out into the blood. Oxygenated blood is returned by the pulmonary vein to the left side of the heart. The tissues of the lungs itself are supplied by segmental arteries from the thoracic aorta.

Lymphatic Drainage

The lymphatic vessels of the lungs and pleura drain mostly into the mediastinal nodes. Part of the pleura can drain to the chain of nodes lying below the sternum, the internal mammary chain. The mediastinal nodes lie around the bronchi, the carina, and the trachea.

Tumours of the Bronchus

Incidence

This is the common form of 'lung cancer'. In England and Wales the number of deaths has increased rapidly. It causes 7% of deaths from all causes and 35% of all cancer deaths. The average age at diagnosis is 55, though it has occurred in patients as young as 15 and as old as 80. Five times as many men as women were affected, but the ratio is diminishing particularly in S.E. England, and now stands at M:F 3.5:1.

Aetiology

The disease has been related to certain occupations. Workers in cobalt and radium mines have shown a high rate more than 50% of them dying of lung cancer. It is believed to be due to inhaling radioactive material in the form of radon. Industrial processes involving nickel, carbonyl, arsenic, haematite, asbestos, and chromate carry an increased risk. However, since these substances have been identified protective measures and screening programmes can be instituted.

Surveys show that heavy cigarette smokers have a greater tendency to develop the disease than light smokers or non-smokers. Those who give up have, after ten years, the same level of risk as non-smokers. In the non-smoking partners of heavy smokers, inhalation of the smoke laden air (passive smoking), is believed to increase the risk by a factor of 2 or 3. Cigar and pipe smokers are considered to be at less risk.

City dwellers at first sight have a higher lung cancer rate. Carcinogens have been isolated from diesel fumes, but if the figures are corrected for cigarette smoking there is little difference between town and country.

Pathology

About 96% of primary lung tumours are bronchial carcinomas. Over half of them originate in one of the larger bronchi, a few in the trachea, the rest in the smaller bronchi or bronchioles, or diffusely throughout the lung. The tumour presents in the bronchus as an ulceration or occasionally a polyp. In the lung there is a firm pale mass containing areas of necrosis and haemorrhage, often also an abcess. Beyond the tumour the lung is collapsed and often infected. Infarction due to interrupted blood supply may also be present.

Most rare of all is a tumour arising from the pleura. Histologically 40-60% are squamous cell types, usually poorly differentiated. About 15% are adenocarcinomas, others are undifferentiated mostly small cell carcinoma (the so-called oat cell).

Very rarely the tumour is a carcinoid.

Spread

Spread is direct through the lung, to the other lung, and to the trachea. Adjacent structures, the pericardium, the heart, the oesophagus may also be invaded. Lymphatic spread occurs early, first to the regional nodes around the bronchi and in the mediastinum, then beyond to the axillary, supraclavicular, and cervical nodes. Downward spread to the para-aortic, iliac, and inguinal groups may occur. Blood spread can give rise to deposits in any site, but the brain, liver, bones, and adrenals are the most commonly affected. Multiple deposits can be found in the pleura as the result of spread across the pleural cavity, transcoelomic spread.

Secondary Tumours

Almost any tumour can metastasise to the lung but most commonly it is those which spread by the blood stream. Seen on X-ray the deposits can appear as discrete rounded shadows (cannon-ball opacities) or as a diffuse mottled shadowing.

Symptomatology

The presentation of this disease can be very varied and can often present considerable diagnostic difficulties. Perhaps one of the most difficult cases to detect is a carcinoma arising in a patient with chronic bronchitis. The first symptom is a change in the character of the cough and the breathing, but this

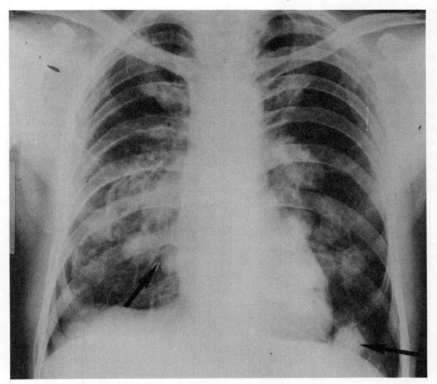

Fig. 13.4.   Lung metastases, osteosarcoma

is seldom noticed by either the patient or his family. Only when symptoms of more advanced disease occur is the change realised in retrospect.

When carcinoma develops in a patient with no previous history of bronchitis the symptoms may be generalised, or localised to the lung and neighbouring structures. There is often a complaint of weight loss, lassitude, and sometimes loss of appetite. Very often the patient tells a story of a seemingly simple cold which fails to clear up and leaves him with a cough and dyspnoea. He may have sputum with either occasional blood staining or frank haemoptysis. Later due to involvement of the recurrent laryngeal nerve hoarseness and stridor can develop. When the pleura is invaded a malignant effusion is formed.

Heart

Invasion of the pericardium or involvement of the cardiac branches of the vagus nerve produces arrhythmias, often auricular fibrillation. A farm worker, who claimed to have been quite well until then, developed 'palpitations'. He was found to have fibrillation, and on investigation had carcinoma of the lung.

A pericardial effusion can also occur, also dysphagia due to invasion of the oesophagus.

Mediastinum

Enlarged mediastinal glands cause symptoms by pressure. Hoarseness as we have already seen can be due to this. The superior vena cava returning blood from the upper part of the body, can be compressed resulting in back pressure, engorgement of the veins, and oedema of the tissues. The patient's face, neck, arms, and upper chest are swollen and cyanotic. The veins are prominent, and in severe cases anastomotic veins over the abdominal wall open up to provide an alternative blood return. This is the syndrome of superior vena caval obstruction.

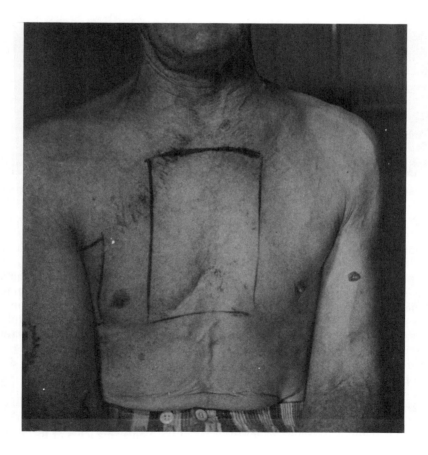

Fig. 13.5.   Early superior vena caval obstruction. Note dilated veins of chest wall, neck and upper arms

Special Sites

Very rarely a tumour can arise as a primary in the trachea. Symptoms are often sudden in onset and severe, the predominant one is stridor. When the pleura is involved there is pain and an effusion causing dyspnoea.

When carcinoma occurs posteriorly near the apex of the lung severe pain in the arms and wasting of the hand muscles is caused. This is due to involvement of the brachial plexus. This plexus consists of nerves supplying the arm and running across to the axilla close to the apex of the lung. In addition the sympathetic nerve chain is caught up in the growth. This causes ptosis (drooping) of the eyelid, constriction of the pupil, and loss of sweating on that side of the face. This last triad of symptoms is known as Horner's syndrome.

The first symptoms of disease are sometimes due to a secondary deposit rather than to the primary tumour. A solitary brain deposit can be excised and only discovered to be a secondary bronchial carcinoma on histological examination.

Skin nodules are usually a late manifestation of the disease but are occasionally a form of presentation. They look like small cherries under the skin.

Generalised Symptoms

Multiple fleeting venous thromboses can develop with any malignant condition and so sometimes occur in association with carcinoma of the bronchus. The usual site for a venous thrombosis is in the leg, but this malignant type is unusual in that it can appear anywhere in the body such as in the arm.

Various hormonal syndromes are associated with small cell (oat cell) carcinomas mostly, but also with a small number of squamous carcinomas and adenocarcinomas. The tumours secrete hormones normally produced elsewhere in the body, these ectopic hormones although they may differ slightly from the natural hormones, are functional and produce syndromes associated with overproduction of the normal hormones. For example, ACTH (adrenocorticotrophic hormone) may be produced in sufficient quantity to cause a Cushing syndrome. Other presentations may be myopathy, neurological deficits, loss of sensation or reflexes, paralyses, mental symptoms. One patient consulted his doctor because of foot drop and weakness of the leg, on investigation he was found to have carcinoma of the bronchus.

These non-metastatic syndromes may arise before the tumour is present, and bear no relation to the severity or extent of the disease.

Hopes that these ectopic hormones could be used as markers of tumour presence have been disappointed because the hormones may be produced in benign conditions, ACTH in association with chronic airways disease, CEA (carcino-embryonic antigen) elevation in smokers, and also because the normal assays may not detect these substances because of their slight differences from normal.

Examination

After a careful history which includes details of smoking habits, occupation and past clinical history, the doctor will examine the chest. This includes not only auscultation of the lungs, but also examination of the heart, the jugular venous pressure, and the rate of the pulse. He will note any signs of superior vena caval obstruction. Already during the history taking he will have assessed dyspnoea, hoarseness, and stridor. The general examination will include a search for signs of wasting, of anaemia, and liver enlargement. Skin nodules are recorded and also any clubbing of the fingers. The lymph node areas are carefully palpated.

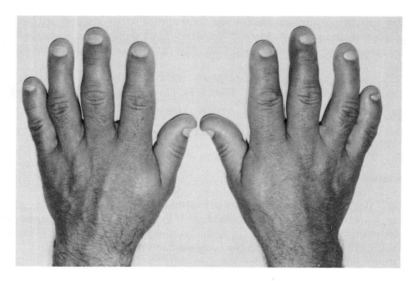

Fig. 13.6.   Fingers showing marked clubbing

The fundi are examined and the reflexes tested. Further detailed neurological testing will follow if indicated. The examination will end with an inspection of the vocal cords to check that they are both moving equally. If a pyrexia is suspected the temperature is taken at some convenient point.

Investigations

Chest X-rays are most important, tomograms will be included as a matter of course, and occasionally a bronchogram is performed. CATscans are particularly useful in investigating the mediastinum. Blood tests, apart from the usual count, may include electrolyte estimations and liver function tests. The sputum is sent for culture and sensitivity if infection is suspected. It is also examined for malignant cells as is also any fluid obtained from pleural aspiration. Radio-active isotopes are now being used for scanning the lung.

In addition a barium swallow may be needed to assess invasion or com-pression of the oesophagus. Thoracoscopy can be used to differentiate between pleural invasion and pleural metastases.

Tests of lung function are useful, particularly if surgery is contemplated. The measurements will indicate if post-operative function will be adequate.

Treatment

Recently the cell type and the staging of the tumour has influenced the choice of treatment, for example surgery has little to offer small cell carcinoma patients. Chemotherapy is more likely to be the preferred method. However, the large number of studies looking at different combinations of treatment methods indicate that, as yet, there is no definite regime; each centre will use its own preferred methods, and the following paragraphs are therefore only guidelines.

Primary Tumours, Surgery

When the patient is fit, has good reserves of lung function, and the tumour is operable, surgery is the treatment of choice for squamous carcinomas and adenocarcinomas. The surgeon decides to operate on the X-ray findings and the bronchoscopic appearances. The number judged operable is small, and at the time of operation it is frequently found that in many, surgery is not possible. Oper-ation involves partial or total removal of the lung. Unfortunately bronchial carcinoma can be present for over a year without causing symptoms, so that by the time diagnosis is made spread has already often occurred.

Primary Tumours, Radiotherapy

Radiation can be given as the primary treatment if a tumour is operable but the condition of the patient makes surgery inadvisable. Otherwise its role lies in palliation or in combination with chemotherapy. One of the drawbacks of its use as a primary treatment is that it may cause pulmonary fibrosis in some individuals giving rise to dyspnoea.

Special situations in which radiation can be particularly helpful are superior vena caval obstruction, haemoptysis, persistent cough and bony metastases.

Primary Tumours, Chemotherapy

It is now generally agreed that surgery is not indicated in the treatment of small cell (oat cell) carcinoma. The tumour metastasises early, and chemotherapy is now regarded as first line therapy, often combined with radiation to the lymph node areas. High dose cyclophosphamide can be used, or various combination regimes.

Chemotherapy has also been used to palliate other types of carcinoma, bleomycin appears to be particularly useful for squamous carcinoma, however watch must be kept for lung fibrosis.

Treatment of Metastases

A solitary brain metastasis can be excised, and this has occasionally happened when the primary has been silent and the secondary deposit diagnosed as a brain tumour. Radiation may be of some use in controlling headache or neurological sequelae, alone or in combination with chemotherapy.

Painful Deposits

Metastases in bone causing pain are treated with radiation. If a pathological fracture occurs treatment is given after surgical fixation.

Secondary Lung Deposits

If a solitary lung metastasis from a tumour elsewhere is found and the patient is fit with no other sign of a recurrence, surgical excision can be considered. In other cases radiation can be given for the relief of symptoms, or where appropriate, radioactive isotopes as for certain thyroid carcinomas, or hormones as for some breast tumours. A decision whether to treat at all will depend upon the overall state of the disease and the condition of the patient.

Effects of Treatment

The effects of radiation on the skin and on the whole body are no different from those described in other chapters. Oesophagitis may cause difficulty towards the end of treatment, meals should then be semi-solid and an anaesthetic mucilage can be very helpful.

Some patients experience after treatment a sudden increase in dyspnoea. Chest X-rays show a diffuse mottling within the treatment area due to a radiation-induced pneumonitis. The condition responds to rest, antibiotics, and prednisone.

A long-term effect in patients who survive may be a fibrosis of irradiated lung tissue. This often produces surprisingly little extra dyspnoea or disability.

Nursing Care

The patient with carcinoma of the lung who is being irradiated is usually in poor condition. He may be so breathless that he needs to be propped up all the time, and all patients require nursing designed to improve their dyspnoea. Inhalations can help in clearing tenacious sputum and bronchodilators are also often prescribed. The physiotherapist may be able to improve the patient's breathing. A patient with a tracheostomy requires suction, and a steam tent will often help his condition. Expectorants are also sometimes prescribed.

When cyanosis is present the use of oxygen would seem to be indicated. In any description of the respiratory centre it is explained that a high oxygen supply as in a tent, may actually depress respiration further. The use of either intermittent oxygen, or a mixture containing 27% oxygen is safer.

Many patients have pain either due to pleural involvement, pressure on nerves, or bony deposits. They will require analgesics given regularly. By maintaining a steady blood level of a drug it is easier to control pain. Larger doses are required to deal with established pain and the interval before relief is longer.

When metastatic deposits have been found in the brain or in the skeleton additional nursing problems can arise. The patient with a cerebral secondary deposit may have some paralysis, and he will then require the type of nursing previously described in the chapter on brain tumours. Similarly the patient with skeletal metastases may require primarily orthopaedic nursing.

If oesophageal obstruction is severe then tube feeding may be necessary until there has been a reduction in the size of tumour. It is often a patient with superior vena caval obstruction who requires this.

When atrial fibrillation is present digitalis is given. The result is usually disappointing. It is rare for either the rhythm or the rate to be improved.

Nurses are often extremely puzzled as to what policy to adopt towards smoking. It should be realised that it is too late to affect the course of the disease. Some patients will stop either because it becomes distasteful or because they feel too ill. Undoubtedly smoking does nothing to improve lung function, but to deprive a patient who gets pleasure and comfort from the habit accomplishes nothing clinically, and affects the patient's morale adversely. For these patients a ban on smoking achieves nothing.

Emergencies

Sudden fitting can occur due to cerebral metastases. The nurse should summon medical aid and apply the usual measures to prevent the patient injuring himself and to maintain the airway.

Haemoptysis unexpected and severe is alarming to the patient. Despite its depressing effect on the respiration doctors usually prescribe morphia. The nurse must try to calm the patient and turn him on to one side if he is faint or becomes unconscious.

Acute dyspnoea due to tracheal obstruction will result in stridor. Tracheotomy may be of no use as it is impossible to get below the obstruction. If the patient can tolerate it a tracheal tube is occasionally passed, but usually all that can be done is to give heavy sedation.

Social Care

These patients and their families face a bleak future. It is unlikely that work will ever be resumed and the financial problems can be considerable. The family can be warned of the outcome by the doctor, but it is the medical social worker who often together with the nurse has to help with the present problems, and make plans to cope with the future. The nurse who has established good relations with the family can contribute much and save valuable time by being able to alert her colleague to any special needs.

Prognosis and Results

Although a few patients can do very well, for the most part, despite intensive efforts to improve treatment, most patients have a poor prognosis. One fifth of patients already have metastases when first seen. Untreated, survival time is about four months. Radiation and chemotherapy extend this, but most patients are dead within a year. Patients who are operable are by definition a special group, 5 year survival is 30%.

Prevention

With such a gloomy prognosis and knowing that this disease is largely preventable, what can be done? Mass X-ray surveys have occasionally uncovered a small operable carcinoma, but in most cases the examination has only revealed cases where the disease is already advanced. This is not a disease which is detectable by present screening methods while it is still treatable.

The chronic bronchitic who smokes could have periodic cytological sputum screening. This might detect malignant change early and avoid the masking of symptoms.

However the most promising measure is to get smoking stopped and air pollution controlled. It is undoubtedly true that when smoking is stopped the risk of contracting the disease progressively falls. Public opinion is now more favourable towards limiting smoking in public. Unfortunately once established smoking is a habit particularly hard to break, and although strenuous efforts are being made to persuade young people not to start, the undoubted consequences seem so far away that the anti-smoking campaign takes on a killjoy aspect. Nevertheless some progress has been made and must continue, for this is one carcinoma that is largely preventable.

If only I could recall as much as I have forgotten,
I would be a wiser man;
If only I could forget what I do know,
I would be even wiser.

14   The Gastro-intestinal Tract, Liver, Biliary System and Pancreas

GASTRO-INTESTINAL TRACT

General Anatomy

The gastro-intestinal tract stretches from the mouth to the anus. It is a muscular tube, specialised to convey, digest, and absorb food. The lining mucosa contains mucous cells and others which secrete chemicals to digest the food. The products of digestion pass through the gut wall. Some of the fat enters the lacteals, passes to the lymphatic duct, into the blood stream, and finally reaches the liver. The rest of the fat enters the portal system and so reaches the liver. Proteins and sugars after breakdown enter the veins and are also conveyed to the liver. The lower bowel, the large intestine, does not digest food but absorbs water.

Oesophagus

About 25 cm long it stretches from the level of the sixth cervical vertebra to the diaphragm, here it becomes the cardia of the stomach. Its sole function is to convey chewed food to the stomach by contraction of its muscular wall. The epithelium is stratified squamous, the blood supply from the aorta, the thyroid and gastric arteries. A rich plexus of lymph nodes surrounds the oesophagus, drainage is initially to the posterior mediastinal nodes, and subsequently upwards to the supraclavicular group or downwards to nodes around the left gastric vessels. Nerve supply is through a plexus of nerves lying on its surface, formed by the right and left vagus nerves.

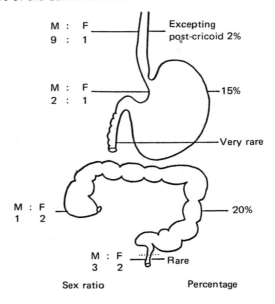

Fig. 14.1.   Incident by site as a percentage of all malignancy

Its length and position cause it to be related to many other structures. Behind the spine and thoracic duct, either in front or at its sides, trachea, thyroid, common carotid arteries and recurrent laryngeal nerves, left bronchus, pericardium, heart, diaphragm.

Tumours

Age, Sex, Site

Carcinoma of the post-cricoid region has been discussed in Chapter 6. In this region there is a marked bias towards women, otherwise 90% of tumours occur in males. The tumour is rare below the age of 50, the usual age is around 65. The commonest site is the middle third, this is closely related to the bifurcation of the trachea and the left bronchus.

Aetiology

With the exception of the post-cricoid area in women, no factors are known, but there have been many suggestions, certain foods, hot drinks, smoking. Rare, but known predisposing factors are leukoplakia, achalasia of the cardia, mucosal ulceration associated with diverticula.

Pathology

Most tumours are squamous carcinomas. Spread is direct, up and down the oesophagus, and through the wall into neighbouring structures in the mediastinum or into the vertebrae. Since the lymphatic drainage is rich, spread can occur easily both up and down the plexus and from there to the cervical or abdominal nodes. Spread by the blood stream occurs late, sites of distant metastases are liver, lung, bone, and brain.

Symptomatology

During the early stages the symptoms are vague and the patient finds it difficult to describe them. He may complain of a sensation behind the sternum, of a cough, or of very slight momentary dysphagia. Later this difficulty in swallowing becomes more definite. The first complaint is of solids sticking, then less solid food is affected, and finally the patient is unable to swallow even liquids. There may be regurgitation leading to spill over into the lungs causing inflammation and infection. As the disease progresses there are signs of wasting and toxic absorption. A secondary anaemia develops and finally cachexia.

If we refer back to the description of anatomy, we can see how easily the closely related structures can be involved. Effusions in the pleura and pericardium may be caused by direct invasion, there will be cough, dyspnoea and cardiac arrythmias. Erosion of the oesophageal wall can cause inflammation of the mediastinum (mediastinitis), with pain, dyspnoea and pyrexia. Haemorrhage, usually fatal, results from invasion of large vessels. A direct abnormal communication between the trachea and the oesophagus can be formed by an erosion. This is a fistula and the patient will develop inflammation and infection giving rise to dyspnoea and cough. Necrotic tissue may actually be coughed up. Jaundice develops late and is a sign of deposits in the liver or the portal glands.

Examination

The clinical history is extremely important in establishing the nature and timing of early symptoms. A story of long-standing anaemia or glossitis may be significant. The general appearance, including signs of wasting or dehydration, is assessed. The nails are examined for thinning, flattening, or spooning. This is koilonychia associated with an iron deficiency anaemia existing for a long time. The mucosae are examined for pallor. The abdomen is palpated for liver enlargement, as the lymph nodes lie deep they are rarely felt. Evidence of cervical enlargement is also sought.

When the mouth is examined particular note is made of any sores at the angles of the mouth or of a shiny atrophic tongue, glossitis. Both these can be signs of iron deficiency anaemia. When hoarseness is present, the larynx must be visualised with the aid of the laryngeal mirror.

Finally an attempt is made to assess the degree of dysphagia. The patient is asked to drink some water. If there is no apparent hold-up soft solids are next offered. All degrees of dysphagia are encountered, from a slight hesitancy to a complete block with regurgitation.

Investigations

The aim of investigation should be to detect the lesion as early as possible. The difficulty lies in the vagueness of the symptoms associated with the early stages. By the time that severe dysphagia is established radical treatment, whether by surgery or radiation, is virtually impossible.

A blood count is important, not only to reveal the presence of an anaemia, but also to decide its nature and cause. It may be sideropenic due to shortage of iron, hypochromic caused by lack of pigment, normocytic the cells being normal size, or microcytic the cells being small. The chest X-ray in addition to being a check for lung metastases, will also show up any widening of the mediastinum due to infiltration of the nodes. If spread outside the oesophagus is suspected, tomograms may be helpful.

To assess the extent of the lesion an X-ray examination is made using radio-opaque medium. It is carefully chosen to minimise the effects if regurgitation and overspill into the lungs occurs. The patient is screened, the radiologist watching the contraction waves very carefully. Any permanent stricture is noted. If too little medium passes it may be necessary to take tomograms of the tumour.

If it is suspected that there is infiltration of the pericardium an E.C.G. may show changes in the normal cardiac pattern. It is rare for these not to be associated with clinical signs.

If involvement of the liver is suspected, then ultrasound and isotope investigations may be used. Since dysphagia will have interfered with nutrition, biochemistry is important and LFTs may be the first indication of liver involvement.

Finally the patient must be examined under anaesthesia and a biopsy obtained. An oesophagoscope is passed, the distance of the stricture from the incisor teeth is measured, the appearance of the tumour noted, and a biopsy taken. If dysphagia is severe, bougies may be passed to dilate the opening or a tube may be put in position.

There is a real danger of perforation occurring during this examination, particularly if necrotic tumour extends through the wall. For this reason only sips of water should be given for at least twelve hours or until the doctor is satisfied all is well. The temperature is watched as mediastinitis due to leakage of oesophageal contents is usually signalled by a pyrexia. The doctor palpates the neck for any signs of surgical emphysema, this is swallowed air which passes into the mediastinum then up the neck and forward to the anterior chest wall.

The combination of the evidence of X-ray studies and the appearance at oesophagoscopy usually enables a decision to be made on treatment. It should be emphasised that this is usually palliative, radical curative surgery or radiotherapy is not often possible.

Treatment

Surgery

In a few cases radical surgery is possible, either initially or after radiation. The operation may be subtotal resection or a total removal including the larynx. This is followed by reconstruction procedures. Both are major undertakings and the general condition and age of the patient must be considered as well as the state of the tumour. Palliative measures include dilatation, insertion of tubes to overcome the stricture, and gastrostomy. Dilatation and tubes allow both food and saliva to be swallowed. A gastrostomy is usually avoided if at all possible. Although the patient can be adequately fed and hydrated he still has distressing symptoms. He is unable to swallow his saliva and is always at the risk of an overspill into the trachea.

Radiation

Although it is usually only palliative treatment that can be given, or a modified course following an operation which is thought to be inadequate, I propose to discuss the problems in planning a radical course of radiotherapy. The oesophagus lies in the body close to vital structures such as the lungs, the vertebral column, and the heart. In the neck it lies behind the trachea in the midline and then passes slightly to the left. In its middle third it returns to the midline, and then runs slightly forward and to the left as it descends to the diaphragm.

Radiation must treat a tubular volume allowing for the alteration in depth and alignment of the oesophagus. The dose to vital structures must be kept as small as possible.

In order to calculate the depth and direction the swallow is repeated with markers on the chest and back when the X-rays are taken. Both anteroposterior and lateral views are taken. From these it is possible to work out the depth at which the oesophagus is lying and also the length and location of the stricture.

It is usual to employ megavoltage radiation. This gives good penetration and spares the skin. Two methods are possible. The radiation beam can be rotated around the patient or fixed multiple fields can be used. The former method is only possible if the area to be treated lies in the same plane. If the back is markedly bent, kyphotic, it is usually not possible to employ rotation.

Close co-operation between doctor and physicist is required. The former indicates by surface markings the extent of the field and any structures to be avoided. Working from an outline of the patient the physicist plots the isodose curves from the number and size of the fields and the direction of the beam. The minimum size of field is eight centimetres long and width four centimetres. The aim is to enclose the tumour in an area of uniform dosage. The doctor has already specified the maximum radiation dose and the length of time over which it is to be given, now he checks the relation of the treatment area to vital structures. Final check X-rays with markers are then taken.

Some centres have a very sophisticated device for checking field position, it is called a simulator. Stated very simply it is an X-ray apparatus coupled with a couch exactly similar to the couch used during treatment. The X-ray tube can be moved to simulate the treatment distance of the chosen therapy machine, and can also be placed in exactly the position from which treatment will be given. Standing behind a protecting screen the doctor can operate the machine and see a form of X-ray picture on a viewing screen. He moves the X-ray tube by remote control and alters the size of the field until he is satisfied. Markers are placed on the skin and an X-ray is then taken, on some machines he can at the same time take a photo with a polaroid camera.

A further refinement is to link simulator and computer so that field sizes, strengths, direction, and isodose curves can all be produced as the patient is set up. Quicker and obviously desirable, but cost is a drawback.

At the first treatment the set-up is checked by the physicist and doctor. Due to the careful planning it is extremely rare for any adjustments to be needed at this stage.

The nursing care of such a patient differs in no way from that already described for pharyngeal and postcricoid carcinoma in Chapter 7. It cannot be stressed too often however that the maintenance of hydration and an adequate diet are of paramount importance. When the stricture is very tight, daily radiation dosage is smaller initially in order to prevent oedema further narrowing the lumen. The immediate complications during treatment are increased dysphagia, mediastinitis, and perforation. The nurse should report any obvious increase in dysphagia, whether symptomatic, that is reported by the patient, or noted by herself, for example development of regurgitation. The doctor must then decide whether this is due to increasing tumour size or to oedema. In the latter case rest from treatment for a few days will enable this to settle, in the former radiation may have to be modified or abandoned. If swallowing becomes completely impossible drip feeding is a temporary measure, but for a permanent by-pass a tube must be inserted into the stomach through the abdominal wall. Retrosternal pain can be a symptom of radiation reaction or a warning of impending perforation. Pyrexia accompanied by a slight increase in the pulse rate may precede perforation, therefore any change in temperature or pulse rate or the development of severe pain should always be reported. If perforation occurs the decision must be made whether to perform gastrostomy and then continue radiating or whether to stop completely. A pleasant but unusual reaction is shrinkage of the tumour. This can result in a tube which has been inserted into the oesophagus becoming loose and being passed on through the bowel. If an X-ray is taken the metal tube may be seen in the bowel.

The bougie method described in Chapter 6 is rarely used now that megavoltage therapy is freely available. Cytotoxic drugs have been used as adjuncts to radiation but the results have been disappointing.

When an oesophageal tube is in position despite vigilance the patient may obtain unsuitable food and block his tube. When this happens he is given aerated drinks or small quantitites of dilute hydrogen peroxide. If the obstructing bolus fails to soften and pass, an oesophageal tube is passed and attempts made to suck the bolus clear. If despite these measures it cannot be cleared, then under full anaesthesia an oesophagoscope is passed and the obstruction removed. For this reason all patients, whether they have a tube or not, must understand and co-operate in dietary measures. Even more important is the education of the family, 'a little bit of what he fancies' may be the prelude to the operating theatre. The doctor begins this process but the nurse and the dietician must continue and maintain it.

Although megavoltage therapy is skin sparing, it is sometimes forgotten that the radiation beam passes through the body so that the skin on the opposite side receives a small exit dose of radiation. Some patients are too ill to lie prone, the posterior fields must be given through the couch so losing the skin-sparing effect. Watch must therefore be kept for signs of skin reaction and the usual methods of care applied.

Follow-up and Prognosis

Apart from examination to assess the general condition and a search for evidence of lymphatic or liver enlargement, reliance must be placed mostly on careful questioning of the patient. Chest X-ray and blood count are performed as a normal routine. If the symptoms suggest the lumen is becoming narrower the question to be answered is whether this is due to tumour progression or fibrosis following radiation. A barium swallow is helpful but often oesophagoscopy is required. If the appearance suggests stricture dilatation by bougie can be carried out at the same time. A long-term complication can be fibrosis of lung tissue. However carefully the treatment is planned some irradiation of lung tissue. is inevitable, but mostly patients do not survive long enough to develop these late complications. Even when surgical resection has been possible the average five-year survival is 5%. Since so few patients are seen at an early stage it is impossible to say whether poor results are due to the nature of the tumour, or whether this is a reflection of the late stage at presentation.

Stomach

Anatomy

Lying immediately below the diaphragm the stomach is essentially a bag. The narrow exit is closed by a ring of circular muscle, the sphincter. The equally narrow entrance, the cardia, has no sphincter but closure is by the mechanical action of the diaphragm and stomach muscles. The body of the stomach is suspended within folds of the peritoneum, is distensible, and moves both with respiration and the position of the body. The two curves of the stomach are known as the greater and lesser curvatures. The covering peritoneum hangs down below the greater curvature as a delicate membrane, the greater omentum. It contains blood vessels, fat and lymph nodes which can be the site of metastases from the stomach or the lower gastro-intestinal tract.

The stomach is intimately related to many structures, this is important in considering the spread of tumours. Related structures include, the left lobe of the liver, the diaphragm, separated by a slit like space, the lesser sac, the pancreas, transverse colon, left kidney and suprarenal, spleen, all lie behind.

Blood Supply, Nerves, Lymphatics

Blood is derived from the coeliac trunk, the splenic and hepatic arteries. Corresponding veins empty into the portal vein carrying blood to the liver.

The vagus nerves supply the stomach.

Lymphatic drainage extends over a wide area and therefore when there is a malignant spread it is almost impossible to excise this whole area. The main groups of nodes lie in the greater omentum, close to the pylorus, near the spleen, and in close relation to the aorta and pancreas.

Physiology

The stomach mucosa contains different types of cells which secrete gastric juice and mucus, and others which secrete hormones which circulate in the blood, and returning to the stomach, modify its secretory activity.

Gastric juice contains hydrochloric acid, peptic enzymes, the intrinsic factor, and mucin. The function of the stomach is to store food and treat it so that further digestion can occur in the rest of the bowel. Food is retained in the stomach for a period depending on the composition of the food and the emotional state of the individual.

Tumours

Aetiology

Many predisposing factors have been suggested. An apparently benign ulcer may show malignant change at the edge, controversy exists as to whether some ulcer treatments contribute to this. Some papillomas and adenomas become malignant. Carcinoma is up to four times as common in patients with pernicious anaemia, believed to be due to metaplasia consequent on atrophic gastritis. It has been suggested there is some link with blood group A.

Various ingested substances such as fried food, alcohol, nicotine, spices have been blamed, and to this list has been added mineral cooking oil and coke fumes. The geographic variation in incidence is definite, in Japan and Scandinavia it is more common, while in Indonesia there is a racial difference between Malays and Chinese.

The possible production of a powerful carcinogen (N nitroso compounds) within the body by the action of gastric juice on foods, has caused much controversy on the role of nitrates present in food naturally or as preservatives. The picture however is not clear cut and, as yet, there is not sufficient convincing evidence on which to form a conclusion.

Age, Sex, Site, Incidence

Although the overall incidence has declined, this is a fairly common tumour causing 15% of all cancer deaths. Twice as many men as women are affected, the average age is between sixty and seventy. Half the tumours are found in the

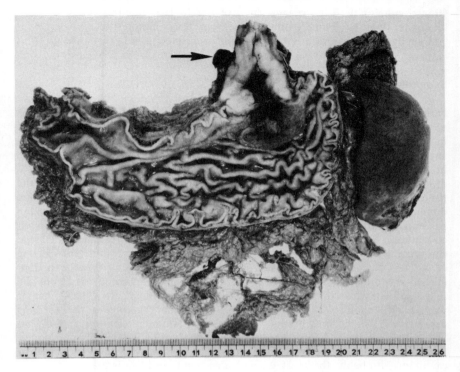

Fig. 14.2.   Carcinoma of the stomach

pyloric region, a quarter along the lesser curvature, and the rest at other sites or diffuse.

Pathology and Spread

The majority arise from the mucosal glands and are therefore adenocarcinomas, very rarely a squamous carcinoma is found. Rarely Hodgkin's and non-Hodgkin's lymphoma can occur. The appearance is variable, polypoid, gelatinous because of much mucus present, diffuse or ulcerated. About 2% are early gastric cancer (EGC) confined to the mucosa and sub mucosa. The diffuse tumour produces rigidity of the stomach wall giving a characteristic X-ray appearance, 'leather bottle stomach'.

Spread is by all known routes. Direct, causes invasion of neighbouring organs, involvement of the colon can produce a gastrocolic fistula. Lymphatic spread involves metastases in the node groups which may in turn invade other organs. Mediastinal or cervical deposits are quite common, particularly the left supravicular group. Blood borne metastases can occur throughout the body, commonly in the liver, lungs and bone. Spread across the peritoneal cavity (transcoelomic) to other organs can give rise to cells looking microscopically like signet rings, Krukenberg tumour, the ovary is a common site.

Usually spread has occurred by the time of diagnosis.

Symptomatology

Patients with this disease often present the same problem as those with carcinoma of the oesophagus, the indefinite nature of early symptoms. Early diagnosis is quite uncommon so that in any man over fifty with vague dyspepsia, unexplained anorexia, or weight loss, the diagnosis should be considered. The anorexia can be curiously selective, it may only be meat which becomes unappetising. Additional symptoms are often related to the site of the tumour. Invasion of the pancreas will produce pain radiating directly through to the back as the predominating symptom. The bowel will be irritated by contents which have bypassed the normal digestive process if a gastrocolic fistula forms, an upset in bowel habit with pain may well result and weight loss will be greater. Gastric emptying will be delayed if the pylorus is invaded, an uncomfortable feeling of fullness is caused by the build-up in stomach contents. Appetite is diminished and projectile vomiting may eventually occur. Haematemesis can be the first sign of trouble, or there may be a complaint of an epigastric mass which is painless but enlarging. Rarely, development of ascites due to peritoneal seedling deposits will be the presentation. Jaundice is a late manifestation, it is due to liver involvement or to obstruction of the bile duct by enlarged lymph nodes.

There is a parallel here with the chronic bronchitic who develops bronchial carcinoma. Probably the most difficult diagnostic problem is presented by the patient with a chronic peptic ulcer in which malignancy develops. The change in symptoms is insidious and most difficult to detect.

Examination and Investigations

A careful clinical history is taken and every effort is made to elicit trivial symptoms which the patient may feel are too slight to mention. During the examination the abdomen is carefully palpated. If the liver is enlarged its character is noted and also the level of the lower edge. When invaded by malignant tissue the liver usually feels very firm and may have a characteristic irregularity or nodularity. The lymph nodes must be carefully palpated, particularly those in the neck. When physical signs are absent investigations may establish the diagnosis. A blood count can reveal severe anaemia.

Other Tests

The examination of the faeces for occult blood is simple. Small haemorrhages from a tumour do not always produce a haematemesis. The blood is altered and passed in the stools.

Direct examination of the stomach can be made at gastroscopy. The flexible instrument first developed by the Japanese enables the investigator to view all parts of the stomach including the fundus. A photographic record can be made. 'Brush' biopsy is now possible, cells are swept off the surface of suspicious areas and sent for microscopy.

Routine biochemistry will include LFTs.

All patients must have a chest X-ray and a barium meal.

Despite intensive investigations the diagnosis may still be uncertain until an exploratory laparatomy is performed.

Typical Case History

A man in his fifties was seen in the surgical out-patients, he had a history of slight weight loss with vague dyspepsia and pain. In the past he had experienced similar symptoms but a barium meal had been negative. On examination there were no abnormal physical findings, the blood count showed no anaemia, and the chest X-ray was normal. This time the barium meal showed the presence of a carcinoma.

Treatment

It will have already been realised that the difficulties of early diagosis render radical curative treatment very difficult. In a patient who is considered to have carcinoma limited to the stomach surgery is the treatment of choice. This will involve radical removal of the growth and a wedge of tissue together with the related lymphatic nodes. Palliative surgery consists of short-circuit operations to overcome obstruction, or local removal of the tumour to prevent recurrent bleeding.

The normal stomach, with the exception of the surface mucosal cells, is extraordinarily resistant to radiation. To be curative a radiation dosage very close to that liable to cause necrosis would be needed, and severe damage would be caused to adjacent structures. For this reason radiation is not employed as the sole means of treatment for carcinoma of the stomach. Hodgkins and non-Hodgkins lymphoma will be treated as such lymphomas elsewhere are managed.

Combined chemotherapy has been used but without much marked impact though it can palliate symptoms. All regimes include 5-FU.

Prognosis

The rare superficial gastric cancer does well, 70–90% 5 year survival. If operable 20% survive 10 years. Most others die within a year.

Hodgkins and non-Hodgkins lymphomas have the same prognosis as those occurring in other sites.

Small Intestine

Carcinoma of this part of the bowel is so rare that even experienced surgeons may have never seen it. Occasionally a lymphoma, usually the non-Hodgkin type, can occur.

The ileum or the appendix can be the site of a carcinoid tumour.

The Colon and Rectum

Anatomy

The colon is four to five feet long and runs from the ileocaecal junction with the small intestine to the point where the rectum joins the anus. It is subdivided for convenience into the caecum and ascending colon, transverse colon, descending colon, the sigmoid U shaped and lying in the pelvis, and rectum. It is sacculated (pouched) in appearance. The lining epithelium is columnar, no digestion occurs, only water absorption.

Blood is supplied by branches of the aorta, the superior and inferior mesenteric arteries. Venous drainage is through the portal system to the liver. Nerve supply is from the vagus. Lymphatic drainage is to nodes lying close to the bowel and then to the groups around the mesenteric arteries.

Tumours

Sex, Age, Incidence

Carcinoma of the colon is twice as common in women as men, but the ratio is reversed M:F 3:2 in the rectum. Nearly 20% of cancer deaths in England and Wales are caused by colorectal cancer. The patient is usually between 55 and 60, but it can occur from childhood onwards particularly in sufferers from familial intestinal polyposis. The condition is uncommon in Africa, Asia and S.America.

Aetiology

Familial intestinal polyposis is a disease which is probably genetically determined. The whole of the large bowel contains polyps, many thousands in number, and almost inevitably malignancy arises in one or more. Other patients who develop polyps but have no family history are also considered to have a high risk of malignant change. The other known predisposing condition is long-standing ulcerative colitis, for when the history is ten years or more the risk of developing carcinoma is five to ten times greater than normal.

The striking geographical incidence pattern led to environmental studies. It has been strongly suggested that Western diet contains less residue and so increased bowel transit time. High fibre diets have become popular but it will be many years before the incidence figures will show whether the link is proven.

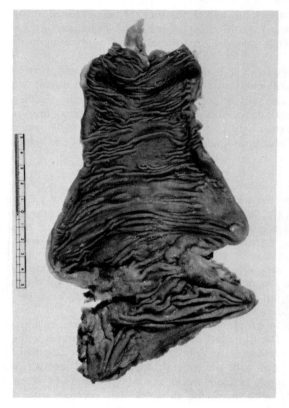

Fig. 14.3.   Carcinoma of the rectum

Site

Half the tumours occur in the rectum and recto-sigmoid area, and a further quarter in the sigmoid colon. The remainder are found largely in the rest of the colon, 4% being multiple, over three quarters of the tumours therefore occur on the left side.

Pathology and Spread

Colon

In appearance the tumour, usually small, is papillary or polypoid with central ulceration, one in ten may be annular and cause stenosis. The microscopic type is usually adenocarcinoma, frequently differentiated to a variable degree and divided into low, average and high grade.

Spread is direct, up and down, and through the wall until it eventually lies outside the bowel. At this stage other organs can become involved.

Transcoloemic spread across the peritoneal cavity can give rise to Krukenberg tumours.

Lymphatic spread is to the regional nodes first, and then more distant sites.

Blood borne metastases can be diffuse, or more usually largely in the liver.

Unusual sites can be involved due to implantation either naturally from malignant cells lodging on damaged surfaces, or artificial, in suture lines.

Other tumours which occur rarely are various malignant connective tissue types, deposits of both kinds of lymphoma, and carcinoid tumours.

Rectum

Carcinoma of the rectum commences as a nodule, the more malignant types ulcerate quickly, while the less malignant grow out into the lumen. Direct spread round the bowel occurs but there is very little up or down. Growth is slow and the formation of a complete ring of tumour may take up to two years, while it may be 18 months before penetration through the wall and the surrounding fascia occurs. At this point it can then spread to the uterus and vagina in the female, and into the bladder, prostate or seminal vesicles in the male. Spread out to the sides can involve a ureter, while backward extension can involve the sacrum and the sacral plexus.

Metastases in lymph nodes are usually microscopic, enlargement is often due to infection. The direction of spread is usually upwards, either to nodes lying close to the rectum or to slightly more distant ones. Spread beyond the lymphatics associated with the superior haemorrhoidal artery is rare until late in the disease. Similarly blood-borne metastases occur late except in the younger patients with more anaplastic tumours. The common sites for this type of metastasis are the liver, lungs, and adrenal glands. Seedling peritoneal deposits are usually associated with a tumour occurring higher in the rectum.

Staging

C.E.Dukes studied specimens both of the colon and rectum removed at operation. He found that the prognosis was affected both by the degree of spread and by the degree of differentiation. The three stages were given the letters A, B, C:

(A) growth limited to the bowel;
(B) growth extending outside the bowel, but no involvement of lymph nodes;
(C) metastases present in lymph nodes;

Dukes found that half the specimens fell into the stage C group.

Symptomatology

The nature of the symptoms, and the timing of their occurrence in relation to the stage of tumour growth, will vary with the site. The faeces are more fluid in the right side of the large bowel and signs of obstruction are delayed. On the left side these symptoms occur fairly early. The patient complains of an altered bowel habit, constipation which is less and less responsive to purgatives alternating with attacks of diarrhoea. There may be lower abdominal pain, at first a dull ache and then this becomes colicky. A lump in the abdomen may be noticed by the patient. This is often hard faeces lying above the stricture rather than the growth itself. Distension can occur and both this and the pain are relieved by passing flatus.

When the primary growth lies in the sigmoid colon pain is usually colicky. There may be an urgent desire to defaecate and the faeces are accompanied by blood and mucus.

Carcinoma of the transverse colon can produce lassitude and anaemia due to intermittent bleeding from the tumour. If a mass is palpable it may be mistaken for a growth occurring in the stomach. On the right side of the colon the most common symptom is an intractable anaemia, diagnosis is difficult as a mass is not always palpable. Indeed carcinoma of the caecum may only be discovered during an operation for appendicitis.

Rectum

The early symptoms of carcinoma in this site are often so slight that a patient does not consult his doctor. Usually bleeding occurs but it can easily be mistaken for bleeding from haemorrhoids. There is nothing diagnostic about the colour, the amount, or the timing of its passage. Altered bowel habit also occurs. Usually the patient complains of constipation, of a feeling that the bowel has not been emptied completely, and of passing flatus and blood-stained mucus. Pain is experienced late in the disease, it is then usually colicky and is severe if there is involvement of the bladder, prostate, or sacral plexus.

Examination and Investigation

During the taking of the history it is important to enquire very carefully into the family history. Those families in which the disease of familial polyposis has occurred are recorded in a central register, but occasionally patients present with this disease who despite careful enquiries would appear to have no known relation with the families already listed. All the members of a family are kept under observation and prophylactic surgery performed in those who develop polyposis. When a sporadic case occurs the rest of the family must be traced and screened.

During the examination search is made for the usual signs of anaemia. Any mass found in the abdomen is carefully palpated to determine its character, whether it is attached to other structures, and if it is palpable bimanually on rectal examination. Enlargement of the liver is sought and if present its degree and type recorded. All the accessible lymph node areas must be examined since, as we have already seen, distant involvement well away from the primary site can occur. Patients who have had long-standing ulcerative colitis may have clubbing of the finger nails; the reason for this is unknown. Even when a mass is found in the abdomen the examination is not complete without sigmoidoscopy. First a rectal examination is made. Any blood or mucus on the examining glove is noted, haemorrhoids may be present. Occasionally a rectal carcinoma may be so low in the bowel that it can be felt by the examining finger. When this is so then the nature of its consistency and the degree of infiltration can be assessed. In a female this can be assisted by vaginal examination at the same time. The sigmoidoscope is then passed to the full extent possible. The obturator is withdrawn, the bowel gently dilated with air, and the instrument gradually withdrawn. The bowel mucosa is inspected, if a tumour is seen its distance from the anal margin is recorded, its appearance noted, and also the presence or absence of blood. A biopsy is then taken and sent for histology.

Even when a tumour is found the routine of investigations is always followed for it cannot be assumed that the visible or palpable growth is the only one present. A blood count to detect the presence and degree of anaemia is performed, and a chest X-ray as a pre-operative check and as a means of excluding pulmonary metastases. Tumour present in the ascending or transverse colon may produce no frank blood per rectum despite persistent bleeding, a test for occult blood in the stools may well be positive in such cases. Barium enema is needed for radiological study of the bowel. A consistent deformity not altered by peristaltic movement is significant. After evacuation of the barium, air is sometimes used to produce better contrast studies, the opaque medium still coats the mucosa and the air distends the bowel. Lesions not easily seen on the ordinary barium enema pictures may be detected in this way. A tumour of the caecum may not be visible on enema studies but show up when a barium meal and follow through is performed. Occasionally the barium can make the symptoms of obstruction temporarily worse. Laboratory study of the clear washings obtained during preparation of the bowel for X-ray examination may reveal malignant cells. Despite all these careful investigations the diagnosis may still be in doubt. The surgeon will then need to perform an exploratory laparotomy. In these cases the patient must be fully prepared, physically and mentally, so that the surgeon can proceed to full resection if necessary. Before the operation when the patient is fully anaesthetised an examination is made. Cystoscopy is also performed to exclude infiltration of the bladder.

Carcinoembryonic Antigen (CEA)

This is an antigen which arises from colonic cancer tissue and foetal endoderm of the gut. Dependent upon staging, site, histology of the tumour and liver function, levels of this antigen may be raised in patients with colorectal cancer, 60–65% are found to have raised levels. Unfortunately CEA levels are also raised in certain benign conditions, particularly cirrhosis. It is therefore no use as a screening test. Neither have early hopes of using the level as an early indicator of recurrence been fulfilled.

The main use of this investigation would appear to be in monitoring response to radiation or chemotherapy. It must be done serially, isolated tests are of little value, rising levels show that tumour regression is not occurring.

Experimental work labelling CEA antibody with radioactive iodine suggests that this may be a method of tumour localisation.

Other Investigations

Depending upon the individual scan it may be necessary to carry out isotope scans, ultra sound examinations, or lymphography.

Treatment

Surgery

Provided that the tumour is still operable surgery is the treatment of choice. The type of operation performed will vary with the site and the degree of spread. In radical surgery the aim is to remove the tumour and the lymphatic drainage of the area. In practical terms this involves the high ligation of the blood vessels supplying the bowel, and the resection of the bowel and the draining nodes in the mesentery. The extent of the clearance will depend upon the tumour, multiple carcinomata may require total colectomy, while for a localised polypoid tumour of the transverse colon limited resection may be sufficient. It must be realised that a tumour of the rectum will always necessitate removal of the rectum and the formation of a colostomy. It is important to grasp that merely to form a colostomy to overcome obstruction may be insufficient if the lesion itself is causing severe pain. The surgeon may decide in this case to perform an abdominoperineal resection. This operation involves dissection by two approaches, the abdominal and the perineal. This can be performed by two teams operating simultaneously, or by one team starting one approach and then moving to the other.

When the disease is judged to be too far advanced, or when the condition of the patient rules out major surgery, then it may be that a colostomy will relieve the symptoms and enable the patient to live a reasonably comfortable life. Many patients have a great fear of this operation. They feel that it is unnatural, that they will become social outcasts, and that this is something which they just cannot accept. It is here that the whole team can work together to prepare a patient mentally. The doctor explains what is involved and the reasons why this is the treatment of choice. If another patient who has had this procedure and is managing the colostomy well can then be introduced and talk about the problems, this is invaluable. Even when this is possible there will be many details which patients may feel are too trivial to be raised, or which they may be too shy to discuss. It is at this point that the nurse can play such a valuable part. A few words when the beds are being made or the daily routine details being taken, can produce a lift in morale out of all proportion to the time spent. It may also provide the doctor with the clue to the psychological management of this particular patient.

Radiotherapy

It used to be considered that radiation had no part to play in primary treatment. However a decrease in the recurrence rate and an increase in five year survivors has been associated with surgery combined with local radiation.

Its use in combination with surgery to treat colonic cancer is as yet experimental, but results are promising.

The questions of timing and the optimum dose schedule have yet to be settled. Palliation of discharge and severe pain, and recurrences, is possible.

Chemotherapy

Adjuvant chemotherapy has not so far fulfilled earlier promise. 5-FU is the most useful drug, so far drug combinations seem not to have improved results, but this may be due to the choice of drugs, for example cyclophosphamide and 5-FU are antagonistic given together. However, some patients respond, and reliable *in vitro* testing of tumour response to cytotoxics might enable such patients to be identified.

Combination with targeting antibodies might in future enable more effective cytotoxic therapy to be given.

Immunotherapy

The stimulation of the patient's immune system by various agents has not produced any major advance either alone or combined with chemotherapy. Some centres claim better results when combining it with radiation.

Screening

Since this is a common cancer a reliable screening programme is desirable. CEA has not fulfilled its promise as a marker, but 75% of rectal carcinomas can be palpated and tests for occult blood are frequently positive in colonic carcinoma patients.

In Germany free screening initially by digital rectal examination, later combined with occult blood testing, has been available since 1971. Figures from one hospital suggest that, despite a low participation rate, the incidence of inoperable colorectal carcinoma has fallen. Tumours with the favourable Dukes' A staging were found in some asymptomatic patients.

If such favourable results continue, hopefully not only will the participation rate increase, but wider use of such screening programmes might make some impact on 'cure' and survival rates.

The Anal Canal

The terminal section of the bowel is lined in the upper part with columnar epithelium and in the lower with squamous. This junction is important since it demarcates the arterial and nervous supply and also the lymphatic drainage. Above this junction the nerve supply is from the autonomic system and is carried in the vagus nerve, venous return is primarily to the portal system, and lymphatic drainage passes ultimately to the lumbar nodes. Below this junction the anus is supplied by segmental spinal nerves, this means that the mucosa is sensitive to pain. The arterial supply is derived from the vessels supplying the skin around the anus, lymphatic drainage is to the inguinal nodes, and venous return is to the internal iliac vessels which form part of the systemic venous system. The venous systems of the upper and lower anus anastamose. This means that if obstruction develops in one system blood can drain back eventually to the heart through the other.

Age, Sex, Aetiology

Compared with colorectal carcinoma this is a rare tumour. The age group is on average five years younger, and slightly more men than women are affected.

Little is known about possible aetiology. Carcinoma has arisen in areas of chronic dermatitis following radiation treatment of severe pruritus. Occasionally malignant change has occurred in an internal pile or infected sinus.

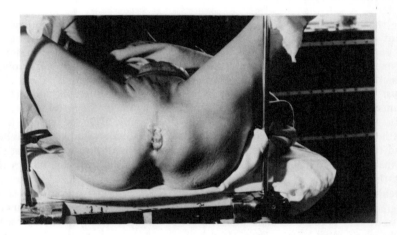

Fig. 14.4.   Carcinoma of the anal margin

Histology and Spread

With rare exceptions carcinoma arises in the anal margin or the squamous epithelium of the anal canal. It is usually a poorly-differentiated squamous carcinoma and behaves similarly to the same type of growth occurring in the skin. Direct spread is to the perineum, perianal skin, and upwards into the rectum. Metastasis by the lymphatics occurs early and can take two routes. From the lower part of the canal and the surrounding skin and tissues spread is to the inguinal nodes. If however the tumour has involved the rectum then the disease can metastasise directly to the lumbar nodes. Blood-borne deposits do not occur until late. Other skin tumours can occur, such as melanoma, basal cell carcinoma, Bowen's disease. They follow the same course as in other sites.

Symptomatology

Because this tumour occurs in a superficial site the patient realises its presence early. Unfortunately despite this fact which leads to early consultation, in many cases spread to the inguinal nodes has already occurred. When the anal skin is invaded the patient will notice an ulcer which fails to heal and gradually extends. If the growth lies further inside the anal canal the complaint may be of discharge and bleeding, this can be mistaken for the symptoms of haemorrhoids. Because of the innervation of the lower part of the canal the lesion will be painful, and this may well be the predominant symptom. Attempts to alter the bowel habit reflect the pain felt on defaecation. In advanced cases the sphincter may be so damaged that incontinence occurs.

Examination and Investigations

After the initial history has been taken the examination will first survey the patient's general condition, and will then concentrate on the assessment of the local condition and of the abdomen. The abdomen is carefully palpated to detect abnormal masses such as a liver enlarged by deposits or a group of involved inguinal nodes. Attention is then concentrated on the tumour. If it is visible it must be measured, recorded either by a sketch or a photograph, and the appearance described. The degree of infiltration is assessed. Since this is such a painful tumour rectal examination may only be possible after the use of a local anaesthetic, the proctoscope must also be passed to check whether there is any spread to the rectum. The most common appearance is that of a growth at the anal margin extending in many cases down between the buttocks. Within the canal the tumour is often annular, and in the upper part it may be indistinguishable from a carcinoma of the rectum.

Sigmoidoscopy and a barium enema X-ray are both necessary. It is unwise to assume that because an anal tumour is seen that it is the only growth present. The diagnosis must be confirmed histologically. A biopsy can be taken at the time of examination using local anaesthetic if necessary.

Treatment

The choice of treatment depends very largely upon the size of the lesion. Radiation reactions in this area are very brisk. The perianal skin is moist and the skin of the natal cleft is easily macerated. Surgical clearance involves extensive surgery and often a permanent colostomy. When the lesion is large and operable surgery is the treatment of choice, for moderate or small lesions radiation can give extremely good results.

Surgery

The operation is a far more radical procedure than might be expected. It involves a wide excision of the skin and resection of the rectum. Block dissection of the nodes is only undertaken at the same time if they are involved. If they become the site of metastases later dissection is carried out then. The patient is left with a permanent colostomy. Early tumours in the anus may not require such extensive therapy, and it may be possible to preserve the sphincters.

Radiation

External radiation therapy produces such severe reactions that it is not used. Some form of implantation is the method of choice, and both primary lesions and localised recurrences after surgery can be treated in this way. To avoid faecal soiling of the implantation site a colostomy may be formed. The patient can be reassured that it is nearly always possible to close this when healing is complete. The needles are placed in a predetermined pattern and left in place for six or seven days. The position is checked by X-rays immediately afterwards, it is most important that any needles lying too close together and producing 'a hot spot' should be removed and reinserted.

The immediate complications of treatment are often severe. The reaction is brisk, radiation filming and moist desquamation develop, and pain is always present, sometimes severe. The implantation site must be kept clean and treated in the same way as any area requiring surgical dressing. A needle site may become infected and occasionally pus forms a pocket and requires drainage.

The late reactions include atrophy of the skin and mucosa with occasional necrosis, telangiectasia, with bleeding, and fibrosis leading to stricture formation. The patient may complain of bleeding, a painful urgency to defaecate, and difficulty in passing the faeces. Necroses usually heal after diathermy coagulation. Strictures if not too extensive, may respond to regular use of a dilator. If bleeding is intractable, then excision and the formation of a permanent colostomy may be necessary. If nodes develop and the local lesion is controlled, block dissection is carried out.

Palliative Treatment

Radiation may be of some use in palliation of advanced tumours, but formation of a permanent colostomy, combined with adequate analgesia and local antiseptics, may be a better method of treatment for some patients.

Some centres have used the cytotoxic agent bleomycin.

Follow-up

After surgery the patient is seen at frequent intervals during the first year and then the period between appointments is gradually lengthened. At each visit a check is made that there is no local recurrence and no spread to the inguinal nodes. When there has been an implant the immediate follow-up will include in addition careful attention to the state of the skin and mucosa. At later appointments the timing of closure of the colostomy is considered and a careful watch kept for late radiation reaction.

Prognosis

If surgical resection is possible 50% of patients have a five year survival, the figure is somewhat higher, 65%, if the tumour is an early one.

Prognosis for the Whole Tract

The prognosis for tumours discussed in this section is summarised in the accompanying diagram.

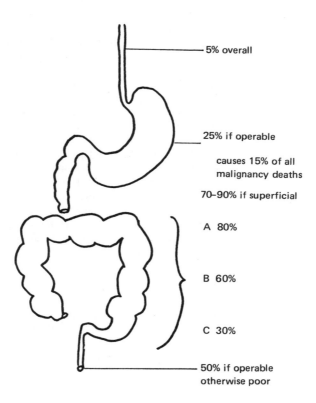

5% overall

25% if operable

causes 15% of all
malignancy deaths

70–90% if superficial

A 80%

B 60%

C 30%

50% if operable
otherwise poor

Fig. 14.5.   Five year survival rates

LIVER, GALL BLADDER AND PANCREAS

Anatomy

Liver

This large organ lies just under the right side of the diaphragm. It can normally only just be palpated at the right costal margin at the end of inspiration. On the backward facing lower surface lies the gall bladder.

The porta hepatis, meaning the gate of the liver, is an important area. Here are found the common hepatic duct carrying bile away from the liver, the hepatic artery carrying oxygenated blood, and the portal vein bringing venous blood from the gut; in these latter two the flow is inwards to the liver. Surrounding these three are lymphatic nodes and ducts.

The cells of the liver are arranged in cords and columns which are formed into lobules, in the centre of these lie veins which drain the liver. Around the margins of the lobule are grouped branches of the hepatic artery, the portal vein, and bile ducts. Kupffer cells which are part of the reticulo-endothelial system (mononuclear phagocyte system), lie along the vascular capillaries.

Due to its position the liver is related not only to the diaphragm but to many of the abdominal structures.

Gall Bladder

This is a pear-shaped sac which contains muscle in its wall. It is joined by the cystic duct to the hepatic duct, together they form the common bile duct which opens into the second part of the duodenum on the duodenal papilla. The common bile duct is closed by the sphincter of Oddi which surrounds the papilla.

Pancreas

Roughly triangular in shape the pancreas is divided into a head which lies in the loop of the duodenum, the body and the tail. The pancreatic duct opens into the duodenum just above the duodenal papilla. Within the pancreas are groups of cells, the islets of Langerhans, which secrete insulin.

Physiology

Liver

This is the great factory of the body. It assists in the breakdown and utilisation of all three main foodstuffs, carbohydrates, fats, and protein. It stores sugar in the form of glycogen and can in various ways regulate the blood glucose level.

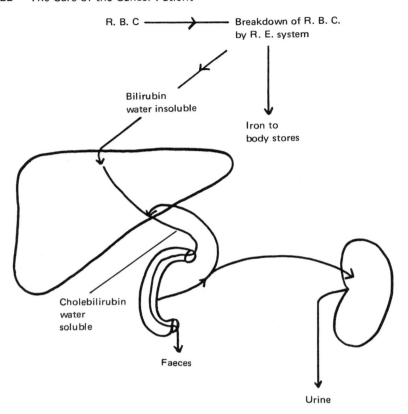

Fig. 14.6.   Formation of the bile pigments

Breakdown of proteins causes the formation of amino acids which cannot be stored, the liver can deaminate these to form urea excreted in the urine. Certain proteins, albumin, fibrinogen, and prothrombin are synthesised in the liver. Fat, probably proteins, Vitamin A, the haematinic principle (probably vitamin B12) and iron are stored. It also acts as a reservoir of blood. Many enzymes are found in the liver, they speed the biochemical reactions by which unwanted substances are either inactivated or changed into an excretable form.

Jaundice

Clinically this is characterised by accumulation of bilirubin in the body tissues staining them yellow. Old red blood cells are broken down by the mononuclear phagocyte system cells and bilirubin is one of the products of this process. At this stage it is insoluble and cannot be excreted in the urine. However, after passage through the liver the bilirubin becomes changed to a soluble form, is stored and concentrated in the gall bladder, and discharged into the duodenum. Slightly altered there, it is mostly excreted in the faeces giving them the charac-

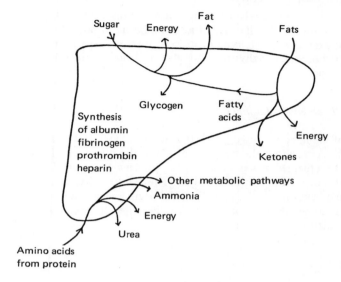

Fig. 14.7.   Some liver functions

teristic colour, a little is re-absorbed to be excreted by the kidneys or again through the liver.

Interruption of this pathway results in accumulation of bilirubin, jaundice. The type of jaundice and the effect on liver function tests (L.F.T.s) varies according to the point at which the interruption occurs.

Prehepatic Jaundice

Any condition which results in excessive breakdown, haemolysis, of red-blood cells, will cause a rise of this prehepatic bilirubin. The liver is unable to deal with this extra load, the kidneys cannot excrete it, and so the level in the blood rises. The bilirubin passes out into the tissues and stains them yellow.

This type of jaundice occurs after a mismatched blood transfusion, in certain types of poisoning, and in the course of the diseases pernicious anaemia and congenital haemolytic anaemia.

Hepatic Jaundice

This type is a little more complicated to understand. Bile flow can be blocked at two points. If the liver cells are damaged or destroyed then bilirubin cannot be changed into cholebilirubin. Consequently bilirubin accumulates in the blood as in the first case. Alternatively the cells may be functioning, but the bile canaliculi are blocked either by pressure from swollen hepatic cells or by destruction by disease. This results in obstructive jaundice. In this case, cholebilirubin will accumulate in the blood, be excreted in the urine, and give the urine a very dark 'tea' colour. When the liver itself is diseased both these types of jaundice can occur and the clinical picture is a mixture of both. Infective hepatitis is a classical example of this type of disease. First prehepatic jaundice is found, then a mixture, and finally the jaundice is usually predominantly of the obstructive type.

Obstructive Posthepatic Jaundice

This type of jaundice is caused by obstruction to the flow of bile away from the liver. It can occur within the liver or outside in the bile ducts. In the ducts the causes can be enlarged nodes or a tumour pressing from outside, stricture of the duct wall, or a stone within the duct. The result is that cholebilirubin does not reach the intestine. It is excreted in the urine giving it a dark colour, while the faeces become putty coloured. This is because cholebilirubin is no longer forming the pigment of the faeces.

Gall Bladder

Bile from the liver is stored in the gall bladder and concentrated. Hormone secretion by the gut causes contraction of the gall bladder and discharge of the bile into the duodenum, here it assists in the digestion of fat.

Pancreas

The pancreas produces enzymes which assist in the breakdown of foods, protein, fats and carbohydrates. These enzymes are carried in the pancreatic juice along the pancreatic duct to the duodenum. Insulin from the β cells of the Islets of Langerhans is secreted into the blood.

Malignant Tumours

Primary Tumours

Incidence

Primary tumours of all three organs are rare in Europeans, although incidence of both liver and pancreatic tumours is increasing. About 1% of cancer deaths are due to tumours of the liver and gall bladder, and 3–4% to tumours of the pancreas. Primary malignancy of the gall bladder occurs more commonly in women. The age of patients is from the mid-fifties onwards, pancreatic carcinoma patients are usually in the lower age range.

In Africa and S.E. Asia the incidence pattern is different. Up to 50% of deaths from malignant disease in S. and E. Africa and S.E. Asia are due to primary tumours of the liver and bile ducts.

Aetiology

Certain factors have been incriminated in the carcinogenesis of liver tumours, cirrhosis whether due to alcohol or faulty nutrition, Hepatitis B infection, myco-toxins particularly aflatoxins, and haemachromatosis. In S.E. Asia parasitic infection is associated with carcinoma of the ducts. A rare sarcoma has been linked to the manufacture of vinyl. Chronic cholecystitis and gallstones are very often associated with a carcinoma, chronic irritation is believed to be the factor.

Symptomatology

The common link between malignancy in these three sites is the effect on the biliary system and the flow of bile. In the liver the formation of bile or its flow may be affected, tumour in the gall bladder or the bile ducts can cause obstruction, and similarly a tumour in the head of the pancreas will result in intractable jaundice due to pressure on the common bile duct.

Other symptoms are pain, loss of appetite, weight loss, lassitude, dyspepsia. Occasionally fever is present, it is low grade and swinging usually.

Due to the role of these organs, many of their biochemical functions may be disordered. LFTs show abnormal results, most commonly bilirubin, alkaline phosphatase and plasma proteins. A rare secreting malignant tumour of the islets of Langerhans can cause raised insulin, glucagon, or secretin levels.

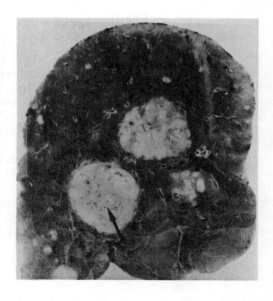

Fig. 14.8.   Liver showing metastatic deposits

Secondary Tumours

The liver is usually the site of these, spread occurring by direct extension, e.g. from the gall bladder, in the blood usually causing scattered metastases, or through the lymphatics to the nodes of the porta hepatis.

Symptomatology

On examination the liver is enlarged, firm and occasionally nodular. The abdomen may feel doughy and enlarged, and on tapping one side the hand on the other side may detect a fluid thrill. This is due to the presence of ascites, fluid in the peritoneal cavity. There are many reasons for its formation, low plasma albumin, peritoneal seedlings, or obstruction to the portal blood flow. In the more severe cases jaundice is present and signs of collateral blood flow may be found. This latter sign is due to blockage of the portal venous return so that anastamoses with the systemic venous return open up. This anastamotic circulation may be seen as enlarged veins over the abdominal wall or around the umbilicus.

The primary carcinoma is not always known. It may be slow growing and unsuspected. By contrast liver metastases grow fast and can kill. A melanoma of the choroid is slow growing and can be removed with apparent cure. Twenty years later the patient can present with jaundice and rapid deterioration due to liver metastases. Despite careful clinical search in other cases the primary may remain undetected and its site only discovered at autopsy. The contrary position can also exist. The liver has great reserves of function so that metastases can remain unsuspected and only be discovered at laparotomy.

Treatment

When it is possible to attempt either radical or palliative treatment of a primary the problem is a surgical one. Radiotherapy is occasionally used when pain is severe and the predominant problem, and high energy electron therapy has been tried in some cases when tumour has caused obstructive jaundice, but on the whole radiation has little to offer. Treatment must be directed to the general care of the whole patient. Occasionally surgical by-pass procedures are justified. They relieve the jaundice and the severe pruritus, making the patient more comfortable in the ensuing months. Chemotherapy has so far made little impact although occasionally a patient has benefited from the use of 5-FU.

Secondary deposits in the liver may respond if part of dissemination from a tumour susceptible to hormone manipulation, radioactive isotopes, or chemotherapy. However the damage inflicted on the liver may already leave residual dysfunction. On the whole liver metastases are a sign of advanced disease.

Prognosis

This is poor. Patients with primary tumours rarely survive more than six months, although if surgically removable the occasional patient has a good prognosis.

For the most part metastatic liver disease has a terminal prognosis.

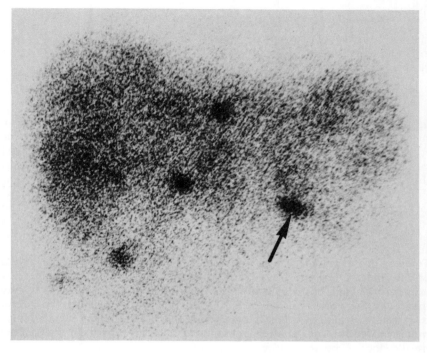

Fig. 14.9.   Liver scan showing metastases

We are born to live not to suffer,
Yet many women suffer and are sacrificed.
They ask only to know that sacrifice is not in vain.
That they may know that we heed and know their plea,
That we shall indeed never sacrifice in vain,
To these women I dedicate this chapter.

15   The Breast

To every doctor whether he be physician, surgeon, or radiotherapist, carcinoma of the breast represents the supreme challenge. Not only is his medical skill tested to the limit, but also his ability to treat the whole patient. To any woman the loss of the breast is a tragedy. She feels her femininity is diminished and she is constantly reminded of her 'mutilation'. Sometimes in a busy clinic, the impact on a woman of the news of impending mastectomy is not fully realised, but usually doctors are well aware of it and can feel as deeply as their patient the burden of this procedure.

The challenge of the disease lies in the inability of medicine to improve materially the survival figures. Despite the major leap forward which followed the perfection of radical mastectomy, the mortality figures have remained virtually unchanged over the last 50 years. This leads us to pose certain questions: is it the nature of the disease itself which is so baffling? Would earlier detection lead to better survival figures? Are the present available methods of treatment effective enough or should we be looking for some revolutionary approach? We know from clinical observation that we are dealing with a growth which can behave in a variety of ways, but we do not yet know all the factors which influence its behaviour. Mammography can detect earlier than clinical palpation, but although it may enable a tumour to be detected while it is still small and therefore at an early stage, the histology may be such that the tumour still behaves aggressively. We need means which will detect malignant cells while they are still confined within the breast, and, as mammography can discover malignancy earlier than palpation, so in its turn this new test will improve on mammography. Even this is not sufficient unless we can also detect cells which may already have disseminated and will become metastatic foci later. We need tests which will search out deposits in bones and other organs while they still consist of a few cells. Only when we can treat a disease localised to the breast, confident that there is no spread, not even of a few cells, can we eradicate the disease. Present methods while effective in controlling the local condition fail to deal with disseminated malignancy.

This chapter has been divided into a number of sections for ease of description. The care of the patient is one such subdivision. Since the subject has so many facets it was felt desirable to gather all the points into one coherent whole, rather than to have small paragraphs scattered throughout the text.

These sections are:

    I.   Basic facts — anatomy, physiology and pathology
   II.   Examination and investigation
  III.   Treatment, surgery, radiation, hormones, chemotherapy
   IV.   Treatment of the advanced case
    V.   Care of the patient
   VI.   Follow-up and prognosis
  VII.   Carcinoma of the male breast

Section I

Incidence and Aetiology

Carcinoma of the breast is the most common malignancy in women, about 11,000 die annually. The cause is unknown, certain factors may play a part, but exactly which are important, in what combination, how they react with the woman's inherited characteristics, cannot be determined, and opinions change. For example breast feeding and early weaning are now regarded as having little influence on carcinogenesis. The previous low rate in Japanese women is rising, probably due to a rising standard in living, and since if these women emigrate to Western style communities the rate among them rises to that of the local population, whatever the factor is, it is likely to be environmental rather than racial. The following is a list of some factors associated with slightly increased risk, nulliparity, early menarche, late menopause, cancer of the breast in another member of the family, mammary dysplasia, radiation of the breast. Other possible factors, but not proven, are diet, psychosomatic patterns, including stress, viruses, immune status, hormone imbalance, and each of these possibly varying in effect on pre- and post-menopausal women. A cause of concern has been the prolonged use of oral contraceptives, but apart from recommendations regarding the ratio of the component steroids, no other action has been considered necessary since, despite large surveys, no positive link has been found with breast carcinoma, indeed there is some evidence of protection against carcinoma of the ovary and uterus. Pregnancy at an early age does appear to confer some protection. However, it would be idle to believe that we have reached a point when a preventative policy can be recommended, particularly in such a fundamental human activity as reproduction.

The age range of maximum incidence is 40–70 although tumour does occur in younger patients, but it is uncommon below the age of 30. Carcinoma of the male breast is very rare, the ratio of incidence male to female being 1:100.

Anatomy

The breast consists of lobules of glandular tissue embedded in fat. It is the fat which gives the breast its rounded shape. Running from the tissues just below the skin to the fascial sheet of the chest wall are fibrous septa. These separate the glandular lobules. The breast overlies the second to sixth ribs and also three muscles. It can be moved freely on the chest wall and is carried upward when the arm is raised. Each lobule is formed of ducts and small sacs lined with secretory epithelium. The ducts join together to form the lactiferous duct which opens on to the nipple.

Blood is supplied by the axillary and internal mammary arteries and by small branches from the intercostal arteries. Venous drainage is by the corresponding veins.

The lymph drainage is to a wide area and is extremely important in carcinoma of the breast. The lymph node groups are:

1. Five groups in the axilla, the highest (apical) receives the drainage from the rest.
2. Internal mammary deep to the junction of ribs and sternum. Lymph passes, then flows on to the subclavian lymph trunk. Since there is communication with the cervical nodes, these can be involved if the main drainage pathways are blocked. Other lymphatic pathways are:

(a) The opposite breast and axilla.
(b) The groin by vessels of the trunk wall.
(c) Peritoneal lymphatics connecting with the lower mammary chain.

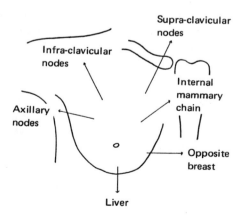

Fig. 15.1.   Lymphatic spread of carcinoma of the breast

Physiology

The breast is rudimentary at birth, development to the adult form takes place at puberty, there is then branching and growth of the duct system. At each menstrual cycle there is further proliferation followed by partial regression, the overall effect is a gradual enlargement in size. During the first half of pregnancy the breasts enlarge, further duct development takes place together with formation of new alveoli. In the second half of pregnancy the epithelial cells swell and secretory activity begins.

The development and activity of the breast is under the control of two hormones, oestrogen and progesterone, working in conjunction with secretions of the thyroid and anterior pituitary gland. Oestrogen and progesterone, in the non-pregnant woman, are secreted by the ovary. The development of the breast at puberty is probably due to the rise in oestrogen levels. During pregnancy the placenta secretes both hormones and acting together these stimulate proliferation of the ducts and the epithelial cells. Lactation is initiated and maintained by prolactin from the anterior pituitary gland, release being controlled by the hypothalamus. At the menopause, ovarian function ceases and therefore its hormone secretion.

The intimate relationship and interplay between the hypothalamus, the hormones of the anterior pituitary gland, the ovary, and the adrenal cortex, and their ultimate effect on the breast is well known but as yet incompletely understood. The importance of this hormone background cannot be over estimated. It has been suggested that disturbance in this balance may initiate malignant change in the breast.

Pathology

Carcinoma develops as a mass in the breast sometimes accompanied by an eczema-like condition of the nipple, Paget's disease. Although some patients first consult their doctor because of an ulceration of the skin, this is not in fact the first but a later stage of the disease. The tumour can occur in any part of the breast including the tail of tissue which extends up towards the axilla. The most common site is the upper, outer quadrant. In appearance the growth can range in size from a half to several centimetres across. The texture varies from soft to extremely hard. Sometimes the breast is hot, swollen and tender, the so-called 'inflammatory' carcinoma.

Histology

There are two microscopic forms of carcinoma, in situ and invasive. The former is of two types, intraduct and lobular. It is important to examine several areas to exclude early invasion. Of the invasive carcinomas most are of the ductal type arising on pre-existing intraduct carcinoma, the others are infiltrating lobular, medullary, mucoid, papillary, and very occasionally metaplastic. The degree of differentiation, grades 1 to 3, influences prognosis together with the degree of spread.

Spread

It is important to realise that the method of spread is very variable and the route will influence the clinical picture.

Direct

The disease spreads through the breast tissue. Ultimately either the skin is invaded and ulcerated, or the muscle and chest wall become attached to the tumour resulting in loss of mobility, or both can occur.

Lymphatic

1. Invasion and blockage of the lymphatics of the dermis results in oedema of the skin and a curious pitting likened to the skin of an orange, 'peau d'orange'. Multiple tumour nodules can develop and provoke a dense fibrotic reaction. The whole breast becomes hard and leathery like a piece of armour, hence the name 'cancer en cuirasse'.
   2. The axillary nodes are involved in about 60% of specimens examined after operation, the internal mammary and supraclavicular groups to a lesser degree.
   Spread to the internal mammary glands is more likely to arise when the tumour is situated in the medial quadrants. Later spread occurs to mediastinal, abdominal, and aortic nodes.

Blood

Spread in the blood stream is common and most women who die of the disease have evidence of it. The lungs, liver, and bones are the most common metastatic sites, but the brain and other organs are not infrequently involved.

Other Methods

Once the tumour has reached the peritoneum or the pleura, spread across the cavity, transcoelomic, can take place. Implantation of cells in the wound at the time of the operation can cause recurrence in the scar. Spread along the lumen of the ducts can also occur.
   An interesting observation is that until a late stage each tumour often characteristically spreads by one or other of the main routes alone, either lymphatic or blood.

Symptomatology

Most women discover the tumour themselves, but an increasing number are being referred from 'well woman clinics'. The patient attends these for a cervical-smear test and part of the routine examination is palpation of the breast. In this way an occasional small lump unnoticed by the patient is detected.

Screening programmes designed to detect tumours at an early stage have been ongoing in the U.S.A. for some time. Pilot surveys being conducted in the United Kingdom will require several years before it is apparent whether they have reduced mortality from the disease, although early results look promising, also in Sweden.

Mass

The usual story is that the woman has noticed a lump while dressing or washing. Occasionally she has examined the breast because she had a knock and so notices a pre-existing mass for the first time. Pain in the breast is not uncommon particularly just before menstruation, it is therefore difficult to pinpoint this as a symptom or malignancy, but some patients do experience a sharp stabbing or pricking pain in the carcinoma, it is not continuous.

Nipple

Changes in the nipple may be the first sign noticed. This can take the form of soreness, cracking, ulceration or itching. In some cases the nipple is drawn in. Discharge, which can be clear or bloodstained, may be seen.

Skin

Patients do not normally notice puckering or dimpling of the skin. Sometimes the skin over the mass is reddened. When ulceration is the first complaint this is a late manifestation. The woman has either ignored, or failed to notice the earlier lump.

Metastases

Occasionally the primary is so small or the breast so large that it is the symptoms caused by metastases which make a patient see her doctor. She may complain of breathlessness, cough, and chest pain caused by metastases in the lungs, of swelling of the arm, a mass in the axilla due to axillary nodes, or pain due to skeletal deposits, the pain being either localised or referred due to pressure on nerves. More rarely the first sign of trouble may be a pathological fracture or signs of cerebral pressure.

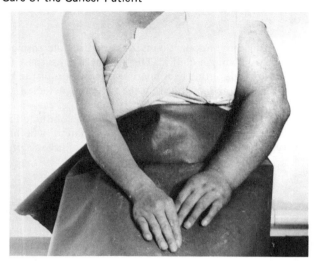

Fig. 15.2.   Oedema of the arm

History and Examination

Whether the woman consults her doctor at once or after an interval of some time she is in a state of fear. Women's magazines carry frequent articles on the disease and the technique of self-examination, and if she has not read them she will have certainly heard much hearsay from her family and friends. Every woman is convinced that a lump in the breast must be cancer. Her primary need is for a reassurance which it is hard to give, no doctor can be certain that this lump is benign until it has been removed. On the other hand she badly needs her confidence restored. Her doctor must steer a careful course between over optimism resulting in false promises, and pessimism which will still further depress her. Probably the first step is to confirm her good sense in seeking advice, and to convey the feeling that she is now sharing her problem with those who can help her.

The history is important. Certain families have a high rate of cancer of the breast and judicious questioning may reveal a pattern likely to be repeated in the patient. The details of any pregnancies and subsquent breast feeding are interesting epidemiologically, but give little guide to the likely behaviour of the tumour. Specific questions on discharge, pain, and nipple retraction must be put.

Examination follows, first the general condition and then the local. On the findings of this examination are based the conclusions on the staging of the tumour using the international symbols, T, N and M with numbers. The details for the breast are repeated on the next page in outline.

Basic scheme:

T. The initial tumour in the breast, size, skin involvement, state of the nipple, fixation to chest wall.
N. Lymph nodes, axillary or supraclavicular. Same or opposite side. Mobile or fixed.
M. Distant metastases.

Modifications are made from time to time.

It must be emphasised that this is a guide only, neither examination nor subsequent operative findings can take account of microscopic foci which may already exist outside the breast, cannot be detected by present means, and completely alter the prognosis.

A simple form of staging based on histological findings and results of investigations designed to discover distant metastases, may be used instead.

Section II

Examination

The breasts are first inspected for any deformity or skin dimpling. Inspection is repeated with the arms raised above the head, and again with the hands pressing in on the hips. These manoeuvres may reveal, or make more obvious,

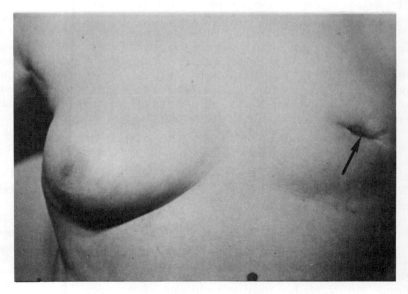

Fig. 15.3.   Indrawn nipple with tethering of the skin

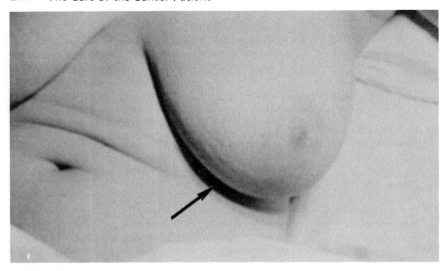

Fig. 15.4.   Peau d'orange

skin tethering or nipple deformity. Then with the patient lying down in a position that spreads the breast evenly over the chest wall, the breast is systematically examined. Both breasts must be checked, also the liver, the axillae, and the neck.

The surgeon repeats the examination and if the mass feels cystic can carry out immediately one investigation, he can attempt aspiration. If the fluid is clear and the lump disappears completely he can be reasonably confident that it is benign. The fluid is sent for cytology and the patient kept under observation. If however the fluid is blood stained, or scanty, or there is only a small decrease in the size of the mass, then this is highly suspicious and operation must be carried out as soon as possible. In some centres a little air is put into the cyst after aspiration, subsequent X-rays will then outline any tumour in the wall and may give some information as to whether it is benign or malignant.

Typical History

Mrs. – , age 45.
    Complaining of a lump in the right breast first noticed while washing a week ago. Painless.

Direct questions. No nipple discharge or deformity. No skin fixation noticed.
No skeletal pain. Still menstruating regularly, no abnormality. Two pregnancies – full term, normal delivery. Not breast fed.
Past history. Nil serious.
Family history. Mother breast removed aged 48 for cancer. Uncle – age 62 cancer of the stomach.

O/E General condition good. No signs of anaemia.
Nipple – slight puckering of the skin in the upper outer quadrant on raising arms. Hard mass 2 cms across. R. upper outer quadrant.
Irregular. Tethered to the skin. Not fixed to the chest wall.
No nodes palpable axilla and neck.
Other breast normal.

Diagnosis – Probably carcinoma. Refer urgently for surgical opinion.

Investigations

These are directed towards discovering whether there is spread beyond the breast and axillary nodes, whether the tumour is operable, and finally to confirming that the tumour is malignant.

Confirmation of malignancy is by biopsy. This may be needle biopsy in the out-patient department, using a local anaesthetic. This has the advantage that early planning of treatment is possible, but the disadvantage that sampling errors may occur in small tumours. More usually part is removed under general anaesthetic for examination, the receptor status can also be determined. The specimen used to be sent for frozen section to obtain immediate results, mastectomy then being carried out if necessary, since it was thought that biopsy would disseminate malignant cells. Since there do not appear to be ill effects from the short delay involved in the normal histology processes, many surgeons now prefer to wait. In this way a woman is spared having to wait until recovery from the anaesthetic to know whether or not she has lost her breast, and the delay enables her to be better prepared if she has to do so.

As we have seen cells can be disseminated giving rise to small foci and yet not cause symptoms, investigations must therefore attempt to detect these foci. It must be admitted that as yet the available tests are comparatively crude. Apart from the routine blood tests and biochemistry reliance is placed mostly on X-rays and isotope scans. Mammography is a technique which X-rays the breast soft tissue. Masses, which are as yet too small to detect clinically, may be seen. The ducts can be outlined by inserting contrast medium into their openings in the nipple. Both breasts are examined, the value of doing this lies in the chance of detecting other masses in the same breast, or another primary in the other breast. Mammography can be useful in those rare cases when a general practitioner feels a mass but the surgeon is unable to do so.

Thermography is used in some centres to supplement the X-ray. A device detects the minute differences in the heat radiated by different tissues and translates this into a pattern of light and dark shades corresponding to the part of the body examined. A carcinoma can appear as a hot or cold spot according to its vascularity.

Since carcinoma of the breast so often metastasises to bone, a skeletal survey must be carried out in addition to the normal chest X-ray. The ribs can be scanned from the chest film, but the vertebral column requires the taking of special views. It is also usual to include the skull and pelvis in the survey. Unfortunately deposits can be present and not show up on the X-ray. When the test is possible,

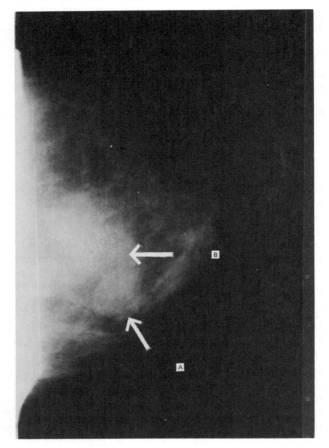

Fig. 15.5.   Mammogram. A. Benign cyst.
B. Carcinoma with calcification flecks

scintiscanning is practised. This is a form of radioactive isotope survey carried out over the skeleton, and also the liver. It enables some deposits not visualised on X-ray to be picked up, but unfortunately still does not detect the very small, few cell deposits.

Of recent years the discovery of hormone receptors in the cells of breast tumours has offered an explanation as to why only some tumours responded to hormone manipulation, a fuller discussion of these receptors is reserved for a later section in this chapter. The assay is performed by a few specialised laboratories in the United Kingdom. A tumour's oestrogen and progesterone receptor content may indicate prognosis, and also be a guide in the choice of therapy if there is recurrence.

The overall state of the patient must never be forgotten in ordering investigations. In very advanced cases, full knowledge will make little difference to the prognosis and in some patients who are already terrified full investigation may do far more harm than good. Apart from the routine clinical examination, blood and biochemistry screens, isotope scans of liver and skeleton and chest X-ray are probably the most useful tests. Carcinoma of the breast can run a protracted course and a doctor must not only exercise medical skill but also his ability to treat the whole human being.

Section III

Treatment

Carcinoma which is less than 2 cms and mobile with or without mobile involved nodes, is the most likely to have a favourable response to initial medical treatment. In staging schedules, these are classed as I and II. Very advanced local disease or distant metastases (stages III and IV) mean that life expectancy is poor, and palliation of symptoms may be more important than mere length of survival, particularly if the side effects of treatment designed to prolong life, actually outweigh the benefits.

There is no one agreed policy of treatment, and the fact that patients may receive different combinations of therapy at different centres, while it is confusing to the lay public, is not indicative of mal-treatment. This is one of the most complicated areas of research. It is bedevilled by changes in tumour definition, varying treatment regimes, and contradictory results. Only studies with very large numbers of patients, the design and execution being carefully controlled, can hope to produce data on which to base conclusions. The tumour manifests so many different behaviour patterns, and is so unpredictable in that very late recurrences are seen (a twenty year interval is not uncommon), that to numbers must be added length of follow-up.

In view of the different treatment policies at present, a patient must be given the opportunity to discuss and question her suggested treatment. It is a matter of supreme importance to her, and many women have read articles in popular magazines which have either given a definite opinion, or left her very confused. On the other hand she may wish for no discussion at all, preferring to leave decisions with her doctor. If it is possible the husband or close relatives should participate in the 'briefing'. The patient is going to need all the support she can get, and it is more likely to be of the right kind if the family is prepared and part of the back-up team. It is most important that if a woman rejects the advised treatment and prefers some other operation or procedure, she should not be made to feel guilty nor that she is taking foolish risks.

The various forms of treatment will be described separately, and then fairly typical treatment policies outlined.

Surgery

Mastectomy   The original operation was devised by Halstead. It is called radical mastectomy and entailed removal of the breast, two underlying muscles, and the axillary lymphatic tissue. It is a mutilating operation and has been modified either by removing other lymph nodes (supra-radical), or by confining the operation to removal of the breast and axillary tail, usually with axillary lymph node clearance or biopsy. The supra-radical mastectomy has been virtually abandoned, but controversy over the merits of each form of modified and simple mastectomy still exists.

Lumpectomy, a wide local excision, is sometimes performed. This retains the breast, but is strictly limited in application as the originators pointed out.

The subcutaneous removal of breast tissue is only suitable for high risk patients or carcinoma in situ, the implantation of the breast prosthesis can be associated with complications.

Patients sometimes request an implant after mastectomy. Some doctors do not feel happy about this, fearing recurrence or new disease, but on balance it will probably do no harm. Although the surgeon may think the cosmetic result poor, the patient may not agree and may feel the boost to her morale outweighs this objection.

Following operation the patient must commence movement of the arm as soon as possible. The physiotherapist can teach the exercises, but it is the task of the nurse to encourage the patient to persist and to repeat that her own efforts will make all the difference to the future freedom of movement. As soon as possible the surgical fitter should see her and measure her for a surgical brassiere. She will not be able to wear it immediately but her morale requires a lightweight temporary one until she can. Every effort should be made to see that the type best suited to her physical and psychological needs is made.

Radiotherapy

This is given over a four to six week period, either as primary treatment, post-operatively, or to treat metastases.

Primary treatment involves radiation of the breast, both internal mammary chains, and the supraclavicular and axillary node groups on the affected side. Post-operatively the node groups and chest wall may be treated, but in some centres not all areas are treated, while in others no radiation is given.

Precautions to be observed are the avoidance of metal containing adhesive tapes, if at all possible surgical dressings should not be secured by elastoplast. If the patient wishes to go away for convalescence before post-operative treatment there is no harm in delay, but when there has been biopsy only then treatment is best started immediately after removal of stitches.

Hormone Manipulation

It is not surprising that in an organ responsive to hormone stimulation tumours are also responsive, growth being stimulated by hormones. In 1896 Beatson reported that oophorectomy had caused marked regression of advanced breast tumours in three women. Since then it has been accepted that about one third of patients would respond to hormone treatment of some kind, but until recently the reason has not been known. Research has now established that the cells of breast carcinoma may have cellular proteins which bind certain steroids, the most important steroids being oestrogen, progesterone, and to a lesser extent androgens. Binding with the steroid causes the receptor to pass into the nucleus of the cell where it can set up RNA synthesis. This in turn leads to increased, or new, protein formation. This protein can cause physiological effects. Cells which have these receptors are called receptor positive, the others negative. Possession of receptors makes the tumours sensitive to hormone manipulation, particularly if both oestrogen and progesterone receptors are present, thereby explaining Beatson's observation. Some authorities also believe that receptor negative tumours recur earlier and patients have worse survival times.

It is for these reasons that it is becoming increasingly common to determine the receptor status of the tumour, and possibly any accessible metastasis.

Methods of Manipulation   These are of two types, surgical or medical. The first involves the ablation of tissues either controlling, or producing, oestrogen and progesterone. The operations are oophorectomy, adrenalectomy, hypophysectomy. The last two are now less commonly performed due to the availability of other methods and to the morbidity which ensued in many patients.

Suppression of production can be achieved by drugs. These can saturate the receptors and compete with oestrogen, e.g. the anti-oestrogen tamoxifen, and possibly also androgens, or synthesis can be depressed by exogenous steroids prednisone) or by adrenal blockers such as aminoglutethimide or similar drugs.

Chemotherapy

Cytotoxic drugs, either singly or in combination can be used to treat breast carcinoma. However there is no general agreement as to the timing nor extent of their use. Many authorities believe that patients with receptor negative tumours should receive chemotherapy as first choice treatment when there is recurrence. Others are less certain, the side effects are not inconsiderable and if symptoms can be controlled by radiation, physical measures, etc., they believe that, since survival time is likely to be short, its quality may be more important than its length. Then too for many women at present the hormone status of the original tumour is unknown, and the assay results from metastases are less consistent, so that a trial of the less arduous regime of hormone manipulation may be preferred. The delay in employing chemotherapy does not seem to diminish its efficacy.

At present there is even more discussion of the role of adjuvant chemotherapy. This involves the use of cytotoxics after initial treatment, the rationale being that these drugs will deal with cells that have disseminated and prevent recurrence. Initial early reports were very favourable, but longer term follow up appears only to show delay in recurrences in pre-menopausal women but no increase in survival time. Many of the young women experience amenorrhoea and it is this effect on the ovaries which is believed by many to be the real reason for delaying recurrence. Currently in the United Kingdom it is not common to use adjuvant therapy except in young women with tumour in axillary nodes, even then many doctors prefer to use simple (single agent) treatment, particularly since statistics show that at least half of them would not develop metastases anyway. In weighing the risk-benefit ratio of this treatment, it must be borne in mind that in addition to considerable toxic effects, there is the added side effect of delay in psychological recovery. Most patients recover from the psychological trauma of the first treatment within a year, but this period is longer when initial treatment is prolonged.

Treatment Policies

1. Modified radical mastectomy (including axillary node clearance), with post-operative radiation if more than four nodes have metastases.
2. Simple mastectomy with biopsy of axillary nodes. Post-operative radiation as in 1.
3. Minimum local treatment for good cosmetic results. +/− post-operative radiation.

Of these three choices the first has been the longest established and therefore long term follow up data are known. As similar long term figures become available they will be compared with them.

Section IV

Treatment of the Advanced Case

The patient with advanced disease can present with ulceration and fungation of the breast, either established or impending, with symptoms due to deposits in the pleura or peritoneum, with pain or fracture from skeletal secondaries, or with neurological symptoms from metastases in the brain. The aim of treatment can no longer be cure but it can be palliation. Every procedure is designed to relieve distressing symptoms such as discharge, to alleviate pain, and to postpone complications such as a pathological fracture. It is necessary therefore to consider both the local and the general condition. Various methods are used either singly or in combination.

It should be noted that advanced carcinoma can be present in the elderly patient and give rise to no symptoms. There is usually a long history indicating slow growth. While in some patients minimum treatment is satisfactory, in others a vigorous policy may be required, particularly since it is no longer believed that elderly patients necessarily do better.

Before treatment the diagnosis must be confirmed and the necessary investigations to determine the degree of spread carried out. Without this base line examination there can be no accurate assessment of progress.

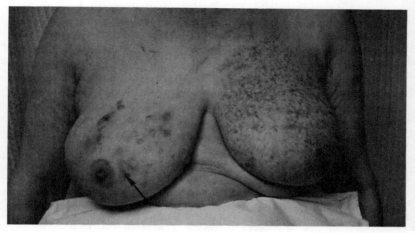

Fig. 15.6.   Metastatic skin nodules in the right breast controlled by hormones

Treatment of Local Problems

Radiation

This will be extremely useful in controlling local symptoms. Despite dissemination the local condition in the breast can respond well. Ulceration, impending or established, will heal or be prevented and the tumour can regress. The pain due to skeletal metastases is rapidly alleviated by radiation and in some cases recalcification can be seen after an interval. Pathological fracture can often be prevented in this way. Other complications can be similarly postponed by treatment. Cerebral secondaries cause severe headache and vomiting which radiation can relieve.

Although the deposits are often multiple, radiotherapy is well worth while for the relief that can be given. Radiation can also be used to suppress the ovaries in a patient unfit or unwilling to undergo surgery. Its effect is less rapid.

Surgery

The surgeon may be able to improve the local condition by a toilet operation. The patient can be relieved of the discharge and foetor of an ulcerating mass. When pathological fracture occurs mobility can often be restored by orthopaedic procedures such as the insertion of a nail, or by a pin and plate. There are some who believe that such procedures should be done prophylactically before fractures actually occur. Although there is a risk of scar implantation, laminectomy (to relieve pressure on nervous tissue) is well worth while when the patient is threatened with paraplegia and incontinence. Even when established, provided that it is done quickly after onset, there may be some improvement. Even if the remaining span of life is short, it is important to maintain the best

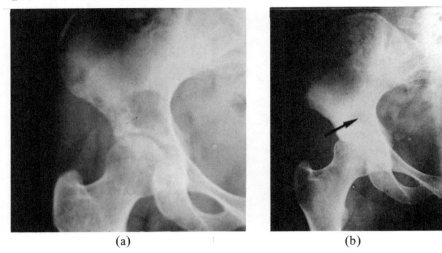

(a)   (b)

Fig 15.7a. Metastasis above R. acetabulum, before treatment.
       b. Metastasis above R. acetabulum, after treatment,
            showing calcification

quality of life possible. That aim is not achieved if a chair bound catheter existence is allowed to occur when it might have been avoided.

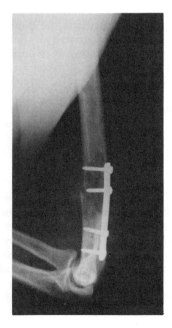

Fig. 15.8.   Fixation of pathological fracture

Radioactive Isotopes

Effusions can sometimes be controlled with this form of radiation. After removing the fluid, a small quantity of radioactive isotope is instilled. It is important that the patient is turned regularly to ensure an even distribution to treat all accessible deposits.

General Treatment

Essentially the choice lies between chemotherapy and hormone manipulation. As we have already seen no harm seems to be caused if chemotherapy is delayed, and in the United Kingdom many centres, even if the tumour's receptor status is known, prefer to try various hormone regimes first. That view is strengthened by the knowledge that even some receptor negative tumours will respond. It should be noticed that before response occurs there may be a 'flare', an exacerbation in some patients.

Premenopausal Patients

For premenopausal women oophorectomy is usually advised, although the advent of the anti-oestrogen tamoxifen may gradually displace surgery. If there is a response then a waiting policy is adopted, and the type of hormone therapy changed at the next recurrence, this may be androgens, adrenal blockers such as aminoglutethimide, progestins, or cortisone.

If hormone manipulation fails, or the disease is rapidly progressive, chemotherapy will be given. In a few centres hormone therapy and cytotoxics have been combined.

It should be noted that androgens may not be tolerated because of virilising effects, the most troublesome being deepening of the voice and growth of facial hair.

Postmenopausal Patients

Except for oophorectomy the same policy can be followed if the woman is more than five years postmenopausal.

Perimenopausal Patients

These are women who are within two to five years of the menopause. They present a difficult problem since they do not, on the whole, do so well. For those who are close to the menopause oophorectomy may be advised, for the rest Tamoxifen will probably be given first, and then the same policy adopted as for the other groups.

Future Policy

It is obvious that there is even less agreement on the policy for the advanced carcinoma than for the operable tumour. Patients who respond to chemotherapy can have a good quality of survival, but those who do not have not only the disease to contend with, but also the side effects of unsuccessful therapy.

Progress awaits not only results of trials, but greater availability of receptor assay, newer more specific less toxic chemotherapy, and predictive tests of a tumour cell's responsiveness to cytotoxic drugs.

The following is the history of a patient treated before the advent of CAT-scanning or the present range of cytotoxic and hormone drugs. It is given not as an example of treatment policy but rather to show that careful management can enable a woman to live a comfortable and useful life.

Mrs. W. — At the age of 42 she developed inoperable carcinoma of the left breast. She was given a course of radiation lasting four weeks, two months later it was noted that no mass was palpable. At this time the periods were still present but irregular.

She remained free of disease for three months but then developed a mass in the right breast and signs of recurrence on the left. She had an oophorectomy, was placed on androgen injections and had irradiation to the right breast. The condition in both breasts regressed and her state remained good for three years.

Three and a half years after her first visit she had several fits. She was seen by a neurologist. A cerebral secondary was diagnosed. A course of radiation to the brain was given and her headache and fits were relieved. Unfortunately epilation proved to be permanent.

Remission was short, a further fit followed and a persistent anaemia developed following a course of cyclophosphamide. Skeletal deposits in the spine, sacrum, pelvis, and femora were found on X-ray. This was five years after her original treatment. Short courses of radiation were given to relieve pain. She was placed on prednisone and later the androgen was discontinued. After six months she was stabilised, able to walk, and live a normal life.

Further pain in the upper spine occurred nine months later and X-ray confirmed skeletal deposits. Radiation relieved the pain and she was given a supporting spinal corset. Her fits recurred six months later. She lapsed into unconsciousness and died eight years after her original diagnosis.

Although she had required repeated treatment, this patient was able to live a normal life, to go away on holiday, and enjoy herself. Her condition was incurable, and while her survival time may not have been lengthened, its quality was good despite her symptoms of recurrence.

Section V

Problems during Treatment

Rehabilitation

From the moment the diagnosis of cancer is made, attention must be paid by everyone in contact with the patient to the process of helping her adjust to her disease, the treatment, and to enabling her to live as full and normal a life as possible. This must of course include the patient's family, as we have already said, but it is an ongoing programme. If the disease is progressive the needs of the patient and the appropriate response change. The patient may experience frustration, fear, anxiety, anger, and may not express these emotions to the most sympathetic doctor but to other members of the team. Responsible reassurance and encouragement are required from everyone. This must be continuous even if the same question or grumble is voiced again and again. Discussion or prognosis and treatment should be reserved for the doctor, patients will take the most innocent replies and place sinister meanings on them, particularly if they differ, however slightly, from what a doctor has said. Persistent worries, emotions, questions should be reported as they may not have been expressed to the medical staff.

In many areas there are groups of women who have had a mastectomy and who are willing to talk to patients who face this problem. This can be a great help to a woman. She not only meets a woman who has coped successfully, but she can ask all the 'silly' questions that she may feel too shy to put to the hospital staff. She can also get advice on the various types of brassiere available and decide which is likely to suit her best.

Radiation

Outpatient If the patient's condition is good and she lives within reasonable distance of the department she can attend as an outpatient, provided that transport can be arranged.

This is often a psychological advantage and helps her to adjust more quickly. It is important that she co-operates by looking after herself well. She must be made to realise that although radiation is only for minutes each day she will feel tired and must rest when she goes home. To have a cup of tea and lie down is not an indulgence but a necessity. She should go to bed early, let the housework slide, and if possible, have her shopping done for her. This is often against all previous habits and the co-operation of the family is badly needed. The husband should be seen by the doctor, the nature of the disease and the treatment explained to him, and the necessity for adequate rest. If there are young children or heavy family responsibilities, either arrangements must be made to cope with them, the help of the medical social worker is most important here, or the woman must be treated as an inpatient. Similarly if she does not tolerate treatment well as an outpatient, she must be admitted.

Inpatient The patient who is well but is an inpatient for social reasons likewise presents few problems. Her one real enemy is probably boredom. Most women have their own remedies, but if necessary the occupational therapist can usually help. Rest in bed after return from treatment should be the rule, even if a woman insists that she does not feel tired.

The importance of building up morale should not by now need emphasising. A woman should be encouraged to make herself attractive, a visit from the hospital hairdresser can be a very good mental tonic. A friendly ear encourages her to chat about her family and plan for her return home.

General   Moist desquamation usually only occurs in the axilla, or, if the breast is still intact and pendulous, in the inframammary fold. Aqueous gentian violet 1% will help to dry this and provide a temporary covering until healing is complete, the patient should be warned that this stings at first. Hydrocortisone cream or spray may also be used.

Nausea is usually experienced in the first 24 hours – this persists in some patients, requiring anti-emetics or vitamin B, pyridoxine. Radiation of the supra-clavicular area affects the throat, and the patient can complain of a sore throat in the third week. Similarly the field over the internal mammary chain can produce dysphagia due to oesophagitis. Although usually temporary and re-covering after treatment stops, a swab should be taken to check for monilial infection. If present nystatin must be given. Weekly blood counts are carried out. If the white-cell count falls too low, below 2,000 mm^3, treatment is intr-rupted for a few days and not resumed until the count has recovered. These reactions are often proportional to fatigue.

Surgery

There must be every encouragement to get the patient to carry out her post-mastectomy exercises. Care must be taken that she does not develop either trick movements to spare her shoulder, or over vigorous movements too early. She needs to be instructed in the care of her arm, particularly if later the compli-cation of lymphoedema occurs. Various operations and compressing splints have been devised for this, but in addition care of the skin and avoidance of trauma are important.

Medical Social Worker

All patients should be seen by the medical social worker. Many can cope with their problems quite satisfactorily with the help of their families. Others may need provision of a home help, aid in making arrangements to care for children, or financial assistance. A woman who is working can be the sole support of elderly relatives and her financial plight can be parlous. Both government and voluntary funds are available to help her, but she often needs the tactful assistance of the medical social worker in making the necessary application.

Care of the Advanced Case

Some patients who are having Stage III tumours treated may be able to have treatment as outpatients. It is important in these cases to be aware that symp-toms of distant metastases not detected by previous investigations may occur quite suddenly. Without dwelling unduly on the subject, watch should be kept for any unusual breathlessness, severe headache, skeletal pain, or deterioration in the general condition. Questions can be asked during casual conversation. The alert nurse or radiographer can be invaluable in early recognition of these symptoms.

Many patients will need admission. The problems they present will vary with each individual. It will probably be most useful to discuss them in separate groups.

Ulceration and Fungation

This is one of the most distressing conditions for the patient. There is discharge, occasionally bleeding, and usually foetor due to infection of the ulcer. Pain is variable and is often surprisingly slight or absent. The ulcer needs gentle, careful cleansing, often two or three times a day. Non-adherent dressings make tending the wound less painful, and traumatising the surface each time is avoided. Elastoplast must not be used to keep the dressings in place, Sellotape or one of the tubular elastic nets can be just as effective. The elastic net dressings can also serve as a supporting brassiere and may do much to relieve pain in a pendulous breast. Occasionally when there is a good deal of necrotic tissue present haemorrhage occurs. Firm pressure is usually all that is needed to stop this. It is frightening to the patient and calm reassurance is very necessary.

Effusions

When tapping of an effusion is necessary for a patient's comfort the opportunity may be taken to attempt control by instilling a cytotoxic drug or a radioactive isotope. Aspiration is continued until there is a dry tap or the patient shows signs of physical distress. The cytotoxic or isotope is then injected and the needle withdrawn. The dressing applied must be waterproof. Apart from the usual observations of pulse and temperature, the patient must be turned regularly every half hour for the next 24 hours to ensure an even distribution. Very rarely an accumulation of a radioactive isotope in one spot has caused necrosis and the formation of a fistula. A physicist always attends if an isotope is being injected, to set up the apparatus, advise on precautions and protection, and monitor for contamination.

Hormones and Steroids

The nursing problems with patients who are receiving hormones or steroids are mostly a matter of vigilance for side effects. When androgen therapy is initiated a course of radiation to a skeletal deposit is often being given in the department, but arrangements should be made for injections to be continued by the community nurse after completion. Nausea should be reported, this can usually be controlled by an anti-emetic, altering the dose, or giving another preparation.

If steroids are being given, or a patient has had either a hypophysectomy or adrenalectomy, the usual response by the adrenals to stress is lost. Profound disturbance can follow, a fall in blood pressure, alteration of the blood electrolytes sodium and potassium, and generalised weakness, shock, and coma. The patient must understand that if she has an infection her tablets must be increased, that she should always carry her steroid card so that if she has an accident or requires an anaesthetic she can be given hydrocortisone injections, and that if she has prolonged vomiting she must call her doctor as she requires injectable hydrocortisone. In hospital any crisis involving these patients must be reported. The case history of one of my patients illustrates the problem and the remedy.

A woman had had a hypophysectomy and was stabilised on steroids. She had extensive ulceration of the chest wall and to speed healing she was given a course of radiation. She lived too far away for daily travel and so was admitted. As she was extremely well she was allowed to go home at weekends. On one Saturday evening she began to vomit and continued to do so at intervals through the night. She felt very ill but did not wish to call her doctor out in the night. The next day her husband was so alarmed that he returned with her to the hospital. When seen by me the following day she was semi-comatose, her pulse was rapid, weak, and thready, and her blood pressure low. An intravenous infusion was immediately set up with dextrose saline and hydrocortisone 100 mg. was given intravenously. Blood was taken for electrolyte analysis, both sodium and potassium were reduced, sodium dangerously so. The fluid was now changed for double-strength saline and two pints were given, the hydrocortisone 100 mg was continued four-hourly, and one gram of potassium was added to one bottle of saline. By the afternoon she was sitting up, and in the evening it was difficult to believe she was the same woman. The infusion was continued slowly overnight with normal saline and discontinued next day. She was a very intelligent woman and was able to grasp the reason for her collapse, she assured me she would not repeat her mistake.

Supportive Measures

These patients represent a range of conditions from those who are comparatively well and leading fairly normal lives, to those who are extremely ill requiring skilled and sympathetic nursing. The care of these patients is a matter of co-operation not only between nurse, doctor and ancillary workers, but also between hospital staff and the family.

Ideally a ward round for all who care for the patient should take place once a week. Failing this every effort must be made to see that everyone knows exactly what the patient and her relatives have been told, what the aim of treatment is, and the prognosis. In the out-patient department the medical social worker will be seen most often, but both the occupational and physiotherapist may be asked for help from time to time.

All who are in contact with the patient should be prepared to listen. A casual remark can give a clue to problems which the patient is too shy or proud to discuss. Symptoms of nausea or mental stress should be reported, the doctor can help both by appropriate medication. The informed nurse or radiographer, knowing the policy of treatment, can continue the physical and mental rehabilitation of the patient by encouraging exercises, rest, and taking the same attitude as the doctor at the first interview.

Physical

Physical aids often keep a patient mobile and can be provided by the Health Service. It may be a stick, a tripod, walking frame, or wheelchair. If the latter is provided it may be necessary for a home visitor to call and assess what rearrangements or alterations to the home are required. They are often simple and financial help can be given if needed. Sometimes rehousing can be arranged, local authorities though under pressure from housing lists are usually very sympathetic. The home nursing of a patient confined to bed can be eased by the provision of a ripple bed.

Patients with vertebral deposits can gain great benefit from a supporting corset or collar. The surgical fitter who is used to dealing with this type of case is invaluable. Endless trouble is taken to see that the fit is correct and the whole appliance though strong is not too heavy.

Social

The social needs of the patient and her family are varied and require time and patience if they are to be met. Financial problems often loom large, and if not solved may make a woman unable to rest or follow the required medical regime. With the consent of the patient employers can be approached, they are usually willing to help and can often arrange lighter work.

If the patient has facilities for making the journey and wishes to do so she should be allowed to return home at weekends. If she is too ill or complications such as fracture are anticipated, this will not be possible. The criteria however should not be too strict. It is often difficult for nurses to understand why patients who are obviously unwell should be allowed out of hospital. If it is realised that the overall prognosis is unlikely to be affected and that the woman's mental well-being and human needs are as important as her physical state, then the decision is easy to understand.

When the family is actually nursing the patient the burden can be very great. The physical task can be prolonged and exacting, the stress of watching deterioration and knowing there can be no cure makes the mental burden even greater. It is important for relief to be available. The community nurse can provide some help, and often the neighbours and volunteers from local groups will sit in and enable the family to have a vital break and rest. A most helpful development has been the provision of specially trained nurses in patients' homes. This is a service funded by voluntary organisations. It is most necessary to foresee and arrange for patients to be admitted to special centres if it becomes impossible to nurse them right up to the end at home. This is discussed more fully in a later chapter.

Post-operative Care

After ablation operations the patient is nursed in accordance with normal surgical procedures, but one or two points are worth making.

Oophorectomy

After oophorectomy the woman usually recovers quickly. The sudden cessation of ovarian activity often means that menopausal symptoms are severe. The oestrogens usually used to control 'hot flushes' are forbidden, they negate the operation and reliance must be placed on sedatives.

Adrenalectomy

Adrenalectomy involves the sudden loss of all the substances secreted by the adrenal cortex and medulla. The patient returns from theatre with an intravenous infusion and a planned regime for hydrocortisone supplements both in the fluid and by intramuscular injection. One of the immediate post-operative complications may be a fall in blood pressure. This is overcome by adding sympathomimetic drugs to the infusion fluid. Estimations of the blood electrolytes must be carried out daily, the composition of the intravenous fluid being adjusted according to the results, fludrocortisone given if necessary later.

Hypophysectomy is usually performed by an ear, nose, and throat surgeon either by a surgical excision or by a radioactive implant. The approach is by the nasal route. Care must be taken to avoid infection as there is always a slight leak of cerebrospinal fluid for a few days. Pitressin is given post-operatively to control the excessive loss of water in the urine due to lack of antidiuretic hormone. Usually this recovers and the injections or snuff can be discontinued. Cortisone supplements are started immediately after operation, later thyroxine may be required and also fludrocortisone to regulate the sodium/potassium ratio.

It is again stressed that patients who have had either of these last two operations require steroid supplements for the rest of their lives. They and their families must be educated to realise the importance of infection and stress so that appropriate measures can be taken.

Section VI

Follow-up

After irradiation is completed the patient is seen one week later, and if she is an outpatient, provided that any reaction is progressing satisfactorily, thereafter at one month, then at three months, and finally six monthly. These appointments can be made alternatively with the surgeon and radiotherapist, or the patient can be seen at a combined clinic. If the woman has been an inpatient she must not be discharged if the reaction is very fierce nor if her home circumstances are unsuitable for adequate rest. If she is allowed to go home the care of the skin and the sequence of the reaction must be carefully explained to her.

At each clinic attendance enquiries are made about general health, and specific questions put on breathlessness, cough, aches and pains. The local site is then examined, the other breast, the lymphatic drainage areas and the liver. If oedema of the arm is present soon after treatment, it is probably due to interference with the pathways in the axilla. If two or three years elapse before its occurrence then it is likely to be due to recurrence in the axillary or supra-clavicular nodes. In the early stages an elastic stocking or an inflatable splint can give some control, but when established there is little that can be done. Very rarely malignant change, usually a lymphosarcoma, can arise in the oede-matous arm.

Every six months a blood count, chest and pelvis X-rays are ordered. Metastases can be present in either site and be quite symptomless. Other X-rays are requested according to the symptoms, once yearly a mammogram of the other breast is performed. Three per cent of women who have had carcinoma of one breast develop a fresh primary in the other. If the breast which was the primary site was not removed this is also X-rayed.

After five years the interval between appointments will be lengthened. Objection is often made to the frequency of visits on the grounds that this arouses so much fear and disturbs the patient. Unfortunately while many recur-rences will occur within the first five years, the disease is unpredictable. Although then no longer curable, much can be done to maintain the quality of life, and this is more easily achieved if recurrence is treated promptly.

Advanced Cases

The timing of appointments will vary in each case. If on hormone or steroid therapy certain blood tests are performed routinely, these are used to assess reactivity of the tumour and therapy response. The type of test depends on the available laboratory facilities. The common ones are for the levels of calcium, and alkaline phosphatase, a rise can indicate reactivity particularly of bone metastases. Other tests estimate glyco-proteins and certain enzymes both as a measure of tumour response and possibly as a guide to future sensitivity.

The same routine at follow-up appointments is followed but adapted ac-cording to the pattern of disease. Hormones and steroids are adjusted, with-drawn, or started as part of a policy individual to each patient.

Chemotherapy

Patients who are receiving cytotoxics must attend for blood counts prior to therapy. Good organisation prevents unnecessary delays and consequent increase in tension.

Prognosis

This is dependent upon two factors, the degree of histological differentiation and the stage at the time of diagnosis.

Patients with intraduct, in situ carcinoma, have a good prognosis, figures of 95% 5 year survival have been quoted. Unfortunately the numbers of such patients are not great. Some tumours disseminate early and despite all treatment there is no response, others progress locally but do not disseminate widely, but the majority seem to grow to about 2 cms and then begin to spread.

Considering all cases treated there is a 5 year survival of 40%, at 10 years 25%. If all the histological grades are considered together those with no lymph node involvement have a 75% 5 year survival, falling to 30% when nodes are infiltrated. However, if the tumour is histological grade I and no lymph nodes are involved the figure rises to 80% or more.

Cure is difficult to assess, particularly since there is no agreement on its exact definition. Patients who survive to 15 years with no recurrence, may still relapse later. It is therefore probably best to use this word with extreme caution.

Summary

What can we say of the present situation? We know some facts about this disease but much remains unknown. Advances can come at any point. Early diagnosis is desirable. Women are being encouraged to carry out self examination of the breast.

Popular press articles and leaflets are available on the technique, but where arrangements can be made for practical instruction the examination is probably better executed. Screening programmes in the U.S.A. have led to claims that the mortality rate has fallen in consequence, but doubts have been expressed about the interpretation of data. Currently in the United Kingdom screening programmes using mammography and clinical examination are being compared with self examination and control groups. Fears about the radiation dose to the breast have been largely overcome by the use of improved techniques which have reduced the dose. The aim is to detect the tumour while it is less than 2 cms and preferably 1 cm or less. At that size there is a good chance that adequate local treatment will cure the local disease, and that spread beyond the lymph nodes is far less likely to have occurred.

The majority of well women in these schemes will not develop breast carcinoma, and the repeated examination may induce anxiety rather than reassurance. If reliable prognostic indicators of a predisposition to carcinoma could be found this would be useful. Some factors are known, but neither alone nor in combination are they able to select with complete accuracy the 'at risk' population. Different tests have been suggested, markers (substances in the blood either in excess or abnormally) and ratios of hormone metabolites, but they have proved largely non-specific or not repeatable when applied to other populations.

We need to know more about the host-tumour relationship. What part does immunity play? When the history has been a long one, is this a reflection of a less malignant type of tumour, or is it due to resistance by the host? Metastases have become active after a recurrence-free period of twenty years or more, what factors are responsible for this?

Present methods of treatment do not appear to have lengthened survival time appreciably. What they have done is to improve its quality. It is unlikely that any refinements of technique alone will advance therapy. Only when the disease is better understood and detected can treatment be logical rather than empirical, and other methods devised. Meanwhile the value of present methods of treatment can be assessed objectively only by clinical trials. This is not unethical since all regimes have proven value. By matching the patients as closely as possible with regard to age and staging and following their subsequent progress, any clear benefit conferred by one particular method should become apparent. Unfortunately such studies must take time, nothing is worse than premature conclusions, particularly if, as a consequence, patients are submitted to unpleasant regimes which are subsequently found to be less effective than originally thought.

In the wildest dreams of our younger days we aspire to master the disease. With advancing years and wisdom, doubt creeps into the crevices of the mind, doubt that as yet the disease is master after all.

Section VII

Carcinoma of the Male Breast

Operable Cases

If operable a mastectomy is performed, this usually entails skin grafting of the operative site. The same radiation policy is followed as in females.

Advanced Cases

Although it has been suggested that the initiation of cancer of the male breast may be due to abnormal sensitivity to normal oestrogen levels, or to high levels of the hormone, once established many tumours appear to be androgen dependent. Orchidectomy often produces striking improvement. In one series regression of tumour was noted in 68% of patients who were castrated. If these measures fail, or there is recurrence, the same kind of therapy choices must be made as for females.

Prognosis

Even operable cases do less well than females. Most patients already have blood borne metastases at the time of consultation.

The pelvis is an arena.
In the peace-time parade,
Each actor plays his part
In harmony, but independent of all others.
In battle, all is changed.
For each becomes dependent upon the actions of all the rest.

16 The Female Reproductive System

Cervix

Carcinoma of the cervix when at a pre-invasive stage may usually be cured by adequate treatment. For this reason intensive screening efforts have been concentrated on it, and figures for the States, and for England and Wales, do show a decline in the number of deaths. Nevertheless the tumour is responsible for about 2.5% of all deaths from malignant disease in the U.K., and there is a trend for it to appear at an earlier age.

Age

The average age of patients is between 40 and 50, but in women found on screening to have pre-invasive cancer, it is around the mid-thirties.

Aetiology

Many suggestions have been made concerning possible carcinogenic agents, none as yet proven, but certain observations lead inevitably to the conclusion that a high risk of developing the disease follows the occurrence of first intercourse at an early age. Statistics show that the disease is more common among women with large families or poor economic and social background, prostitutes, certain racial or religious communities, or when there is early intercourse, or multiple partners. By contrast the disease is rare in nuns and Jewish women. It has been stated that all women over the age of 16 who have sexual activity in their teens enter the high-risk group. These facts must be borne in mind when planning screening programmes. A few cases arise in a cervical polyp or in relation to chronic cervicitis or a laceration, but these predisposing conditions are not given the importance once attached to them. An interim survey has not established any link between oral contraceptives and the disease, nevertheless a close watch needs to be kept on the situation.

The discovery that type 2 herpes simplex virus was frequently found associated with carcinoma of the cervix led to popular journalism identifying the virus as the cause of cervical cancer. This has not definitely been proved. It certainly causes genital herpes, a condition which can be severe in some patients. If a vaccine for this is developed, its use may supply the proof at present lacking. Other possible carcinogens are the male smegma, and sperm DNA, and some investigators have suggested that the sexual habits of the male partner may be of some importance.

The close link with sexual activity has led the condition to be labelled 'venereal' by some. While it is true that women treated for sexually transmitted diseases may be at risk and should perhaps be subsequently screened, the label could be counter productive by making women hesitate about a 'smear' test for fear of being thought promiscuous.

Anatomy

The uterus and ovaries lie within the true pelvis. Probably one of the most important facts to grasp is the close relationship to other structures, in front the bladder, on either side the ureter, and behind the rectum. The covering epithelium of the cavity of the uterus and the cervix is in continuity with that of the vagina.

Uterus

The uterus consisting of fundus, body, and cervix, is a midline structure, pear-shaped and about three inches long. Normally it is bent forward, anteverted, over the bladder and is separated from it only by the peritoneum which covers it and sweeps forward on to the upper surface of the bladder. It is suspended within a fold of peritoneum which runs across the pelvis from side to side, this is the broad ligament. The round ligaments run from the uterus to the inguinal canal and are attached to the labia majores. The uterus narrows to a waist, the isthmus, and continues downwards as the cervix. The vagina circles the cervix at its mid point. Internally the uterine cavity continues into the cervix as the cervical canal, the junction is called the internal cervical os. The external os is situated where the canal opens into the vagina, in women who have not borne children it is round but becomes slit-like after childbirth.

The epithelium of the uterus is cuboidal forming simple tubular glands. At the internal os this becomes columnar and the glands branching. The vaginal cervix is covered with a stratified squamous epithelium continuous with that of the vagina. Under the microscope a definite junction between the columnar and squamous epithelium can be seen.

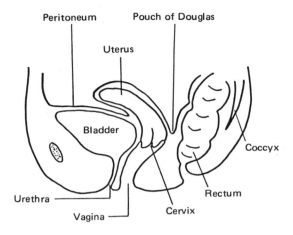

Fig. 16.1.   Female pelvic organs

Relations

We have already seen that the uterus normally rests on the bladder, behind there is a pouch lined by peritoneum, the pouch of Douglas. It separates the uterus from the rectum and often contains loops of intestine. Lying half-an-inch laterally from the upper part of the cervix on each side is the ureter. If a ureteric stone is present at this point it can be felt on vaginal examination.

Fallopian Tubes

Lying in the free edge of the broad ligament are the fallopian tubes, they open into the upper part of the uterus on either side. At the other end they open into the peritoneal cavity and have delicate finger-like processes, fimbriae, closely related to the ovary. When the ovum is shed it passes into the tube and is propelled along to the cavity of the uterus.

Ovaries

The ovaries, almond-shaped, and about one-and-a-half inches long are attached to the back of the broad ligament by a small mesentery. Although usually described as lying on the side wall of the pelvis their position is extremely variable, and they can be found quite normally in the pouch of Douglas.

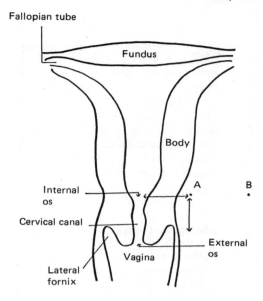

Fig. 16.2.   Longitudinal section of the uterus

Vagina

The vagina in its upper part surrounds the cervix forming a well. This is divided for convenience into fornices, anterior, posterior, and lateral. The vagina runs down and forward through the pelvic floor to open into the vestibule. Like the uterus its relationship to other organs is most important. In front the bladder and the urethra within the anterior vaginal wall, behind, the anal canal and above this the rectum and the pouch of Douglas, on either side muscles, fascia, and in the upper part, the ureters.

Blood Supply

The uterus is supplied by a branch of the internal iliac artery, the uterine artery. This artery also supplies the cervix and the upper part of the vagina and anastamoses with the ovarian artery. The vagina is supplied by branches derived ultimately from the internal iliac artery. The ovarian artery arises directly from the aorta.

The venous drainage is as follows:

Uterus — to the internal iliac veins but also communicating with the veins of the bladder and vagina.
Ovary — right side to the inferior vena cava. Left side to the left renal vein.
Vagina — to the internal iliac veins.

Lymphatic Drainage

This is complex but important. The ovarian lymphatics pass to the aortic group of nodes, but the uterus, body and cervix, and the vagina have varied drainage routes. The fundus of the uterus together with the fallopian tubes drains mainly along the same path as the ovary, but a few lymphatics run with the round ligament to the inguinal nodes. The cervix drains in three ways, sideways along the broad ligament to the external iliac nodes on the pelvic wall, along the line of the uterine vessels to the internal iliac nodes, and backwards to the nodes lying close to the sacrum. The lymphatic drainage of the vagina varies according to three zones, the upper third drains to the external and internal iliac nodes, the middle to the internal iliac nodes, and the lower to the superficial inguinal nodes.

Carcinoma of the Cervix, Pathology and Spread

Most tumours of the cervix arise at the junction of the squamous and columnar epithelium and are squamous cell carcinomata. Those which arise in the upper part are occasionally adenocarcinomata, but mostly they are squamous developing in epithelium which has changed from columnar, squamous metaplasia. Very rarely a secondary tumour occurs, a secondary from a breast carcinoma has been recorded. Spread is initially directly throughout the cervix, uterus, uterine appendages and vagina, then on to the bladder and rectum. Later lymphatic metastases to the pelvic nodes occur. Late in the disease distant blood-borne metastases arise.

From the descriptions and diagrams of the anatomy and lymphatic drainage it is easy to see why neighbouring structures are so frequently involved by tumour, and indeed why tumour arising in these structures so often invades the cervix and vagina. Lymphatic spread will surround the ureters early causing obstruction, hydronephrosis, and renal failure. Death from pyelonephritis and uraemia is common.

Staging is used to try and assess the extent of spread, but it is no more than a guide since microscopic metastases may be present in a lymph node which otherwise appears healthy. Stage 0 is the stage at which every clinician hopes to detect the carcinoma. It is called the pre-invasive stage, is symptomless, and is only detectable microscopically. The basement membrane of the epithelium is intact but the cells are atypical. Many of these carcinoma in situ fail to progress to frank malignancy, but of those that do some may take 10 to 12 years to do so, while others develop rapidly.

Stage I   Indicates spread to the cervix only (divided into two types, a and b.)

Stage II   There is spread to the fornices of the vagina, the upper vagina and the tissues such as the broad ligament.

Stage III   The spread extends out to the pelvic wall, up into the body of the uterus, down into the lower vagina and pelvic lymph nodes are involved.

Stage IV   Neighbouring structures are invaded. There is evidence of distant metastases.

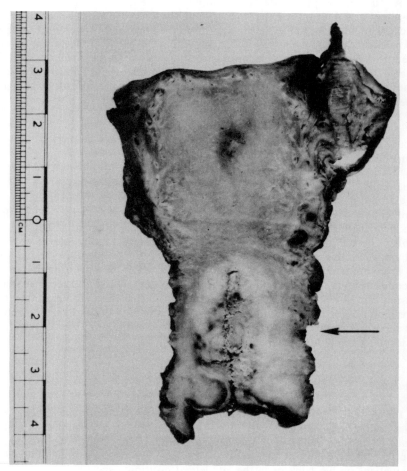

Fig. 16.3.   Carcinoma of the cervix

Symptomatology

At the pre-invasive stage there are no symptoms at all, the woman is well and has no reason to believe she has a tumour. The first symptom to occur, as the growth becomes invasive, is painless bleeding. At first this is only slight and irregular, possibly associated with coitus (intercourse) or menstruation. When the periods are present this can be mistaken for irregular menstruation, particularly if the menopause is expected, irregular bleeding is often wrongly thought to be associated with this. Bleeding is followed by discharge, at first thin and then copious and often offensive, this can be due to infection of the growth or to obstruction of the uterine canal with pus pocketing in the uterus, pyometra.

As the disease progresses all symptoms become more severe. Pain makes its appearance and denotes extension beyond the cervix. This pain can be in the back, the abdomen, the legs as sciatica, or in the knee, and is due to involvement of ligaments or direct pressure on nerves within the pelvis. If ulceration into the bladder or rectum occurs, incontinence of faeces or urine develops with discharge into the vagina. Although bleeding is often severe enough to require transfusion for the correction of anaemia, it rarely causes death, uraemia or pyelonephritis are the usual causes.

Screening

The realisation that carcinoma often preceded symptoms by many years led to a search for a method that would detect the tumour at this early stage. All epithelial surfaces shed cells, and when stains were discovered which would show up abnormalities in desquamated cells a true screening programme became possible. The method is of course the cervical smear, and there are now many clinics where this service can be obtained.

Probably it is best to take a scrape from the whole external os with a special wooden spatula, Ayres scrape. This should be done where full medical examination can be made also. It should be appreciated that this cytological screening is essentially for the symptomless woman. Invasive growths may be too necrotic to shed malignant cells, and if reliance is placed entirely on cytology in these cases frank carcinoma may be missed.

Method

If the patient's history is not known by the family doctor or she is being seen at a well woman clinic, a careful history is taken and a general examination made to exclude malignancy in other sites, notably the breast. The information should include details of the menstrual cycle and contraceptive measures. With the patient on her back or in the left lateral position a speculum is passed into the vagina to visualise the cervix and a scraping taken. The material is spread on a labelled slide and placed in fixative immediately. The minimum of lubrication should be used and any blood or discharge gently removed first, the test is not performed during menstruation. Vaginal and rectal examination follows including a bimanual. The inguinal nodes must also be examined. The smear is reported as positive, negative, or suspicious. In every 1,000 women screened, five will have positive smears and eleven will be suspicious. In the case of the latter, the patient must have repeat cytology at regular and frequent intervals, positive smears indicate a need for full investigation and biopsy. There is as yet no method by which one can predict which lesions will remain static, which will regress, or which will become invasive.

Population for Screening

Who should be included in the screening programme? The official policy is to encourage all women over the age of 35 to be examined. A brief review of the high risk group leads us to suppose that all women over 16 who are sexually active, married women, pregnant women, and women attending gynaecological clinics should be screened. The programme has been previously hampered by lack of financial resources and a shortage of trained personnel, but the age limit of 35 tends to ignore the fact that many younger women have carcinoma in situ or invasive cancer and so may die before reaching this minimum age. When automation is available then screening of the whole adult population of women will be possible.

It is also important that the test should be carried out by a doctor who will subsequently make a pelvic examination. It has already been pointed out that invasive cancer may not always give a positive smear, and if no examination is made there may be a failure of detection.

Education

There is little doubt that despite the enthusiasm of many women, and the fall in the death rate in the over 35 group, there is still much to be done. The women who are most at risk often do not attend clinics. Many employers co-operate and allow their women workers to attend talks and have the test performed during working time. It is most necessary that facilities for doing the test are available at the same time, these women will rarely attend again if they cannot have their test at the first visit. Women who have a negative smear should have the first repeat at 12 months in order to try and pick up any whose first test was a false negative. Thereafter ideally it should be an annual procedure, but with the present resources available a reasonable compromise is once every three years. The suspicious smear is repeated in three to four weeks, and if still suspicious, every three months as long as these results are obtained. This may have to continue for life. Patients with positive smears are submitted to further investigation and treatment.

What can be expected from such screening programmes? It must be realised that many pre-invasive cancers probably never progress to malignancy, some may regress, other malignancies may never pass through this early stage, while yet others are incurable by the available methods whatever the stage of the disease. Although these facts must be accepted, of equal importance are the statistics drawn from the results of earlier screening programmes. In British Columbia the incidence of invasive cancer fell from 28.4 to 19.7 per 100,000 while in the population screened new disease was only at the rate of 4.5 per 100,000 compared with 20 per 100,000 in the unscreened population. In addition after nine years the mortality figures began to decline, only time will show if this trend continues, particularly in view of the increasing incidence in women under 35.

A very positive gain from the screening programme has been a change in the attitude of women. Every woman who has a smear knows that this is a test for cancer. She hopes that it will be negative, but knows that even if she has the disease help can be given her. The doctor is now able because of this to discuss the subject freely with his patient, in time this new attitude should begin to transfer to malignancy of other organs, and as women survive due to having treatment, fear will diminish. The advantage of having the smear taken in the clinic by trained personnel is the trust which is built up, and the chance to widen the examination to include other systems.

Further Examination and Investigations

Exactly the same examination procedure is followed initially as after the cervical smear. When growth is clinically obvious there is usually little doubt of malignancy. The constant finding is the amount of bleeding which takes place on gentle contact. On the vaginal cervix the early lesion appears as a nodule, a small ulcer, or a small area looking like an erosion. As the growth develops it can be described as looking like a cauliflower or an ulcer with hard, raised, everted edges. Carcinoma within the cervical canal may show no abnormality on examination in the early stages. It may only be discovered on curettage for irregular bleeding. Later the cervix becomes hard and enlarged, sloughing occurs, and deep excavation is found.

Occasionally other conditions such as cervicitis, erosion, or tuberculosis may be mistaken for carcinoma. The diagnosis is easily settled by biopsy.

Investigations

A blood count must be performed to assess the presence of anaemia and its degree. Blood biochemistry is necessary as a gross measure of kidney function prior to I.V.P. A chest X-ray is important before anaesthesia to establish freedom from pulmonary metastases. Further investigation will vary according to the findings at the initial examination.

Positive Smear, No Clinical Findings

If the smear merely shows dysplasia some centres will place the patient on a close follow up regime, treating the areas with cryosurgery, laser therapy, or diathermy, and repeating the smears every three months. Others will proceed to biopsy as for a positive smear. The former policy may particularly be preferred if the patient is young and anxious about fertility.

Colposcopy

A colposcope is a binocular microscope which enables the cervix to be examined under magnification. Lugol's iodine or acetic acid may be used to show up abnormal areas to be biopsied.

X-rays

Very early, involvement of lymph nodes near the ureter can occur. It is essential therefore to X-ray the kidneys, the ureters, and the bladder by means of an I.V.P. With modern contrast media and techniques it is rare now for retrograde pyelography (passing catheters into the ureter from the bladder) to be necessary. In some centres a radioactive scan of the kidneys is also performed. As part of the preparation for these investigations an M.S.U. for culture and sensitivity is taken.

E.U.A. and Biopsy

When these investigations are complete the final procedure is an examination under anaesthesia and biopsy. Not only are the cervix, vagina, and pelvic floor fully examined, but a cytoscopy and sigmoidoscopy are done at this time. Finally a biopsy is taken, this can be either a punch biopsy of areas indicated by previous tests, or a cone biopsy. Cone biopsy removes the external os together with a cone of tissue, previous coloscopy makes it possible to tailor the cone according to the findings.

Histology

If the cone biopsy shows carcinoma in situ, many centres take no further surgical steps but keep the patient on three-month follow-up. If microinvasive carcinoma is found, policy varies. Some centres follow the same policy as for carcinoma in situ, others advise a more radical operation.

Positive Smear with Clinical Findings

Additional Investigations

The same investigations as for the other group of patients are made but not colposcopy. Instead pelvic ultrasound or CATscans will be done and a lymphogram. It is extremely important to know if there is any evidence of lymphatic spread, and so lymphography should always be carried out. Unsuspected involvement of lymph nodes may well alter the staging and render necessary a change in the planned treatment. Barium enema, arteriography, phlebography, skeletal survey may be required if signs or symptoms suggest spread of the disease not shown on other investigations.

E.U.A. and Biopsy

Examination under anaesthesia as already described is performed. Punch biopsy is carried out. The assessment of any pelvic spread is vital, for on this will depend the type and extent of treatment.

Established Case with Symptoms

The same investigations are carried out as for the patient with only a positive smear and clinical findings. If carcinoma within the canal is diagnosed, then dilatation and curettage of the uterus and canal must be performed to exclude a uterine growth invading the canal. The curettings from each site must be placed in labelled bottles and the sites noted on the request for histology.

Smears and Pregnancy

Since smears are performed in the ante-natal clinic it is inevitable that some will be reported as suspicious or positive. The former are followed two- to three-monthly during pregnancy and thereafter as already described. The patient with a positive smear presents a more difficult problem. The question to be answered is whether this is invasive carcinoma. Simple inspection of the cervix is of little help since during pregnancy it often looks unhealthy. Colposcopy using Schiller's test can be used as a guide to punch biopsy, cone biopsy carries a high risk of haemorrhage, abortion, or difficulty in subsequent labour due to scarring. Frank invasive carcinoma is a different problem, close-to-term treatment can be postponed until after delivery, earlier in pregnancy it will be a matter for clinical judgment, whether to terminate pregnancy and proceed to surgery, or to adopt a policy of close observation and wait until term. These decisions cannot be taken by the doctor alone. There must be full discussion with the patient and her husband and decisions made with their full agreement.

Treatment

The regime adopted will depend upon the clinical staging. The surgery available varies from local excision to radical procedures such as pelvic exenteration. No opinion is expressed as to their relative value, each has been proven and much will depend upon the past experiences of the surgeon concerned. Definite answers will only be available when comparative trials, as for carcinoma of the breast, have reached adequate numbers and follow-up periods to allow valid conclusions to be drawn.

Treatment Policy

Stage 0. Carcinoma in situ. Cone biopsy, or total hysterectomy with a cuff of vagina.
Stages I and II. Total hysterectomy with a cuff of vagina, ± removal of nearby nodes, or Wertheim hysterectomy or radiation.
Stage III. Occasionally surgery, usually radiotherapy, surgery for palliation.
Stage IV. Radiotherapy. Surgery for palliation.
All cases submitted for curative treatment should have regular follow-up with cytological smears.

Cone Biopsy

This operation is often preferred for the woman who has not completed her family. It is also regarded by some authorities as curative. It is a procedure that has however both immediate and late complications. The operation must be performed in hospital and the patient kept in for observation afterwards for a few days. The most important immediate complications are haemorrhage and to a lesser extent infection. Later the woman can experience irregular or heavy bleeding, pain on intercourse, or difficulty in subsequent labour owing to an incompetent or stenosed cervix. Inflammation in the parametria is maximal 14 days after biopsy, if hysterectomy is to be carried out it should be postponed for at least one month.

Hysterectomy

Total hysterectomy involves the removal of both the uterus and the cervix. It is now usual to take also a cuff of vagina since it is here that recurrences tend to occur.

Extended

Since lymphatic spread occurs so often, some surgeons attempt to remove the tubes and ovaries together with the local nodes.

Wertheim

This is a very radical procedure and even in skilled hands the morbidity is high and mortality is 3–4%. The aim is to remove all the lymphatic tissue, the rationale being that even in late disease spread is often confined within the pelvis. The bladder, ureters, rectum, large nerves and vessels together with enough peritoneum to cover the pelvic floor are left, all other pelvic tissues including most of the vagina are removed.

Pelvic Exenteration

This operation is only considered in a few cases. It is performed when invasion of the rectum or bladder, or both, has occurred, but distant metastases have not been found. The uterus, bladder and vagina are removed, the ureters being implanted into the sigmoid colon. If the rectum also has to be removed a colostomy is formed. The ureters are either implanted into the colon above this, or into a bladder made from a loop of ileum, a separate opening on the abdominal wall, urinostomy, is then required.

Radiotherapy

This is given in two ways, contact therapy by means of a radioactive source which is left in place for a few hours and then removed, and externally by conventional or megavoltage therapy to the pelvis. The reason for the split treatment is that it is impossible to deliver the same dose to the whole pelvis as that required locally at the cervix, the tolerance of normal tissues would be exceeded. The aim is to deliver a high local dose by intracavitary radiation and bring up the dose at the pelvic side walls by external radiation.

Radioactive Source

A source can treat a small block of tissue, placed in the uterus and fornices of the vagina it delivers a high local dose. A point 2 cm from the midline of the cervical canal and 2 cm above the lateral fornix is known as point A, and at this spot the ureters cross the uterine vessels. The source is left in place long enough, in separate applications, to give a dose at point A sufficient to destroy the tumour, but not enough to cause necrosis and fistula formation. Two centimetres further out laterally is the pelvic wall, point B. Because radiation falls off with distance, the dose at point B is less, so this is supplemented with external radiation. Due allowance is made for the small amount which will reach point A and raise the dose further. Insertions are made at an interval of a week and may be two or three in number.

External Radiation

The field includes the pelvis and the vagina. Shielding is used to cut off radiation from the central area previously treated. Treatment can be by conventional or megavoltage therapy and will last four to six weeks. The timing in relation to insertions varies entirely according to the centre, in some it will precede, in others it will be given in an interval or after insertions are completed.

Insertion

Different centres use varying sources, but all are designed to deliver a dosage according to the basic principles. To prevent slipping and misalignment of the source, special spacers to fix them or keep them apart can be employed. Attention has been directed towards protecting the operator from the radiation to which he is exposed. Machines have been developed whereby catheters are put in position and then the sources brought up through these into place by remote control.

The method described here is one developed in Stockholm and still regarded as standard in many centres. The preparation of the patient will be described in the section on nursing care at the end of the chapter. One point only will be mentioned here. Close attention must be paid to the temperature and the total white-cell count before insertion. A slight elevation of either or both may be the only indication of a pyometra. Since foul discharge is often present in these patients, and there is also the risk of discovering an unexpected pyometra, they are normally left until the end of the theatre list.

Method

After the patient is anaesthetised and prepared, the bladder is catheterised and emptied. The doctor carries out an E.U.A. then changes gloves for the insertion.

The cervix is grasped under direct vision with volsellum forceps and the canal is located with a sound. When the canal is stenosed or obscured by growth this may not be easy. Dilators of increasing size are passed. If a pyometra is discovered, no attempt is made to make an insertion. The uterus is drained, if necessary a drain is placed in position, and the patient is returned to the ward.

The source in the form of a tube and two boxes has been sterilised, and if it is not being inserted under remote control, is kept in a protective container until needed. Each source is threaded for easy recovery.

The doctor picks up the tube in long handled forceps, an assistant withdraws the last dilator and the tube is slipped into position. A box, with its thin end in the antero-posterior plane, is placed in each fornix. The strings are held out of the way and the vagina packed with gauze. Care is taken to keep the boxes separated and pack them off from the rectum behind. A probe connected to a radiation monitoring device is passed into the rectum, and if the dose is too high the vagina is repacked or the sources changed.

Before return to the ward X-rays of the pelvis are taken. This checks that the sources are correctly placed and have not slipped, and also whether the position of the uterus is grossly abnormal. If it is the radiation plans can be altered to take account of this.

In the Ward

Back in the ward the catheter is connected to a continuous drainage bag. A portable protective screen is wheeled up over the bed. The operation notices will indicate when the source is due for removal, usually after 24 or 48 hours. Meanwhile the patient is placed on a light diet with plenty of fluids and kept in bed. An hour before removal is due, an injection of a strong analges such as pethidine is given. The vulva is then cleansed and the pack gently withdrawn. The patient is asked to breathe deeply and relax. The strings are identified and with gentle traction each source usually slips out. It is grasped with long-handled forceps and placed in a protective container, a little peroxide solution is usually added. If there is any difficulty the patient is taken to theatre and the sources removed after full anaesthesia, this is a very rare occurrence. The catheter is withdrawn last of all.

Chemotherapy

This is not a primary treatment. No cytotoxic drug specific to carcinoma of the cervix has been discovered, and no existing substance has been shown to have any clear advantage over any other.

Advanced Case and Recurrence

Stage III carcinoma is treated with radiation. The combination of external and intracavitary sources is employed. The advanced stage IV growth requires palliation of symptoms. If bleeding is severe a 48-hour radioactive insertion, probably boxes only, can often provide some relief. Occasionally whole-pelvis radiation is justified, but more often good nursing and adequate analgesia are the only measures justifiable.

The elderly patient who presents with a malignancy of the cervix often has a more slowly-growing type of tumour. Both for advanced and stage I and II growths, provided the patient is fit for anaesthesia, a 48-hour radium insertion is usually sufficient to afford palliation of symptoms for the natural span of life.

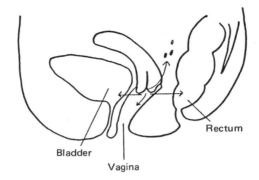

Fig. 16.4.   Spread of carcinoma of the uterus

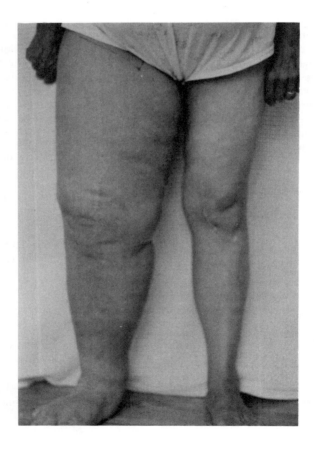

Fig. 16.5.   Oedema of the leg due to pelvic obstruction by carcinoma

Palliative Surgery

When faecal incontinence, or conversely obstruction of the bowel develops, a relieving colostomy can be fashioned. The operation is short and can be performed in all but the very ill patient.

Urinary incontinence is a much more difficult problem. Re-implantation of the ureters is a lengthy operation and there is little hope of repairing the fistula. Insertion of a catheter may be sufficient to keep the bladder empty particularly if it is inserted early before the fistula becomes too large.

Pain

When pain is intractable and analgesics have lost their effect, relief can be obtained by interrupting the pain pathways. Formerly this was done by injecting alcohol around the nerves and ganglia, or by cutting the tract in the cord carrying the sensation of pain at the appropriate level; this is called cordotomy. It is now possible by intrathecal injections of phenol to achieve the same effect without operating, but if bilateral there is a risk of permanent faecal or urinary incontinence. When this is already established the risk is obviously non-existent, but in a patient who is still able to get about and reasonably well apart from the pain, the arguments for and against must be carefully considered.

Oedema of the Legs

When this is due to lymphatic obstruction little can be done. Elastic stockings give some relief occasionally, but the benefit is usually temporary. If the obstruction is venous then the use of stockings is often more helpful unless the return from the pelvic veins is completely blocked.

Recurrence

Lower vaginal recurrence is treated by an insertion. Boxes placed in tandem one above the other in a vertical line, or occasionally needles mounted in a rubber corrugated drain, can be packed into place against the lesion. If the whole vagina has been fully radiated no further therapy can be given. Similarly since the pelvis receives the maximum dosage tolerated by normal tissues no further treatment is possible. Occasionally extensive surgery, pelvic exenteration, is justified. In some instances nodes seen on lymphogram to be clear may later become involved, the radio-opaque dye remains in the nodes for several months and changes can be seen. If these nodes are outside the previously treated area, they can be irradiated. Effusions in the peritoneal or pleural cavities are dealt with in the normal way.

Cervical Stump Carcinoma

This is now more rarely seen since subtotal hysterectomy leaving the cervix behind is performed less and less. Treatment is by radiation omitting the intra-uterine tube.

Follow-up

At each visit a smear is taken and a full examination is made. If the patient has given a history of any symptoms the appropriate investigations are ordered.

Prognosis

Untreated about 90% of patients die within three years of diagnosis (invasive carcinoma). For the rest, if treated, stages Ia and Ib have a five years survival of virtually 100% and 75%, while for stage III and IV the figures are 25% and 5% respectively. Death is usually due to renal failure consequent on obstruction of the urinary tract by disease.

CARCINOMA OF THE UTERUS

Age and Incidence

Although the body and fundus form with the cervix the whole uterus, carcinoma in this area differs in many respects from that occurring in the cervix. The age group affected is older, the peak age of incidence being 55, and the death rate is lower, about 1,000 annually, or 1% of all deaths from malignant disease. The women affected also differ, it is commonest in the unmarried or the childless; of the married women, about 50% have never been pregnant. Cancer of the cervix is twice as common as malignancy of the body of the uterus.

Aetiology

Where there is hyperplasia, overgrowth of the lining of the uterus (endometrium) there is a tendency for carcinoma to develop, and current opinion inclines to the view that tumours arise as a result of hormone imbalance, particularly oestrogen stimulation. Some surveys have linked prolonged oestrogen administration to palliate menopausal symptoms with later development of carcinoma, but this may be an association of menopausal disorders requiring oestrogen therapy, being then associated with an incipient cancer. Certain rare tumours of the ovary secrete oestrogen and induce hyperplasia of the endometrium, carcinoma then developing later. Obesity and diabetes are also related to increased incidence. Fibroids may be found at the same time as carcinoma, but are not a predisposing factor.

Menstrual Cycle

Uterus	*Ovary*	*Hormone*
Day 1-5 menstruation and repair of endometrium	Graafian follicle	Rising level of oestrogen
Day 6-14 proliferation of endometrium	Graafian follicle	Oestrogen
Day 14	Ovulation	Oestrogen
	Follicle → corpus luteum	progesterone
Day 15-28 proliferation and thickening of endometrium	Corpus luteum	Oestrogen progesterone
Day 1 Menstruation Fall in oestrogen and progesterone	Degeneration of corpus luteum	

Very recent work has postulated a difference in the age at which gonads and adrenals become mature resulting in a hormone imbalance, and thereby leading to cancer induction.

Hormones and the Menstrual Cycle

The menstrual cycle is initiated and controlled by the hormones secreted by the ovary, but the ovary in turn is both stimulated by, and in its turn stimulates, the hypothalamic pituitary axis. The hypothalamus is itself in turn receiving impulses from the higher centres of the cortex. This explains why girls taking up new careers such as nursing, may have amenorrhoea. Due to emotional stress the cortex acting through the hypothalamus upsets pituitary secretion and hence menstruation. The gonadotrophins of the pituitary (these are substances acting on the gonads) are follicle stimulating hormone, F.S.H., and L.H., luteinising hormone. These substances between them cause development of the Graafian follicle and its secretion of oestrogen, the shedding of the ovum, ovulation, the transformation of the follicle into the corpus luteum secreting both oestrogen and progesterone, and finally the degeneration of the corpus luteum with a fall in progesterone. In turn ovarian hormones stimulate or depress the secretion of gonadotrophins by the rise or fall of their blood levels.

Pathology

The majority of tumours are adenocarcinomas, most being well-differentiated. In appearance the growth is papillary or solid and can fill the entire uterine cavity. Very rarely a sarcoma can occur. This can sometimes be the result of malignant change in a benign fibroid, and it has also been noted to develop in some cases many years after a radiation-induced artificial menopause.

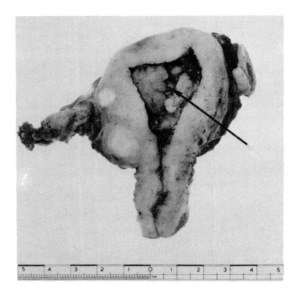

Fig. 16.6.   Carcinoma of the uterus

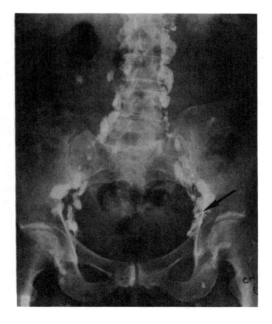

Fig. 16.7.   Lymphogram. Metastases in the pelvic nodes.
Carcinoma of the uterus

Spread

Direct

The tumour spreads through the wall of the uterus eventually involving the peritoneum, or downwards into the cervix. Deposits can arise in the ovaries, omentum, and other organs.

Lymphatic

This happens late in the disease. Spread is along the line of the ovarian vessels to pelvic and later the aortic nodes. Isolated deposits which occur in the vagina or close to the external urethral meatus may result from cells shed in to lymph vessels or veins.

Distant Spread

This is rare but can occur more often than in carcinoma of the cervix. Liver, lungs or pleura can be involved.

Distant and lymphatic spread is usually associated with less well differentiated and anaplastic tumours.

Symptoms

In women who have passed the menopause the usual symptom is post-menopausal bleeding. If menstruation is still taking place, there is irregular bleeding between periods. Discharge may be present, at first watery, but later profuse and often offensive. Pain accompanies the late stage of the disease and indicates extensive spread. Due to the deposits on the peritoneum, ascites can form and give rise to abdominal distension. Occasionally the initial complaint is of oedema of one or both legs, the swelling, unlike postural oedema, never completely subsiding when at rest. Thrombosis of veins in the legs may also be seen. Both these symptoms are due to pressure by the uterus on veins or lymphatics within the pelvis obstructing the return from the legs.

The symptom of post-menopausal bleeding is unusual enough for a woman to consult her doctor early, this may account in part for the rather better prognosis since the disease is therefore treated sooner. The patient at most risk is the one who is at the menopause and interprets irregular bleeding as a menopausal symptom.

Examination

It is not necessary to repeat the details of the physical examination. It differs in no way from that already described in the section on the cervix. It will only be emphasised here that the general examination must never be omitted and assessment is always made bimanually of the pelvis.

The patient is also questioned about taking any 'pills' for menopausal symptoms. Stilboestrol or one of the other oestrogens may have been prescribed, and if this is stopped or taken irregularly, uterine bleeding due to oestrogen withdrawal can occur.

In the old when the growth is fungating, the uterus may not be enlarged, but as a rule size is uniformly increased. If fibroids are detected it cannot be assumed that they are the sole cause of enlargement since carcinoma may also be present.

Investigations

These are the same as for the woman who has had positive clinical findings on examination for carcinoma of the cervix. There are however one or two extra tests which may be done.

A smear can be taken from the posterior fornix. Although not as useful in detecting carcinoma of the body of the uterus compared with the smear from the os for malignancy of the cervix, it is possible to obtain positive results in some cases. Blood should be sent for sugar estimation, particularly if the patient is obese, complains of thirst, or alternatively has lost weight. There seems to be some tendency for the obese diabetic to develop this disease.

E.U.A. and Biopsy

In addition to complete examination of the uterus and associated organs, cystoscopy and sigmoidoscopy are performed. Even if it is suspected that bleeding is due to fibroids or to the use of a synthetic oestrogen, diagnostic dilatation and curettage must be performed. If pyometra is found, then as previously described, the uterus is drained and the patient returned to the ward, curettage being postponed until infection has settled. If it is possible to proceed the canal is dilated and a sound passed to assess the depth and capacity of the uterus. Curettings are then taken from the whole of the uterus and canal, these must be carefully labelled according to site.

Treatment

Radical

Attempts are made to stage the tumour, this can be done by assessing the spread clinically, and histologically by considering the degree of differentiation and the mitotic activity of the cells.

Provided that the growth is operable, the treatment of choice is surgery. The operation is either total hysterectomy with removal of the fallopian tubes, ovaries, and a cuff of vagina, or a Wertheim hysterectomy. In some centres a post-operative course of radiation is given, particularly if, at surgery, spread is found in the immediate vicinity of the uterus (parametrial). The whole pelvis is irradiated and it is usual to carry out insertions using vaginal boxes in order to treat the vagina adequately. This is because when metastases occur after surgery, they frequently do so in the vaginal vault.

If surgery is not possible or the patient is unfit or refuses operation, treatment can be carried out by radiation completely. The same principles apply as in the case of the cervix. Insertions are made to give a high dose at point A and the dose at the pelvic side walls supplemented by using external therapy. Variations from the previously described technique may be found. The vaginal boxes may be placed in tandem, one below the other, to irradiate the whole of the vagina, or an older technique packing the whole uterine cavity with smaller tubes, Heyman's technique.

Palliative

In advanced cases, or when there are recurrences, treatment is tailored to the individual needs. The mainstay of primary treatment for the advanced case is radiation. For recurrences, megavoltage therapy may sometimes be used, vaginal deposits may be suitable for a radioactive implant, and surgery can palliate obstruction. The most hopeful treatment for recurrences at the moment is hormone therapy.

Hormones

The explanation why a progestin has a favourable influence on uterine carcinoma must obviously be connected with the normal progesterone control of the uterus,

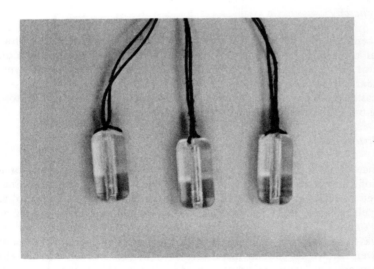

Fig. 16.8.   Small radioactive tubes. Heyman's technique

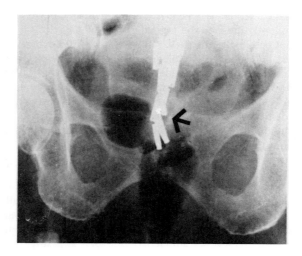

Fig. 16.9.   X-ray uterine tubes. Heyman's technique

but the exact mode of action is as yet unknown. There is no doubt however that it is effective. It can now be given orally or intramuscularly and although large doses are required, the side effects are few, some oedema, occasionally nausea, but they may in fact never be seen.

Chemotherapy

Some centres are attempting to use chemotherapy combined with a progestin to treat recurrences and advanced tumours. There is no clear evidence on the merits of single compared with combination cytotoxic regimes. As yet this treatment is experimental.

Occasionally alone or in combination with radioactive isotopes, cytotoxics may be put in the abdominal cavity after paracentesis.

Case History

A woman of 59 had undergone a hysterectomy four years previously for carcinoma of the uterus. She had not received post-operative radiation. She was admitted to hospital with symptoms of urinary retention and found to have a large vault recurrence. She was given a full course of radiation with good regression of the tumour. Eighteen months later she had a fall and fractured her femur. This was found to be a fracture through a metastatic deposit. On X-ray her lungs were shown to contain metastases as well, the shadows had the characteristic cannon-ball appearance of secondary deposits. She was given a course of radiation to the fracture site, after a pin and plate operation, and placed on a progestin. Within six weeks the chest X-ray showed marked improvement. She was maintained for a further 18 months on hormone therapy, but eventually the disease escaped from control and she died from metastatic disease.

Follow-up

The timing of appointments is basically similar to that already described in the section on cervix. Both the local and general conditions are reviewed and examined. If symptoms or signs of recurrence are found, admission for full investigation, E.U.A. and biopsy is necessary.

Prognosis

Radical treatment of this disease gives good results. At five years 80% of those patients whose tumours could be given radical treatment are alive.

Chorion Epithelioma

This extremely rare tumour is included in this discussion because it is an example of a normal biological process failing to stop and instead 'running amok', and also because of the striking success of chemotherapy. In Chapter 1 it was remarked that the trophoblasts of the placenta invade the uterine wall and then stop, controlled by some unknown biological mechanism. This tumour results from a failure of that control. The trophoblasts become hyperplastic and invasive and the cells of the chorionic villi become atypical. The benign form of this tumour is the hydatidiform mole which arises during pregnancy.

Over half the chorion epitheliomas arise in hydatidiform moles, one quarter in abortions, and almost as many in normal pregnancies. Although rare in white races, it is more common among Middle-Eastern peoples and in Taiwan and the Philippines.

Symptoms

The most common symptom is haemorrhage which results in anaemia. Pain may be present, and in late cases cough and haemoptysis due to deposits in the lungs. Fever and rigors are not uncommon. If this tumour develops during pregnancy the uterus is larger than expected for the week of gestation and the pregnancy test is positive at a very high dilution. Spread is by the blood stream and occurs early, a common site is the lung. Local spread is to the vagina, vulva, and broad ligaments.

Investigations

These are designed to determine the site and degree of spread.

The placenta produces human chorionic gonadotrophin and this is present at high levels in the blood when the disease is active. It can therefore be used as a marker both for the progress of therapy and to screen for recurrence.

Treatment

Surgery

Initially the uterus is emptied by a D. and C. to control bleeding. Very occasionally a hysterectomy may be carried out at the end of treatment if there is bulky residual disease.

Chemotherapy

Methotrexate has revolutionised treatment. The malignant rapidly dividing cell is susceptible, and multiplication is slowed or halted. Normal cells in a high state of activity are also vulnerable, and the toxic effects are explicable on this basis, gastro-intestinal symptoms, soreness of the mouth, vomiting, diarrhoea, and spontaneous bruising, and bleeding due to bone-marrow depression. These effects can be reversed by discontinuing, lowering the dosage, or giving folinic acid. Other substances which occasionally are used after methotrexate are cyclophosphamide, vincristine, and actinomycin D. Since the depressant effects on the marrow are severe, and the number of cases small, treatment is given in specialised centres.

Results

As high a remission rate as 90% has been achieved, and even when there is severe and widespread disease up to 75% remission rates have been quoted.

CARCINOMA OF THE OVARY

Anatomy

The ovary has no peritoneal covering but it does have a covering of cubical epithelium. The bulk of the ovary is made up of a connective tissue framework, stroma, which contains parenchymal cells capable of developing along varying lines. Some cells develop as Graafian follicles. These follicles contain the ovum which is shed at the mid-point of the menstrual cycle and conveyed through the fallopian tube to the uterus. After the follicle has ruptured, cells from one of its layers proliferate to form the corpus luteum. After the menopause, the ovary becomes small and shrivelled and the follicles disappear.

Age and Incidence

The age range is from 30 to 60, but the average age is about 45. The disease is slightly more common than carcinoma of the cervix causing about 3% of all deaths from malignant disease.

Aetiology

No specific factors have been suggested. Many malignant tumours have corresponding benign counterparts, and it is thought that malignant change may take place in some of them.

Pathology

Many systems of classification have been devised, but that produced by the W.H.O. is now the one most used internationally. The group containing the most commonly occurring tumours is called 'common epithelial tumours', and they probably all arise from the surface mesothelium of the ovary. Within each group there are further sub-divisions according to histological type. In this group the more common are serous, and mucinous tumours, both of them having benign counterparts.

Endometrioid Adenocarcinoma

Areas of squamous metaplasia are frequently found, but quite a proportion of the tumours are well differentiated. About a third of the patients have a co-existing carcinoma of the uterus, and a smaller number either endometriosis of the ovary, or hyperplasia of the endometrium.

Hormone Secreting – Special Tumours

Granulosa cell and thecoma   The origin of these tumours is uncertain, but the first resembles histologically the granulosa cell layer of the Graafian follicle, the second may arise from areas of hyperplasia in the cortical stroma of the ovary. Tumours formed from them on the whole behave in a benign way, but 30% recur after removal and a few metastasise. Most secrete oestrogen and induce endometrial hyperplasia. As already pointed out in the last section, this can lead to uterine carcinoma.

Androblastoma   (formerly Arrhenoblastoma). This is a very rare tumour usually occurring between 20 and 30 years of age, but this varies with the histological type. Some tumours are endocrinologically active producing androgen, or occasionally oestrogen. A small proportion show malignant behaviour.

Other Tumours

Dysgerminoma   A rare tumour in Caucasians but more common in Japan and India. It is thought to arise from primitive germ cells. There ia a wide age range but it most commonly occurs in the third and fourth decades. It spreads by the lymphatics and blood stream, at the time of operation one quarter of cases have evidence of local spread. It is very sensitive to radiation.

Benign Dermoid Cyst   A benign dermoid cyst is a tumour which contains cells representing all three germ layers of the embryo, and so bone, teeth and lung and skin may be found in it. When there is a neoplastic change in this tumour it becomes a malignant teratoma of the ovary.

Spread

Direct. Through the ovary to adjacent structures such as the uterus or intestines.
Peritoneal. Multiple peritoneal deposits giving rise to ascites.
Lymphatic. Both pelvic and abdominal nodes are involved frequently. The only
    exception is the mucinous type of tumour.
Blood. This is rare and usually occurs in the late disease.

Secondary Tumours

The ovary is frequently the site of metastases from other primary sites, particularly gastro-intestinal tract, breast, uterus and cervix. These metastases account for 5–10% of ovarian tumours.

Symptoms

Early

These are unfortunately extremely vague or completely absent in the early stages, and by the time abdominal distension or pain is present metastases have usually occurred. In some cases there is a history of vague epigastric discomfort and pain, and this can last for as long as two years. Vaginal bleeding is not usually caused by the ovarian growth unless there are metastases in the uterine endometrium or the tumour is secreting oestrogen.

Late

In the late stages nausea, vomiting, general wasting, and oedema of the lower limbs occur. This last symptom is due to obstruction by the tumour of the pelvic veins and lymphatics. Bowel obstruction can also develop because of invasion by the growth.

Most women consult their doctors because of pain or abdominal swelling. In some a cyst causes torsion of the ovary and necessitates emergency laparotomy, the malignancy is only discovered on routine histology.

The insidious nature of symptoms is best illustrated by the story of one patient. She was in her late thirties and noticed that the waist band of her skirt had become tight. As she had only recently had it dry cleaned she attributed this to shrinkage. Only when the fit became tighter still did she realise that it was her abdomen that was enlarged. On close questioning she admitted to a vague feeling of lethargy for six months and occasional left-sided abdominal discomfort. The abdomen was enlarged to the size of a 24-weeks' pregnancy. At laparotomy an ovarian tumour about eight inches in diameter was found. It was attached to the pelvic side wall and its removal caused brisk arterial haemorrhage necessitating the rapid transfusion of three pints of blood. The malignant nature of the tumour was obvious on naked-eye inspection and was confirmed by histology.

Examination

Although usually unhelpful, a careful history must be taken. This is particularly so in the case of the woman admitted as an emergency with a provisional diagnosis of appendicitis. She may have had previous attacks of pain which arouse the suspicion that her symptoms are due to intermittent torsion of the ovary caused by a cyst. The histologist must in these cases cut sections throughout the tumour to avoid missing one small area of malignant change.

General Examination

On palpating the abdomen a mass may be felt, it sounds dull on percussion. An attempt is made to get below it and slip the fingers into the pelvic brim, this will not be possible if it is fixed in the pelvis or to an abdominal structure. Unless very small, the tumour is not as a rule mobile. Signs of ascites are sought, a fluid thrill, or shifting dullness. With the patient on her back, fluid lies in the flanks, percussion is dull here, resonant in the centre. If the woman now turns on her side, the fluid accumulates on one side and dullness is all on that side, the uppermost flank now sounding resonant. If the patient is obese, there may be no abdominal signs, and even in the thin woman, none may be found.

The pelvic examination is usually more helpful as a mass can be felt, and provided that it is not fixed to it, the uterus can be moved separately. The pouch of Douglas may contain hard fixed tumour and the position of the uterus may be altered. The texture and surface of the tumour can often be felt more readily on rectal examination, parts of the tumour may be tender.

Other signs of malignancy are occasionally ulceration in the vagina, oedema of the legs and the vagina, and thrombosis of the veins of the leg. Lymph nodes in the groins, supraclavicular fossae and the axilla must be routinely palpated.

Complications

Rarely an ovarian tumour may become impacted in the pelvis and cause retention of urine. This is more likely to happen with the benign type.

Rupture

Malignant cystic tumours can rupture either into the peritoneal cavity or into another viscus. Rupture may be precipitated by a blow or other trauma. If rupture occurs into the peritoneal cavity the symptoms may be only those of gradually increasing ascites. If there is bleeding, peritoneal irritation occurs giving pain and abdominal rigidity. The pulse rate is rapid and the patient may be shocked. If rupture occurs into the bladder or bowel and the cyst becomes infected, the patient is febrile often with a high swinging temperature. Pyrexia of itself does not indicate infection, advanced disease is often accompanied by this.

Investigations

The final diagnosis must await laparotomy and histology, but certain tests can be done in an attempt to establish the nature of the mass. The routine blood count and chest X-ray, also abdominal and pelvic ultra sound must be performed. Other blood tests include urea, electrolytes, and possibly liver function tests. In the absence of carcinoma of the uterus cells are occasionally found in the posterior fornix, but more often, particularly with some of the early tumours, cells can be seen in fluid obtained by cul-de-sac puncture. This procedure involves puncture of the posterior fornix and aspiration of fluid from the pouch of Douglas. Plain X-rays of the abdomen occasionally show calcification in the tumour and distortion of the bowel may sometimes be seen on barium enema. An I.V.P. and lymphogram must now be regarded as routine investigations. If there is any reason to suspect that the tumour is a secondary, then a mammogram and full X-ray investigation of the gastro-intestinal tract should be undertaken. Finally before laparotomy, any anaemia should be corrected by transfusion.

The patient who presents as an emergency due to torsion or rupture of a tumour can only have a minimum of investigations. These must include blood tests and X-ray and ultra sound.

Preparation of the Patient

If there is good reason to suspect a malignant tumour of the ovary, then there is a chance that extensive surgery may be required. As many of these women are still in the child-bearing years the possibility must be discussed with the patient and her husband. It has been argued that this can cause great emotional stress, leaving the woman to worry about the nature of her disease. This is a matter for individual decision in each case. What is certain is that no radical surgery should be contemplated in an unprepared patient.

Surgery

Laparotomy

An E.U.A., cystoscopy, and sigmoidoscopy precedes the laparotomy. When the abdomen is opened the diagnosis is usually clear but the gastro-intestinal tract must be carefully examined to exclude any tumour there.

If the case is advanced, as much tumour as is possible is removed. This is contrary to the usual rules for malignant surgery which forbid partial removal, but the patient is rendered so much more comfortable that it is justified. It also leaves less bulk to be irradiated.

If the tumour is confined to the ovary, most surgeons remove the other ovary and also the uterus and tubes. Some centres advocate leaving the uterus since in their experience it has not often been involved by metastases. If the uterus is left behind, then curettage to exclude tumour must be performed. The most difficult case is that in which there is only a small malignant tumour of one ovary, and the patient is young and has not yet completed her family. Occasionally it is justified to restrict resection to the affected ovary, but usually since the other ovary is often the site of a microscopic deposit, the full operation must be carried out.

If malignancy is discovered only on histology, though the decision is a hard one, surgeons usually re-open the abdomen and complete the full procedure.

Further Treatment

Any further treatment that is given will depend upon the extent of spread of the tumour (staging) and its histological grading, again 1 to 4.

Staging

1. Tumour confined to ovary/ovaries.
2. Spread only in the pelvis.
3. Spread throughout the abdomen except the liver.
4. Distant metastases or liver involvement.

It is unfortunately true that while surgery is the treatment of choice, only 20% of these tumours are completely removable, most of the other 80% will prove technically inoperable. In 35% deposits have already appeared in the peritoneum and omentum.

While not a radiosensitive tumour, a combination of radiation and surgery followed by chemotherapy does seem to have improved results at three years. However optimism must be restrained as numbers treated are as yet too small for valid conclusions to be drawn.

Radiation

Method   If the uterus has been left it can be used as a carrier. Radiation is then given by a combination of megavoltage therapy to the whole pelvis combined with two insertions of a tube and boxes. Even when the uterus has been removed, if there is a mass palpable per vagina, boxes can be used at the vault.

Many centres now treat both abdomen and pelvis, this involves a large area of the body. In some cases when the bulk of residual tumour is large, it may be better to substitute chemotherapy and reserve radiation for local treatment. Radiation therapy lasts from four to eight weeks according to the method and dosage employed.

Chemotherapy

Attempts are continuing to culture tumour cells and test their sensitivity to various cytotoxic drugs. This procedure is as yet experimental, but would be of great value for this tumour if successful. Single drug therapy was the usual method for years, but now combination therapy, including cis-platin, is becoming more widely used. The combined drugs are given at intervals of 3 to 4 weeks, six or more times. As yet it is not clear exactly what benefits will be achieved. Chemotherapy probably reduces the size of bulky tumour better than radiation, but the length of remission and the chances of cure are still being evaluated.

Immunotherapy

The results of treatment up to now have not been very good. Research into methods of stimulating the body's immune defences has therefore been applied to this tumour. The usual specific and non-specific methods have been used. Recently interest has been aroused by the use of tumour antibody labelled with a radioactive isotope, to treat widespread metastases causing effusions. As yet, though interesting, such treatments are experimental and confined to special centres.

Second Look Laparotomy

In some centres a second laparotomy is recommended after treatment. The reason for the procedure is twofold. If there appears to be no response to chemotherapy the decision to stop can be confirmed, while if tumour bulk has been reduced, removal may now be possible.

Treatment Policy

Since policy does vary and there is as yet no one regime which has been shown to be the best, the following is a summary of a very common treatment plan:

Stage 1.   Surgery. If complete removal and low grade histology no further treatment. If high grade histology, post-operative radiation.

Stage 2.   Surgery + post-operative radiation. If residual tumour bulk large, chemotherapy may also be given.

Stages 3 and 4.   Surgery. Stage 3 minimal residual tumour or complete removal, give post-operative radiation + chemotherapy. Stage 4 or bulky residual tumour, post-operative chemotherapy.

Radioactive Isotopes

These are used sometimes in an attempt to control ascites. They are instilled after paracentesis. The results achieved are variable.

Special Tumours

These are rare tumours and may appear to be of low or doubtful malignancy. The usual treatment is surgery followed by radiotherapy.

Palliation

Both surgery and radiotherapy are employed as indicated to relieve symptoms due to spread of the disease. The procedures have already been described.

Follow-up

This is basically the same as for carcinoma of the uterus. When recurrence or extension of the disease involving the peritoneum is found, the most urgent need is usually for paracentesis.

Prognosis

The prognosis is entirely dependent upon the stage and histological grading of the tumour. Stage I tumours of low grade malignancy have a good prognosis and 5 yrs survival figures of 62% have been quoted. On the other hand once spread outside the ovary has begun, the survival rates fall rapidly with staging, ranging from 10% to 30%, with no five year survivors if there are distant metastases.

CARCINOMA OF THE FALLOPIAN TUBE, THE VULVA AND THE VAGINA

These tumours are rare. The treatment of the first is by surgery followed by radiation, the prognosis is very poor. Carcinoma of the vulva is treated primarily by surgery. Since lymphatic spread occurs early, the operation is radical involving total vulvectomy with block dissection of the superficial inguinal and external iliac nodes. When no nodes are involved, survival rates of 86% at five years are quoted. Primary tumours of the vagina have a poor prognosis. The close relation to the bladder and rectum means that surgery must often be very radical. Intracavitary radiation has also been used. With either method results are poor.

Nursing Care, Late Complications of Radiation

These are described first, for although they are medical problems a nurse who is in the outpatient clinic may be told by the patient of symptoms which point to their existence. As they often relate to the most intimate part of her married life a woman may feel unable to talk to the doctor about them.

Vagina

Adhesions nearly always occur in the vagina. If intercourse is regular and recommences after treatment, these may be avoided, but later narrowing of the vagina can occur due to fibrosis. Pain on intercourse (dyspareunia) and slight bleeding can follow. In these circumstances vaginal dilators may be required, and the situation must be discussed with the patient and her husband. It is axiomatic that recurrence as a cause of the bleeding must first be excluded.

Discharge may also occur. If not due to recurrence this may be the earliest sign of necrosis of the vaginal wall. If ulceration arises a fistula with the bladder or occasionally the rectum can follow. If very early, diathermy coagulation may initiate healing, but the established fistula will require diversionary operations.

Bowel

The small intestine and the large bowel inevitably receive some radiation. If a hysterectomy has preceded therapy a loop of small bowel may be held down in the pouch of Douglas by adhesions. The rest of the small intestine being freely mobile will be less affected, but a fixed loop will receive a maximum dose, and the result may be a permanently altered bowel habit, usually diarrhoea. The mainstay of treatment is an antispasmodic, to prevent over activity of the bowel smooth muscle, and careful diets. The patient herself will learn by trial and error that some foods are best avoided.

The junction of the rectum and sigmoid colon is in many patients tethered by a very short mesentery. When radioactive insertion followed by external treatment is given, this point is particularly vulnerable. Some months after completion of treatment, the patient may complain of rectal bleeding, often severe. After examination to exclude recurrence it may be necessary to fashion a temporary defunctioning colostomy. With rest and the use of prednisolone retention enemas the ulceration usually heals and the colostomy can be closed.

Skin

If conventional therapy has been used epilation of the pubic hair is usually permanent. The skin may show telangectasia and fibrosis. Even with megavoltage therapy a leathery thickening of the subcutaneous tissues can follow. In severe cases the skin can break down and a large necrotic ulcer form. This becomes infected and healing difficult. Very careful nursing can clean up the infection and the necrotic debris ready for skin grafting. Avoidance of trauma and infection in the post-operative period is vital.

Urinary Tract

The urethra, the bladder and the lower part of the ureters are all vulnerable and can be the site of late reactions. The bladder mucosa can atrophy and telangectasia can develop. At first cystitis due to irritation of the mucosa occurs.

This can be followed by severe haematuria which can cause anaemia requiring transfusion for its correction. In these circumstances a transient infection which would ordinarily probably resolve without symptoms is sufficient to precipitate bleeding. After the exclusion of recurrence it is usual to adopt an expectant policy. The patient is advised to have a high intake of fluid, this dilutes the urine making it less irritant to the damaged mucosa. If haematuria becomes too frequent or the bladder becomes greatly contracted due to fibrosis, ureteric transplant may be required. Stenosis of both the urethra and the ureter can occur. Periodic urethral dilatation is usually sufficient to maintain an adequate stream. Ureteric stenosis is a more difficult problem, it may not be detected until obstruction to the kidney outflow has produced hydronephrosis. The help of a urologist must be sought, remedial surgery can range from total nephrectomy to local excision of the stenosis and reimplantation of the ureter in the bladder.

Bone

When radiation is applied laterally to the pelvis, it passes through the head and neck of the femur. Very rarely this can produce a weakening of the bone and later spontaneous fracture.

Cervical Smear

The tray will contain a bivalve vaginal speculum, lubrication, gloves, two containers for the slides, two slides and the Ayres spatula. It is a small point but well-fitting gloves are not only more comfortable for the doctor but make examination easier. Before the examination begins the nurse should mark the slides with the patient's name and the date and make out the cytology request form. When the smear is being taken a good light is essential and the nurse can help by holding a torch at the correct angle. It is usual to spread the smear on two slides. These should be placed at once in the containers. Patients may have a little bleeding after the examination and will feel more comfortable if they are given a protecting pad.

Insertions

It is important to admit the patient at least two days before insertion, earlier if transfusion for anaemia is required. This period enables a woman to get to know the nursing staff and be mentally prepared for the procedure. This interval is also necessary before any of the operations described in the earlier part of the chapter, it must however not be too long or fear and doubts will have time to build up.

Preparation

It is again emphasised that careful attention must be paid to the temperature and white-cell count. Raised levels combined with an elevated E.S.R. may be the only indication of a pyometra.

If transfusion is required it is probably best to give packed cells. It is more difficult to make sure the infusion runs satisfactorily, but for many patients it is less of a load on the circulatory system.

For a satisfactory E.U.A. and for the patient's comfort while the insertion is in place, the bowel should be empty. This can be best accomplished by giving an enema the night before. This is particularly necessary if due to pain the intake of codeine or codeine compounds has been high.

Ward Care

On the return to the ward, before the screen is wheeled up, the position of the pack must be checked to ensure that the source has not shifted. The temperature and pulse must be charted four hourly. It is very rare for the uterus to be perforated during insertion, but if it is, peritonitis can follow and this is signalled by a rising pulse rate and pyrexia, pain as a diagnostic sign is more variable. In fact any undue pain should be reported. Patients experience irritation of the bladder both during the insertion and after, but severe pain is rare, and is usually a symptom of a complication such as perforation or haematoma formation in the broad ligament following over-enthusiastic dilatation. As every nurse is aware, a patient with an indwelling catheter is at risk from urinary tract infection. Following insertion bladder drainage is continuous and strict asepsis must be observed when emptying the collecting bag. The patient is encouraged to drink plenty of fluids both for comfort, the urine is dilute and less irritating, and for dilution of the concentration of any bacteria that unfortunately reach the bladder.

There is usually no bowel action while the source is in place but it should be as effortless as possible if it does occur. To this end liquid paraffin is usually given. The diet is light.

Analgesics should be given in adequate dosage and some sedation is usually necessary at night.

After Insertion

When the catheter is removed it is a wise precaution to send a specimen of urine for culture and sensitivity. The presence of any infection can then be detected early, it is difficult otherwise to separate the symptoms of radiation cystitis from those of urinary infection.

Unless the general condition is poor, patients can usually return home between insertions. The woman's morale benefits. She should of course be told to report immediately any profuse bleeding, severe pain, or pyrexia. The patient with advanced disease may require to be kept in hospital. If the growth is extensive and necrotic there is a risk of severe haemorrhage which may require vaginal packing.

Vaginal Haemorrhage

Extensive growths may at any time during treatment give rise to haemorrhage. If this is severe it is alarming to the patient. It will usually respond to vaginal packing. In an emergency this can be done in the ward after giving omnopon or pethidine, but it is usually better for this procedure to be carried out in theatre where both the light and facilities are better.

Radioactive Needles

On those rare occasions when these are used, all the precautions already described in the section on the tongue are taken with regard to checking. When the implant is in the vagina or vulva, an indwelling catheter is used for bladder drainage.

Post-operative

The usual surgical problems following laparotomy are found with these patients, indeed some may prove more troublesome because of the complications of malignant disease, fixation, infiltration, obstruction. It should not be forgotten that in the case of a pelvic operation there is a tendency for retention of urine to occur, and again this may be aggravated by the special conditions of malignancy.

Chemotherapy

Patients suffering from chorior carcinoma are treated in a special centre. The specialised tests can be carried out there, and the staff are used to the problems that may arise during treatment. Combined chemotherapy usually involves a short stay in hospital so that side effects can be treated and minimised. If single agents are used this can be carried out on an outpatient basis.

Radiation

A few patients may be able to tolerate treatment as outpatients. They need to live within easy travelling distance of the hospital, have adequate arrangements for someone else to look after the family and household responsibilities, and be willing to follow the instructions given on rest and diet. Even when the woman and her family are completely co-operative, it may become necessary to admit her during treatment.

The areas to be irradiated are large, particularly when ovarian carcinoma is being treated. The absorbed dose of radiation is high especially if the patient is obese. In these cases the dose may have to be reduced, both the daily fraction given and the overall total.

Certain reactions are almost inevitable and it is only their degree that varies. These effects can be divided into local and general.

Local Effects

Skin

Despite the use of megavoltage therapy, some skin reaction occurs in the natal cleft and the groins, in the obese patient it can be severe. The skin in these sites tends to be moist and moist desquamation almost invariably follows reaction. The usual treatment is prescribed. The inpatient is not discharged until this is well under control, particularly if the home conditions are unsatisfactory.

Colostomy

The area around the colostomy can cause very difficult nursing problems. Towards the end of treatment the bowel action is loose and can be very irritating to the skin. If the colostomy has to be included in the field, the skin being moist reacts badly. The combination of maceration and irritation can cause great pain and discomfort. The help of a specially trained stoma nurse is desirable. Efforts should be made to apply treatments to protect the skin around the stoma before radiation begins.

Bladder

Radiation cystitis cannot be avoided. Patients should be encouraged to drink plenty of fluids. An M.S.U. must be sent for culture and sensitivity, infection may already be present, and even when initial culture is negative, the patient is certainly more liable to become infected. A mixture containing potassium citrate will render the urine alkaline temporarily and so make it less irritant to the bladder mucosa. If however there is any suspicion of renal damage, this is probably better witheld as the kidney may not be able to deal with the extra potassium load. Frequency can be relieved with an antispasmodic.

Bowel

Diarrhoea almost always occurs and patients must be encouraged to persist with treatment when it develops. They can be told that when radiation is finished the diarrhoea will gradually begin to decrease and is unlikely to be a permanent condition. The timing of this symptom is usually the third or fourth week of treatment, but if there has been surgery, it occurs earlier, usually towards the end of the second week.

Measures are taken to relieve symptoms. The nurse must not be disappointed that they are never completely successful, cessation of treatment is the only cure, and in severe cases, rest from treatment for several days may be necessary. Kaolin mixtures, anti-spasmodics, plenty of fluids, and a careful diet will all help to lessen the severity of symptoms, but above all the patient requires quiet supportive encouragement. An adequate intake of fluids and diet are very necessary or the condition will be aggravated by depletion of electrolytes. Rarely the condition may progress to paralytic ileus requiring intravenous infusion and gastric suction.

A stool specimen must be sent for culture and sensitivity. It cannot be assumed that this is a radiation reaction, infection can also occur. The blood count, both for haemoglobin and white cells must be kept under observation, and also the levels of sodium and potassium. The levels of these two electrolytes are particularly liable to fall when vomiting or diarrhoea is severe. If oral intake is possible, they can be corrected by dietary supplements, otherwise intravenous fluids are used.

If bleeding occurs, this must be investigated as it may be due to secondary deposits.

It must not be presumed to be due to radiation reaction unless investigations are negative. Haemorrhoids may bleed when diarrhoea is severe and hydrocortisone suppositories and ointment will be of benefit. Bleeding from the bowel may require interruption or cessation of treatment, prednisolone retention enemas can be helpful.

Vagina

Severe erythema can arise during treatment and dysuria may be due to this. Hydrocortisone sprays or ointments will give some relief but must be combined with complete bed rest, this is particularly necessary when the patient is obese.

General Effects

General systemic effects can make their appearance as early as the first week of treatment. We do not know the mechanism by which they are caused, and though prophylactic regimes of vitamin complexes and anti-emetics have been tried, their success has been variable.

Blood

The most vulnerable element is the white cell. If the count falls suddenly, treatment must be stopped. It usually recovers spontaneously, but steroid supplements can be required. Platelet and red-cell counts fall late in treatment if at all, it must be stressed that iron supplements are too slow in action, and transfusion is required. If the platelet count is dangerously low, then fresh blood is required.

Vomiting

A certain amount of nausea is inevitable and this is usually accompanied by loss of appetite. An anti-emetic is usually successful provided that rest and the fluid and food intake are adequate. When vomiting occurs treatment is temporarily stopped, and if necessary intravenous fluids and gastric suction begun. Any patient on steroids must have the dose raised during this time.

General Measures

It must be conceded that with a few exceptions, most patients suffer discomfort during the treatment. Its degree is variable and often depends upon the co-operation of the patient in taking adequate rest and maintaining her dietary intake.

The nurse while expecting reactions should not implant this thought in the patient's mind, for when she expects to be sick or to have other reactions they will certainly occur and often be that much more severe. By insisting on a sensible daily routine and by being sympathetic, reassuring, but firm when reactions occur, the nursing staff will do much to minimise the inevitable discomforts and reactions.

By now it will be realised that morale is a most important factor. The occupational therapist can be invaluable in providing light simple occupation for those in need of it. The patient's library will cater for the avid reader, and the visits of the hairdresser can give a necessary fillip to morale. A tactful sister can divert and neutralise the sitting-room bore who by long narrations of her own or others' symptoms can have a disastrous effect on the other patients.

In all this trying period the support of a woman's family is most important. Few relatives fail to co-operate if the facts are simply and clearly explained. Without being harassed by family problems the patient can be kept in touch with day-to-day family affairs and so prevented from feeling cut off.

Encouragement will help her to persist and endure when symptoms become severe. The management of a patient remaining at home while on treatment is guided by the same principles. All those in contact with her must be continuously alert for symptoms which may indicate a need for admission, and must reinforce constantly the main points of a sensible daily routine.

The attitude should be a positive one. The patient should be led to realise that she can be an active member of the therapy team. By her co-operation she can affect her own reactions and the course of her treatment.

17   The Male Reproductive System

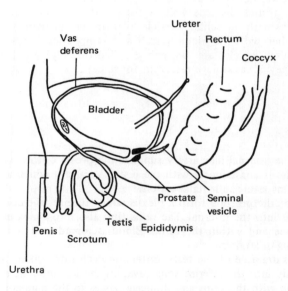

Fig 17.1   Relations of the male reproductive organs and urethra

Anatomy

Prostate

This organ surrounds the urethra as it leaves the bladder and this part is called
the prostatic urethra. The prostate has been described as being the shape and
size of a chestnut. Most of it lies behind the urethra only a small rim of tissue

lying in front. Above is the neck of the bladder, below the tip rests on the external sphincter of the bladder. On either side are the fibres of muscles which run from the pubis to the rectum, in front lies the symphysis pubis and behind the rectum. The prostate can be palpated on rectal examination. A median groove divides it into right and left lobes. A further median lobe is marked off by the two ejaculatory ducts which open into the prostatic urethra.

Scrotum, Testes and Epididymis

The scrotum forms a pouch of loose tissue in which lie the testes, each with its epididymis. The left testis lies at a slightly lower level than the right. In renal or heart failure the scrotum readily becomes oedematous because of its dependent position and the laxity of the tissues. Running along the posterior border of the testis is a duct, the epididymis, the tail lies at the lower pole of the testis where it becomes the vas deferens. This tube runs up through the scrotum, along the inguinal canal, round the side wall of the pelvis and then turns towards the bladder, it joins with the seminal vesicle to form the ejaculatory duct. The vas deferens together with the blood vessels and lymphatics forms the spermatic cord. The seminal vesicles are two paired coiled tubes lying below the base of the bladder. They act as storage reservoirs for semen.

Blood Supply

A branch of the internal iliac artery supplies the prostate, the vas deferens, and the epididymis. It anastomoses with the testicular artery which arises from the aorta at the same level as the renal vessels.

The veins of the prostate form a plexus which receives the dorsal vein of the penis. It drains into the internal iliac veins, and also into a plexus lying in front of the vertebrae and within the canal. Blood is forced into this latter plexus during coughing or straining.

The venous drainage of the testis differs on each side. On the right the vein empties directly into the inferior vena cava, on the left into the renal vein. The lymphatics run with the veins and drainage passes to the para-aortic nodes. On the left there may also be some drainage to the nodes below the left renal vein. The lymphatics of each side communicate freely across the midline and also with the nodes lying around the aorta in the mediastinum.

Nerve Supply

The testis is supplied by the sympathetic nervous system through the spinal nerve T.10.

Microscopic Structure

Prostate

The prostate consists of muscular and glandular tissue enclosed in a capsule. The glands secrete a slightly acid fluid containing phosphatase, this drains by ducts into the urethra.

Testis

The testis is covered by a white capsule and is divided into two or three hundred lobules each containing one to three seminiferous tubules. These tubules join to form about 12 efferent ducts, which in turn join again forming the epididymis. Lying between the seminiferous tubules are the interstitial cells. Spermatozoa (sperm) are formed in the tubules, they lie in a thin fluid and are propelled along the efferent ducts into the epididymis. The interstitial cells are grouped around blood vessels and secrete the male hormone testosterone. The semen is formed of spermatozoa and secretions from the epididymis, the seminal vesicles, the prostate, and small glands opening into the urethra. Semen is discharged into the prostatic urethra and then ejaculated by the penis during coitus. Reflex nervous stimulation closes off the sphincter and prevents reflux of semen into the bladder.

Physiology

Just as in the female the ovary was related to the hypothalamus and the anterior pituitary through an interplay of hormones, so also is the testis. The exact mode of action of the pituitary gonadotrophins is uncertain. Luteinising hormone, L.H., maintains the activity of the interstitial cells producing testosterone. This hormone is responsible for the development and maintenance of the secondary sex characteristics and also stimulates formation of sperm. Follicle stimulating hormone is believed to maintain the level of spermatogenic activity.

Male hormones are called androgens. Two less-potent androgens are secreted by the adrenals, they belong to a chemical group called the 17-ketosteroids.

Prostate

The secretion of acid phosphatase by the gland is maintained by testosterone. There is thus a sharp increase in the concentration of the enzyme in the prostate at puberty. There is normally no discharge of phosphatase from the prostate into the blood, when the blood level is raised it is usually diagnostic of metastasising carcinoma of the prostate.

Descent of the Testis

In the embryo the testis is formed from a ridge of tissue at the level of the adult kidney, which explains the high origin of the testicular vessels. It descends finally reaching its adult position in the ninth month of pregnancy. As it descends it carries with it its blood vessels and lymphatics. To reach the scrotum, it passes along the inguinal canal through openings in the abdominal fascia called the internal and external rings. The descent of the testis can be arrested at any point and this occurs in about 2% of males. After puberty, the higher temperature to which an undescended testis is subjected renders it sterile, and also more liable to malignant disease.

CARCINOMA OF THE PROSTATE

Age and Incidence

This is a disease which is rare below the age of 50 but increases with age. With more men living longer it has therefore seemed to be on the increase. It accounts for about 4% of all deaths from malignant disease.

Aetiology

In nearly all men over the age of 50 the prostate becomes enlarged. This is due to a benign nodular hyperplasia, the normal tissue is compressed by this over-growth into a narrow rim, or false capsule to the gland. It is suggested that this is due to decreased androgen secretion with increasing age resulting in an imbalance between oestrogens and androgens. Conversely carcinoma is thought to arise in a situation in which the hormone balance is disturbed by excess androgen formation. Most malignant tumours are certainly hormone-dependent and are inhibited by depressing the level of androgens. Over the age of 50 an increasing percentage of prostate specimens removed at operation or post mortem are shown on section to contain microscopic foci of cancer. At the age of 50 it is 15% rising to about 80% over the next three decades. This is a rate far in excess of cases which become clinically obvious. There is thus much food for thought. What factors cause this latent carcinoma to progress, finally producing signs and symptoms? For the research worker the answer will provide one more clue to the solution of the problem of carcinogenesis.

Pathology

The majority of these tumours are adenocarcinomas, anaplastic growths are rare. The degree of differentiation varies. In some it is so high that it is not easy to distinguish carcinoma from benign hyperplasia and it is only invasion of blood vessels, lymphatics, or the capsule which establishes the diagnosis. Normally the prostate feels hard and firm and is not greatly enlarged, but if benign hyperplasia is also present these characteristics are obscured.

Spread

Direct

This is through the gland and capsule particularly posteriorly. Penetration of the capsule is followed by invasion of the bladder, seminal vesicles, and rectum.

Lymphatic

This occurs commonly. Nodes involved are the iliac and aortic groups. Occasionally spread to the mediastinum is found.

Blood

In 70% of cases there are bony metastases and often these determine the clinical presentation rather than the primary. The communication between the prostatic venous plexus and the prevertebral venous plexus probably accounts for the very frequent spread to the spine. The pelvis and upper ends of the femora are also common sites of metastases. On X-ray these secondary deposits are sclerotic in type. The bone appears denser. Blood spread to the liver and lungs can also occur.

Symptoms

These depend entirely on whether they are caused by the primary tumour or by metastases.

Primary

Some enlargement of the gland occurs and if the median lobe is chiefly involved, urinary symptoms occur. Reference to the anatomy section will make it obvious that the flow of urine from the bladder will be impeded. Since this also occurs with benign hyperplasia the symptoms are the same. There is increasing difficulty in micturition. There is hesitancy in starting, the stream is slow and poor, and there is a terminal dribble. The bladder cannot empty completely as the opening of the urethra is carried above the lowest level of the bladder and so retention occurs. This gives a sensation of incomplete emptying and frequency follows. As chronic retention progresses there is a dribbling overflow incontinence. Due to retention many patients acquire a urinary infection. Some authorities believe overflow incontinence to be more common in malignant disease. It is certain that invasion of the external sphincter of the bladder makes the incontinence worse. Often patients are admitted as an emergency when complete acute retention occurs. Occasionally extension towards the rectum causes difficulty on defaecation and stricture formation. Invasion of the rectal wall with ulcer and fistula formation is rare, but in a very few cases biopsy of a supposed rectal cancer has shown it to be in fact a prostate carcinoma. Haematuria is more commonly associated with benign hyperplasia.

Secondary

The type and site of metastases will determine the nature of the symptoms, particularly if those related to the urinary system are not present.

Lymph Nodes

As the nodes invaded early lie deep, they are not usually palpable. However a diffuse involvement may obstruct the lymphatic drainage of the lower limbs. Oedema follows, usually on one side only. It has already been pointed out that there is free communication with mediastinal lymphatics so that a hard enlargement of the supraclavicular or axillary nodes may be the presenting system. Occasionally superficial inguinal nodes are also affected.

Bones

The metastases are osteoblastic, they form dense bone and frequently cause severe pain due to pressure on nerves. Since the sacrum, pelvis, and lumbar vertebrae are so often involved, pain is frequently referred to the buttocks, the lower back, and radiating down the thighs (sciatica). In other bones involved a mass may be palpable, skull, ribs, clavicle, while pathological fracture can occur, particularly in the two former bones. Lesions in the skull can cause cranial nerve palsies by pressure, and collapse of an involved vertebra will give symptoms of spinal-cord compression. Widespread involvement of bones containing blood-forming marrow produces a severe anaemia.

Other Sites

In the late stage deposits may be found in the skin, liver and lungs. The testis and breast have also been recorded as involved.

Such advanced disease presents a clinical picture of cachexia, severe anaemia, and unremitting pain.

Examination

After a careful history which deals particularly with urinary symptoms, the examination is first directed to the general condition. Signs of wasting and anaemia are sought. The abdomen is carefully palpated and liver enlargement noted. It is rare, even in the very thin patient, to be able to feel enlarged nodes in the abdomen. The other lymphatic sites are then examined. Finally rectal examination is made. The prostate is assessed as to size, texture, regularity and fixation. Any pelvic extension is noted. In the lateral position complete palpation is not always possible even using the bimanual technique. Many doctors prefer to have the patient lying on his back with the knees flexed.

Investigations

An M.S.U. must be sent for culture and sensitivity as so often patients with chronic retention have a superimposed urinary infection. If culture is positive, the appropriate antibiotic is given.

Blood Tests

The routine haemoglobin and white-blood count is performed, any anaemia must be corrected. Blood is also sent for estimation of electrolytes, urea and both phosphatases. In the case of the latter the sample should not be taken until 24 hours after rectal examination, as this may have caused a temporary elevation of the serum level. The test is modified to exclude enzyme derived from bone involved by Paget's disease. If there is any reason to suppose that the liver is invaded, liver function tests are included in the blood investigations. Urea and electrolyte values may be abnormal if the urinary obstruction has caused back pressure on the kidneys and renal damage. This more often occurs when there is benign hyperplasia.

Cytology

Fluid expressed from the prostate by careful massage can be examined for malignant cells. The test should not be carried out until three days after rectal examination.

X-rays

The chest must be examined and a skeletal survey done of suspicious areas on isotope bone scan. An I.V.P. will assess the kidneys, ureter and bladder. Rarely vesiculography and urethrography were used to determine the extent of a tumour already detected clinically. Both examinations involve instilling a water soluble radio-opaque medium, the former into the vas deferens, the latter into the urethra. Increasingly ultrasound is being used to diagnose and follow progress during treatment.

Lymphography

The abdominal nodes can only be examined this way.

Bone-marrow Aspiration

Even when there is no X-ray evidence of metastases aspiration of bone marrow from the ileum or sternum can reveal malignant cells. Some authorities consider that this should always be done when radical prostatectomy is planned.

Biopsy

Lymph-node Excision

An enlarged node can be removed easily if accessible. It is often a great help in confirming the diagnosis.

Bone Biopsy

Only certain sites are suitable and it is possible to miss the affected area. Material obtained by these two methods can be examined for acid phosphatase content. If the diagnosis is in doubt, this can lead to discovery of the primary in the prostate, but it must be remembered that secondaries from other sites can give positive results.

Prostate Biopsy

Occasionally tumour tissue is found in the gland removed because of symptoms and signs of hyperplasia, but when carcinoma is diagnosed clinically biopsy is needed for histological confirmation. Three methods are used, needle, open and transurethral.

Cystoscopy

It is important to examine the bladder. In late cases any deformity or invasion of the bladder can be seen. With the instrument in position rectal examination is made easier and induration or fixation more readily appreciated. As the prostatic urethra is traversed there is often a grating sensation when carcinoma is present.

Treatment

During the last few years it has become more usual to consider radiotherapy even for early cases. Surgery often interferes with sexual function so that radiation can be a useful alternative. Modern machines enable more precise localisation of radiation fields, and experience has enabled doctors to reduce associated side effects.

The type of treatment chosen will depend upon the patient's health, age and the extent of the tumour. In early cases the choice may be surgery or radiotherapy. Older, less fit patients may be given radiotherapy, hormones, or a combination of both. Advanced cases similarly receive radiation and hormones. Early results from trials suggest that chemotherapy may not only benefit patients with advanced disease, but combined with hormones can perhaps be used with advantage earlier in the disease.

Surgery

Radical prostatectomy is the treatment of choice in those cases in which invasion of the anatomical capsule has not occurred and in which there is no evidence of metastases. The operation is carried out either through an abdominal or perineal approach. To avoid retrograde infection along the vas from the urethra, both tubes are sectioned and ligated.

Palliative

Transurethral resection can give useful palliation of urinary symptoms. The obstruction is removed. This can be particularly valuable when hormones alone cannot achieve rapid relief.

Radiotherapy

Radiation can give as good results in early cases as surgery, with the advantage that decreased potency is found in fewer patients, 30-40%. Careful localisation is necessary in planning, to avoid unnecessarily high doses to the rectum and the anterior bladder wall. To keep as much of the bladder wall as possible out of the treatment area, the patient is treated with a full bladder, the course of treatment lasts four to six weeks. Previous surgery or local extension of the tumour, as well as total radiation dose, all influence the incidence of late side effects. These may be related to the bladder and urethra, or the bowel. Late recurrence of symptoms related to these areas must always be investigated, since they may be due to tumour spread rather than radiation effects.

Palliative

Radiation can also be used to treat local recurrences or painful metastases. It will often bring quick relief when hormone therapy is slow in taking effect.

Hormone Therapy

About 80% of tumours are stimulated by testosterone from the testis and hormones from the adrenals. Successful therapy to depress these levels, or alter the androgen oestrogen ratio, can cause marked regression of the tumour and dramatic relief of metastatic and urinary symptoms.

Surgical

As the testes are the source of androgens their removal abolishes one stimulus to the prostatic carcinoma. The operation usually performed is subcapsular orchidectomy. A synthetic prosthesis can be inserted and the organisation around it simulates a testis, this is aesthetically more acceptable.

Oestrogens

Synthetic female hormones, oestrogens, are administered. The side effects are nausea, gastric upset, oedema of the ankles. Genital hypoplasia, pigmentation of the nipples and enlargement of the breasts can be produced and embarrass some patients. Hepatic failure and jaundice are rare. A phosphorylated diethyl-stilboestrol, Honvan, does not cause hypertrophy of the breasts. It is activated by the acid phosphatase of the carcinoma cells and therefore tends to have local action only. It is given at first intravenously and later orally.

Long term thrombo-embolic effects have led to some questioning of the use of oestrogens. Recently oestrogen has been chemically combined with a cyto-toxic. The mode of action is not entirely clear, but it is possible that the oestrogen 'targets' on the tumour thereby concentrating the chemotherapy in the malignant tissue. It is also suggested that it may be possible in future to link hormones or cytotoxics to monoclonal antibodies specific to the tumour.

Hormone therapy, whether surgical or by oestrogens, is the treatment of choice when widespread metastases are present. The methods can be used sequentially or as combined therapy.

Relapse after these two forms of treatment can sometimes be controlled by the stopping of adrenal androgens. This is accomplished by suppression of adrenal activity. A variety of methods are available, medically by small amounts of oral cortisone, surgically by adrenalectomy or hypophysectomy. The surgical procedures are major and often the condition of the patient precludes them. Radiation hypophysectomy is difficult to achieve.

The introduction of drugs which block adrenal synthesis of sex hormones offers a method of 'medical' adrenalectomy, as yet this approach is still under evaluation. Similarly antiandrogens which compete with testosterone for receptor sites, and long acting releasing hormones which block the pituitary receptors and so reduce the output of gonadotrophins, are both being investigated.

Chemotherapy

More attention is now being paid to the use of either single agents or combined therapy. As yet the treatment is experimental, but if early reports are substantiated, there could well be a place for chemotherapy either alone, or in combination with hormones, in the treatment of advanced disease.

Follow-up

Patients receiving radiotherapy may get skin reaction in the natal cleft requiring an early follow-up appointment. Otherwise the spacing of appointments will be governed by the clinical condition. Rectal examination, X-ray of the chest, isotope scan of the skeleton, acid phosphatase determinations, and blood counts are the mainstay of the investigations, with increasingly the use of ultra sound to visualise the pelvic disease.

Nursing Care

The principles are the same as those outlined in the previous chapter. Should spinal-cord compression develop, then the techniques outlined in the chapter on spinal tumours must be used. The treatment of carcinoma of the prostate usually involves loss of libido and sexual potency. Although many of the patients are old and have already experienced a natural decrease in these functions, others may find these changes profoundly disturbing. These patients require very sympathetic handling and often need tranquilisers or anti-depressant drugs.

Prognosis

With changing methods of treatment it is too early to give survival rates. When disease is localised surgery gives good control, and claims are now made that radiotherapy can equal this.

When metastases are present, a 25% 5 years survival rate is quoted for treated cases.

In older patients hormonal treatment can establish a long period of control, but in younger patients 'escape' tends to occur earlier.

One of the problems in assessing 'cure' and survival rates, is that many patients are old and may die from intercurrent disease rather than prostatic tumour.

CARCINOMA OF THE SEMINAL VESICLE

This is a very rare disease. It is not usually diagnosed until inoperable. Surgery is the treatment of choice when possible, but in either case the prognosis is poor.

CARCINOMA OF THE SCROTUM

This disease is exceedingly rare causing only 0.25% of male deaths from malignant disease. It is interesting historically as its association with an occupation, chimney sweeping, was first described by Potts at the end of the eighteenth century. Aetiological factors now are exposure to derivatives of petroleum and coal tar associated with poor hygiene.

It occurs usually in the age range 50–70, and the fear that it is venereal in origin leads many patients to delay seeking advice until the disease is well advanced. The histology is that of squamous cell carcinoma, and in appearance it may be ulcerative or proliferative. Inguinal lymph nodes may be enlarged, either due to infection or to metastatic deposits. Treatment of choice is surgery. Block dissection of operable nodes is carried out later. Alternatively radiation can be used both for nodes and also in certain cases for the primary tumour.

Provided the tumour is localised, results are good. Invasion and fixation of the testes or inguinal nodes worsen the prognosis. Secondary involvement of the scrotum can occur due to spread from malignant tumours of the testis and epididymis.

CARCINOMA OF THE TESTIS

Aetiology

During the description of anatomy it was pointed out that malignancy develops more commonly in the undescended testis. The risk is up to 35 times greater in the ectopic than in the normal testis. The association with trauma or mumps is now believed to be incidental.

Types of Tumour

The main types of tumour occurring are seminoma, teratoma, and combined tumours. The teratoma is now usually referred to as non-seminomatous germ cell tumour, (N.S.G.C.T.). The seminoma arises from seminiferous epithelium, while the teratoma probably originates in the germ cells, the combined tumour contains both tumours, either separately or mingled. Teratomas are subdivided into four groups according to histology. Although discussion will use the general term teratoma, the sub-groups are given, together with abbreviations, as these names may be encountered:

Teratoma differentiated (T.D.), or teratoma mature.
Malignant teratoma intermediate (M.T.I.)
Embryonal carcinoma, or malignant teratoma undifferentiated (M.T.U.)
Malignant teratoma trophoblastic (M.T.T.)

Age and Incidence

Although rare, 0.5% of male deaths from cancer, it is the most common form of malignancy in young men.

The age range is wide, but seminomas commonly occur about the age of forty, 50% are under 50 years old, while teratoma has a peak incidence around 30, 48% are between 20 and 29. Seminoma accounts for 40% of testicular tumours, teratoma 32%.

Pathology and Spread

Seminoma

The testis is enlarged by a pale, firm, pinkish tumour which very rarely penetrates the white capsule (tunica albuginea). Under the microscope the tumour consists of irregular lobules of round or oval cells, no tubules are formed.

Spread

Direct   The tumour usually remains confined to the testis, but can spread to the epididymis or spermatic cord.

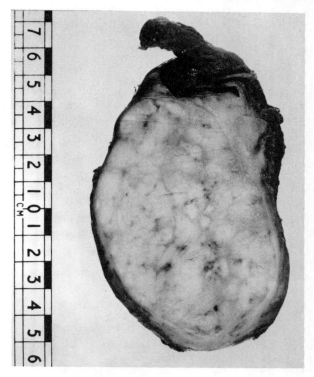

Fig. 17.2.   Seminoma

Lymphatic   This is found in three quarters of fatal cases. The para-aortic nodes are most usually invaded, but spread can be higher to the chest and supra-clavicular areas.

Blood   This is found usually late in the disease. The most common sites are the lungs and liver, but other organs such as the brain can be involved.

Teratoma

The tumour often has a nodular surface, is partly cystic, partly solid, and frequently contains areas of necrosis. The cell type ranges from fully differentiated to anaplastic, trophoblastic. The more differentiated tumours may contain tissue resembling that of any organ in the body. Due to its origin a teratoma can secrete either one, or both of two chemical substances, alphafoetoprotein (A.F.P.) and beta human chorionic gonadotrophin (H.C.G.) The first although present in other tissues is characteristic of foetal liver, the second is normally secreted by the placenta.

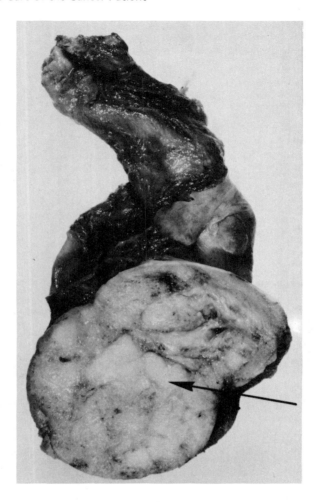

Fig. 17.3.   Non-seminomatous germ cell tumour (teratoma)

Spread

Direct   This is usually only within the testis.

Lymphatic   This is less common than from the seminoma. The nodes, when involved, are para-aortic and pelvic.

Blood   With the more malignant types this can occur early and deposits are found usually in the liver and lungs.

Combined Tumour

The appearances are usually predominantly of a teratoma with a distinct focus of seminoma.

Lymphatic Spread

It should be noted that drainage can occur to the opposite side of the lymphatic chain, particularly from right-sided tumours, so that cross metastases can occur. Since the lymphatic drainage follows the venous drainage, right-sided tumours drain predominantly to nodes along the right iliac veins and vena cava, left-sided to nodes along the aorta. Some left-sided tumours also metastasise along the spermatic lymphatics and will tend to cause deposits in nodes just below the left renal vein. Blockage of the lymphatics can cause retrograde spread.

Symptoms

By far the commonest symptom is painless enlargement of the testis. The progression is slow and the tumour may be well advanced before the patient notices anything wrong. Occasionally the presentation is more dramatic with sudden pain, swelling, and reddening of the skin. This looks like an inflammatory condition. Very rarely the first symptom may be the enlargement of a supra-clavicular node or the symptoms of an intra-abdominal tumour.

The symptoms when an ectopic abdominal testis becomes malignant will either be those of an intra-abdominal tumour, or those of metastatic deposits in nodes or the liver and lungs. It is usually a seminoma.

Examination and Investigations

After the history and general examination, local examination of the testis, followed by lymphatic palpation is carried out. Both testes must be examined. The testis feels enlarged and firm, in the early stages it is difficult to distinguish between it and the tumour. The cord is often thickened by lymphatic deposits. The diagnosis is usually obvious but occasionally the swelling of a hydrocoele or haematocoele can obscure the testis. Other conditions which can sometimes mimic malignancy are inflammation, haematocoele, and a gumma due to tertiary syphillis now very rare. If carcinoma is suspected scrotal biopsy must not be done because of the risk of dissemination.

Blood Tests

These will include full blood count, LFTs, serum calcium, urea, and electrolytes, assay of the blood levels of **AFP** and **HCG**. A serological test for syphilis should also be performed if this disease is suspected.

X-rays

Routine X-rays include the chest and I.V.P. The kidneys are only affected when nodes are grossly enlarged, but if skin markers are used the examination is useful in locating protection for the kidneys during radiotherapy.

Routine lymphography by injection of lymphatics in the feet is employed. This will show up involved nodes in the pelvis and para-aortic areas. In addition if teratoma is suspected, whole lung tomography, CATscans of lungs, liver and retroperitoneum may be carried out. Occasionally an inferior venocavogram is required.

Other Investigations

Ultrasound and isotope scans of the liver and retroperitoneum may be made. Renal function is assessed.

If it is thought that a patient is likely to receive bleomycin, lung function tests are needed. This gives a baseline against which to compare tests during cytotoxic therapy, and so obtain early warning of lung damage.

A young man may not have completed his family. In this case, provided that both sperm morphology and count are normal, it is possible to bank sperm for future artificial insemination of his partner. Chemotherapy or radiation to the other testis may cause sterility or defective spermatogenesis.

The aim of this barrage of investigations is to discover the nature of the tumour and the degree of spread. On the findings depend the staging of the tumour and decisions on treatment. When there is obvious widespread disease the investigation regime will be restricted.

Treatment

Seminoma

Surgery

Simple orchidectomy and removal of the cord up to the internal inguinal ring is first carried out. It is important that ligation of the cord with its blood vessels and lymphatics is done before the testis is handled. This prevents the dissemination of malignant cells. Since the patient is usually young or middle aged, both he and his wife must be mentally prepared for the operation. It should be explained that removal is necessary and that the testis is almost certainly sterile. If there are any accessible suspicious nodes these will be biopsied, and some centres will also operate to sample the abdominal nodes.

Subsequent treatment is given according to staging.

I.   Tumour confined to testis, no evidence of spread.
II. Spread to abdominal lymph nodes.
III. Spread to lymph nodes in the chest or distant metastases, or both.

Radiation

The seminoma is very radio sensitive. Post-operatively the pelvic nodes on the same side, and the central and para-aortic nodes are treated. Only if there is evidence on lymphography that there is cross spread, or that low para-aortic nodes are diseased, would the nodes on the opposite side be treated. The remaining testis is shielded.

The scrotum and inguinal nodes on the affected side are only treated if spread to the scrotum has occurred. Stage III patients were formerly treated by radiotherapy. There is now a tendency to use chemotherapy, particularly if metastases are in areas extremely sensitive to radiation.

Recurrences These can be treated by radiation or chemotherapy, the choice probably depends both on the same considerations as for Stage III patients, and the quality of life likely to be obtained.

More sharply defined radiation beams enable the kidneys to be shielded yet give an adequate dose to nodes. In the very rare event that it is necessary to include substantial kidney tissue in the radiation fields, the dose to these areas must be limited.

Chemotherapy

Similar regimes to those used for teratoma are used.

Teratoma

Improvement in investigative methods enabling more accurate staging, and the advent of new cytotoxic drugs seem to be making an impact on survival rates, the outlook for teratoma used to be far worse than for seminoma. Again treatment is dependent upon staging.

I.   Tumour confined to testis, all tests including AFP and HCG negative.
II. Spread to abdominal lymph nodes.
III. Spread to lymph nodes in the chest or distant metastases or both.

Various modifications of this staging have been made including separation of those with distant metastases into a stage IV. Sub-division of each stage into subgroups by nodal volume, lung and liver status can also be made. The marked improvement effected by chemotherapy is likely to cause these more detailed stagings to be used, thus enabling more precise tailoring of drug regimes to each patient.

Whatever the stage, prognosis is adversely affected if the tumour is large and markers (AFP and HCG) are present.

Surgery

As for seminoma. In the United States a further operation to remove all the nodes from the retroperitoneum is performed. This is a major procedure and may impair sexual function through nerve damage. Radiation is preferred in Britain.

Radiation

The decision as to the use of post-operative radiation is governed by staging. Stage I patients receive post-operative radiation as described for seminoma. Studies are going on to attempt identification of a sub-group which may only need orchidectomy, and conversely others for whom chemotherapy might be more appropriate.

For Stage II patients the sequence chemotherapy or radiation, has been based on the tumour size. Bulky disease (Stage IIb) responds less well to radiation, and toxicity may be increased if radical radiation is followed by cytotoxic drugs. The practice in Britain has been to treat Stage IIb disease with chemotherapy followed by radiation, and less bulky disease (Stage IIa) by radiation only, reserving chemotherapy for any further metastases. However currently it is being considered whether two courses of chemotherapy should be given prior to localised radiation in Stage IIa.

Chemotherapy

This is the treatment of choice for Stage III patients. It involves admission to hospital for five days for up to four times, weekly injections of one of the drugs for 12 weeks, and then maintenance injections of another for up to two years. It is called the Einhorn regime and includes cis-platin.

Following treatment, surgery or radiation may be necessary to deal with residual tumour.

Special Centres

The number of patients suffering from testicular tumours is small. In view of this and the specialised nature of investigation and treatment, such patients are probably best managed at a small number of centres with expertise in this field, particularly since 83% have Stage I or Stage II tumours which are potentially curable.

Follow-up

Frequent follow-up is necessary during the first year, investigations to detect any recurrence will be done and these must include estimation of the levels of the two chemical markers. Just as a fall during treatment shows tumour response, so a rise after treatment indicates renewed tumour activity. Thereafter depending upon the treatment given, and the prognosis, intervals between appointments will be lengthened.

Prognosis

This is good for seminoma, 85–90% of treated patients with early tumours survive 3 years and recurrence after this period is unusual.

The figures for teratoma are much more difficult to assess in view of the changing regimes, overall, all stages, it is probably about 50% at 3 years. However claims have been made that in patients with advanced disease, not previously treated, chemotherapy can produce a sustained response in at least half. In the future it is anticipated that survival figures should improve.

OTHER TUMOURS

Tumours of the interstitial cells are usually benign. In children precocious puberty may occur, gynaecomastia in adults. Occasionally lymphoma of the testis may be found in older patients, it is treated as elsewhere in the body. Other tumours of the testis and epididymis are very rare, only a small number are malignant.

Each man lives within a fortress,
Believing that his neighbours' walls can be breached,
But never his own.

18   The Urinary Tract

Embryology

The urinary tract is concerned first with the formation of urine and then its storage and excretion. Malignant tumours in various parts of the system although arising in adjacent areas differ not only in the frequency of their incidence, but also in their pathology and behaviour. This becomes easier to understand, and certainly more interesting, when the development of the system in the embryo is considered.

Three Germ Layers

In the embryo cell division begins after fertilisation. Eventually three layers of cells are present, ectoderm, mesoderm, and endoderm. From these all the organs of the body are formed, this process of organogenesis is complete by the twelfth week of pregnancy. It is from the mesoderm that the kidney is formed.

Formation of the Bladder and Urethra

The bladder and the female urethra are formed from the urogenital sinus derived from endoderm. The first, prostatic part of the male urethra has a similar origin, the second is formed by the fusion of genital swellings and elongation of the swelling giving rise to the penis, and the third is formed by ectodermal cells.

Formation of the Kidney and Ureter

The urine secreting part of the kidney, the nephron, arises from mesoderm. The nephrons together with connective tissue and blood vessels form the renal medulla and cortex. Tissue budding off from the urogenital sinus forms the renal pelvis, the ureter, and the collecting ducts of the kidney. The lower end of the bud passes through the bladder wall opening into the bladder at the trigone which is formed from mesoderm. The rest of the bladder derives from endoderm.

Anatomy

Kidney

Normally paired, the kidneys lie in a groove on either side of the spine behind the peritoneum. They extend from the twelfth thoracic vertebra to the third lumbar, the right lying slightly lower than the left. Above and behind is the diaphragm, in front are the abdominal contents. The suprarenal gland, shaped like a cocked hat, fits like a cap on top of each kidney, but both anatomically and functionally it is separate from it.

On the medial side of each kidney is a depression, the hilum, nerves, blood vessels, lymphatics and ureter enter and leave here.

Inside the kidney the ureter is opened out into the pelvis which is split into a number of calyces. A papilla of renal tissue carrying the collecting ducts dips into each calyx.

The renal artery arises from the aorta, and the vein runs directly to the inferior vena cava. Nerve supply is from the sympathetic system. Lymphatic drainage is to nodes at the hilum and then the para-aortic group.

Nephron

The basic unit of the kidney is the nephron, this can only be seen with the aid of the microscope. It is the system which forms and secretes urine, in the process retaining useful materials required by the body.

Glomerular Tuft

A division of the renal artery, an arteriole, forms a knot of capillaries, the glomerular tuft. From this tuft, a vessel runs down to the first part of the nephron tubule, breaks up into a network of capillaries, and then forms a venule. This eventually joins others and drains into the renal vein.

Bowman's Capsule

The glomerular tuft is pushed into the blind end of the nephron so that the nephron forms a cap around it. This part of the nephron has a wall one cell thick with pores between each cell, it is called Bowman's capsule. Capillary tuft and capsule together form a Malpighian body. The nephron runs from the capsule as a convoluted tubule, the proximal tubule. It then forms a straight hairpin loop, with ascending and descending limbs (the straight loop of Henle) before again becoming convoluted, the distal convoluted tubule. Finally the nephron tubule opens into a collecting duct. This duct joins with others and discharges urine into the pelvis of the kidney at the renal papilla.

If the kidney is cut longtudinally it will be seen that there are two clear zones of tissue, the outer is called the cortex and the inner the medulla. The glomeruli and convoluted tubules mostly lie in the cortex, the straight loop of Henle and the collecting ducts in the medulla. The epithelium of the nephron tubules is cuboidal. Each kidney contains about one million nephrons.

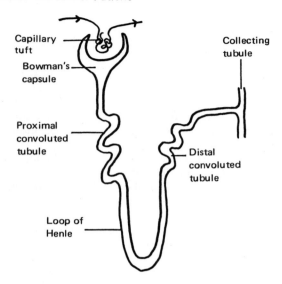

Capillary tuft

Bowman's capsule

Collecting tubule

Proximal convoluted tubule

Distal convoluted tubule

Loop of Henle

Fig. 18.1.   Diagram of nephron

Ureter

The ureter narrows as it leaves the kidney, running down beside the spine to the pelvic brim. Its course is then round the pelvic wall, forward towards the midline, finally entering the bladder at an oblique angle. In the male it lies above the seminal vesicle and is crossed by the vas deferens, while in the female it lies above the lateral fornix of the vagina closely related to a lymphatic node draining the cervix.

Muscle in the ureter wall contracts propelling urine along it. Blood supply is from various arteries lying along its course. The lining is transitional epithelium.

Bladder

In common with the kidneys and ureters the bladder lies behind and below the peritoneum of the abdominal cavity. When empty it is shaped rather like the bow end of a boat lying keel upwards, the bow or point being just behind the symphysis pubis. Above the bladder is the peritoneum, small intestine, colon, and in the female the uterus. On either side lie muscles, while behind are the rectum, in the male the seminal vesicles and the last part of the vasa deferentia, and in the female the vagina and the upper part of the cervix.

The bladder is lined with transitional epithelium. In the resting state this looks many cells thick, but when stretched out is seen in fact to be only a single-cell layer. The strong muscular wall is arranged in criss-cross bundles of fibres which condense at the opening of the urethra into a circular sphincter, the internal urethral sphincter.

The blood supply is from branches of the internal iliac artieries. The veins form a plexus draining into the internal iliac vein. Nodes in the iliac and para-aortic groups receive the lymphatic drainage.

Urethra

Female   The female urethra runs down from the bladder in front of the vagina opening at the external meatus one inch behind the clitoris.

Male   For convenience the urethra is divided into three parts, prostatic, membranous, and spongy. The first runs down through the anterior prostate receiving the prostatic and ejaculatory ducts. The second pierces the fibres of the external urethral sphincter. Thereafter it runs forward and down, unless the penis is erect during coitus.

Sphincters, Epithelium

The internal urethral sphincter is not under conscious control and in the female its fibres are less well developed. There is conscious control of the external sphincter. The bladder transitional cell lining is carried into the urethra, then becomes columnar, finally it is squamous at the external meatus.

Penis

The skin is loose, and has no adipose (fatty) tissue. Folded back on itself (prepuce) at the distal end it overhangs the glans, and is removed in the operation of circumcision. The penis contains the longest portion of the urethra. It is erectile and the male organ of coitus. Erection occurs when three masses of erectile tissue become engorged with blood. Blood supply is from the internal iliac artery, venous drainage is by the prostatic plexus and deep dorsal vein. Nerves derived from the sacral nerves serve both erection, through the sympathetic system, and sensation.

Physiology

Kidney

The overall function of the kidney is to excrete waste products, and maintain the body water and salts in balance.

Bowman's capsule behaves like a sieve. Large entities such as blood cells and plasma proteins are retained in the capillary, the blood liquid and dissolved substances such as glucose, salts, urea, pass out into the nephron to form the filtrate. The cells of the tubule wall extract glucose, salt, potassium, passing them back into the blood, and excrete waste products of metabolism and drugs, and finally absorb water to produce the concentrated urine. The varying functions of the tubule are regulated by blood levels and by certain hormones.

About 170 litres of filtrate are formed daily, but 99% is reabsorbed, so that daily urine volume is about 1.7 litres. In old terms this is equivalent to about 298 pint bottles and about 3 pints respectively. Water reabsorbation in the distal convoluted tubules is controlled by anti-diuretic hormone (A.D.H.) stored in the posterior pituitary. Without this there is copious urine and continuous thirst, the clinical condition of diabetes insipidus.

Bladder

About 290 cm^3 (half a pint) is the comfortable capacity of the bladder. In the infant, in response to a full bladder, micturition is effected by a reflex arc through the spinal cord, with no conscious control. With training voluntary control of the external sphincter is established by the cerebral cortex. A paraplegic patient usually has retention first, then the infantile pattern may become established. Some patients achieve a form of control, by stimulating the reflex arc with some cutaneous sensation such as stroking the abdominal skin.

CARCINOMA OF THE KIDNEY

Since a special chapter is to be devoted to tumours in children discussion of Wilm's tumour will be postponed and not included here.

Pathology

This is a tumour of kidney tissue and is generally agreed to arise from tubular cells. It is an adenocarcinoma and originates in the cortex. The term hyper-nephroma is no longer used since it was based on a theory of origin no longer acceptable. This postulated the existence of ectopic foci of adrenal cells which then became malignant.

The tumour is vascular taking the form of rounded masses. When cut across areas of necrosis, calcification, haemorrhage, and golden-yellow tissue can be seen. The cells range from well-differentiated resembling tubular epithelium, to the poorly-differentiated. On the histology a grading is given and this indicates the malignant potential of the growth. Grade I, well-differentiated, has a low potential, while for the poorly-differentiated Grade III, the potential is high. The prognosis must of course take into account the evidence of invasion of the renal vein and distant metastases.

Spread is initially direct through the kidney including the renal pelvis and the surrounding capsule and sac. Blood-borne metastases occur early, they are found commonly in the bones, lungs, and brain. In 30% of cases there is spread to the para-aortic nodes and later more distant groups.

Sex, Age and Incidence

The tumour is seldom seen in patients under 40, the peak incidence is in the sixth decade. Men are affected twice as commonly as women. It is not a common tumour accounting for only 1% of all malignant tumours, but it makes up 80% of the total of renal tumours.

Aetiology

It has been observed that the kidney which contains an adenoma often has associated chronic inflammatory and arteriosclerotic changes. It has therefore been suggested that these changes may predispose to malignancy.

CARCINOMA OF THE RENAL PELVIS AND URETER

Aetiology

This tumour arises from an epithelium which is transitional and the same as the bladder. It has therefore many characteristics similar to bladder carcinoma, among them the aetiological factors.

Industrial Exposure

Workers in certain industries such as dye, rubber and cables, coal tar, have in the past had exposure to chemicals which after metabolism were excreted in the urine as beta-naphthylamine. A known carcinogen, it appears to need urine to become active. A policy of restriction of the processes and screening of workers is now followed.

Squamous metaplasia in response to irritation caused by calculi, may progress to malignancy. Bladder cancer, and to a lesser extent, kidney cancer, is more frequent in smokers.

Self medication with large quantities of phenacetin containing analgesics has been linked with carcinoma of the renal pelvis.

Age, Sex and Incidence

These are far less common tumours than those of the kidney tissue, forming only 12% of the total of renal tumours. They are found in patients aged from 50 to 70 and men are three times more likely to be affected than women.

About half of the pelvic tumours are multiple but involvement of both kidneys is rare.

Pathology

In appearance the growth may be papillary with or without infiltration of the adjacent tissues, infiltrating, or solid. The last two types infiltrate diffusely into the kidney and also give a pale irregular thickening of the pelvis and calyces.

The cell type is transitional in about 80% of the cases. The differentiation ranges from the regular 'papilloma' type through to the highly-invasive solid

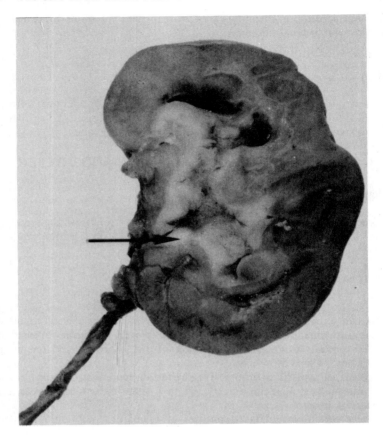

Fig. 18.2.   Carcinoma of the pelvis of the kidney

tumour. The rest of the growths are squamous, and of these in one-third of cases there is an associated calculus. They are highly invasive.

Spread

Direct spread to the kidney and surrounding tissues occurs. In nearly half further tumours appear in the ureter or bladder, and it is not clear whether these are multiple primary growths or the result of spread by implantation or by lymphatics around the ureter. Lymphatic spread to the para-aortic nodes is common. Although invasion of the renal vein is not usually seen, metastases in the lungs and other distant sites occur quite frequently with the infiltrative type of tumour.

Symptomatology

The symptoms are virtually the same for both types of tumour, differing only in their degree, timing, and severity. It is unfortunate that often they do not appear until late in the course of the disease or are dismissed as trivial by the patient. For convenience they will be divided into three groups, primary site, obstruction and metastases.

Primary Site

Haematuria and pain   The severity, and the timing in the course of the disease, of these two symptoms, vary with the site of the tumour. Bleeding usually occurs first and the amount can be very small or profuse. The patient is often quite well between attacks. Pain does not always accompany bleeding. Indeed until the tissues surrounding the kidney are involved there may be little or no pain. When the tumour is in the kidney tissue pain is usually felt in the loin or epigastrium, while with tumours of the renal pelvis or ureter pain is mostly due to clots obstructing the ureter. This latter type is very severe and colicky in nature.

Obstruction

Permanent obstruction of the ureter producing hydronephrosis is more often caused by tumours of the pelvis and ureter than by malignancy of the kidney tissue. The symptoms produced are often vague and do not indicate directly renal disease, in some cases they may be completely absent. If infection occurs the symptoms will mimic those of pyelitis. Very rarely the left testicular vein is obstructed by growth invading the renal vein. In these circumstances a varicocoele of the left testis may develop.

Distant Sites

In about a quarter of cases the first symptoms are those due to distant metastases. These can be very variable, a pathological fracture, cerebral symptoms, haemoptysis, or ulceration due to an enlarging skin nodule. One of my patients presented with vaginal bleeding. On examination she was found to have an obviously malignant deposit, but there was no evidence on clinical examination to suggest a primary site. Biopsy showed it to be a secondary deposit from an adenocarcinoma of the kidney.

Other Symptoms

If there are no symptoms of metastases and the primary tumour is silent, there may be little to suggest the true diagnosis. In these cases the symptoms are vague and can include those of lethargy, weight loss, anaemia, hypertension, and uraemia.

Differential Diagnosis

Haematuria, pain, or swelling in the loin can be produced by many other diseases of the kidney or adjacent structures, or they may be symptoms of a systemic disease. It may well be that despite exhaustive investigation the diagnosis is only established at exploratory operation.

Examination and Investigation

Careful questioning can reveal symptoms preceding those of which the patient is complaining and dismissed by him as trivial. The routine recording of present and past occupation may also provide the first clue to the diagnosis. After a general examination including the lymphatic areas, the abdomen and loin are carefully palpated. In normal subjects of slim build only the lower pole of the right kidney can be palpated and this at the end of inspiration. It is not surprising therefore that tumour is only detectable in about half the cases, in others it is very small or the patient is obese. When palpable it is felt below the twelfth rib, moves with respiration, and may feel hard or irregular. Occasionally an advanced tumour produces a bulge in the loin. Tumours of the ureter are rarely felt as they occur in its lower part and therefore lie deep in the pelvis.

Investigation

Blood Tests

As always a full blood count must be performed, anaemia may be present and occasionally the eosinophil count is raised. A full electrolyte analysis should include urea, calcium, and phosphorus. Calcium may be raised while the phosphate level is low.

Urine

Examination of the urine will include testing for blood. Cytological screening may identify malignant cells shed from the renal pelvis or ureter, but it is less likely for them to be found if the tumour is in the kidney tissue. A specimen of urine must also be sent for culture and sensitivity. Infection may be present and is particularly likely to occur if there is any obstruction.

X-ray

Plain   Plain X-rays of the abdomen may give a soft-tissue shadow of the kidneys and occasionally suspicious calcification can be seen. Other X-rays performed are, chest with tomography or CATscan, abdominal CATscan. When CATscanning cannot be performed ultra sound of the abdomen may be substituted.

Radio-opaque   By injecting intravenously a material which is excreted by the kidneys and opaque to X-rays, the urinary tract can be visualised. It used to be thought that if the blood urea was high this examination, I.V.P., was not only useless but dangerous. Now with modern opaque media it can often be performed and rarely fails to show some detail. If the pictures are inadequate, catheters are passed into the ureters at cystoscopy and radio-opaque medium injected, retrograde pyelography. This examination is particularly useful when a carcinoma of the ureter is suspected, any stricture which is found is regarded as malignant until proven otherwise.

The appearances of the pyelogram vary with the situation of the tumour. The changes in appearance can vary from a slight irregularity to a complete obliteration of the normal pattern. In the ureter the appearance is usually that of a stricture or an irregularity of the outline.

The state of the blood vessels in the kidney can be examined by injecting radio-opaque medium directly into the renal artery or into the inferior vena cava. The normal pattern can be distorted or obliterated, or invasion of the renal vein or inferior vena cava may be seen.

Cystoscopy

When the site of bleeding is uncertain, cystoscopy is performed while bleeding is still present. It can then be established whether the blood is coming from the lower urinary tract or the upper. If it is from the upper the side can be identified.

Radioactive Isotope Scan

Certain radioactive isotopes are concentrated in the kidney. Isotope as well as X-ray scans of the skeleton are performed. Scanners are placed over the kidneys, the rise in radioactivity is plotted as a curve, and a dot scan is also recorded. Because tumours of the kidney substance often have necrotic and avascular areas, the usual scan pattern may be disturbed.

When it is strongly suspected that a cyst or solid tumour is malignant, needle biopsy is contraindicated due to risk of disseminated cells. When cyst puncture is done cytology of the fluid must be performed.

Occasionally diagnosis is only established at operation, this is particularly true for the ureter.

When symptoms are due to metastases, biopsy may establish the kidneys are the primary site.

Treatment

Surgery

When the tumour is operable surgery is the treatment of choice. The opposite kidney must be functioning normally and there should be no metastases in the chest. The scope of the operation varies from nephrectomy with removal of lymph nodes and the whole renal vein if invaded, to nephrectomy with removal of the ureter and a cone of bladder.

Even when the disease is advanced operation may occasionally be useful in relieving pain, haematuria, and toxic symptoms. A solitary metastasis is not necessarily a bar to operation. When the deposit has been stationary for some time surgery has been successful.

In some centres, under X-ray control, catheters have been used to introduce various emboli into the renal artery, or into obviously abnormal arteries. The aim is to cause infarcts of the tissue supplied. Such techniques could make surgery less difficult and affect tumour growth, but they are, as yet, experimental.

Palliative

Secondary deposits may cause symptoms which can be relieved by surgery. A pathological fracture may require fixation, or a solitary skin metastasis can be excised. Quite often secondary deposits can appear years after removal of the primary tumour, in these circumstances even major procedures such as a lobectomy can prove worth while.

Radiotherapy

Since this is basically a surgical problem, the use of radiation as a primary method of treatment is confined to patients unfit for surgery or to those with inoperable tumours. Palliative radiation of secondaries is extremely valuable, particularly in relieving the pain of metastases. The place of radiotherapy as an adjunct to surgery is less well defined. In a few cases radiation has reduced the tumour to an operable size allowing surgery to take place after a three-week interval. Post-operative radiation is now usually given in selected cases, particularly when the renal vein or the capsule is invaded. Recurrences after excision are also treated by radiation.

Megavoltage therapy is used for treatment of the primary site, the course lasting five or six weeks. The fields used must be large and in order to cover the immediate lymphatic drainage must cross the midline. Normally two opposed anterior and posterior fields are used. Since the fields cross the midline the medial part is shielded off at 4000 or 4500 rads. to protect the spinal cord. In planning and placing fields, it is usual to carry out an I.V.P. with skin markers in position. This identifies the relation of the field to the other kidney, and ensures that the renal bed and the scar on the treated side are adequately covered. If at operation the surgeon puts in clips to define the tumour or kidney limits this is a most useful aid to planning.

Chemotherapy and Hormones

Cytotoxic drugs have been used to treat inoperable and widespread disease, but no magic improvements have been seen and chemotherapy is not commonly used.

Some patients, usually males, have been helped by the use of progestins.

Unfortunately prediction of response is not possible and so selection of suitable patients is difficult, particularly in view of possible acceleration of the disease in some.

Nursing Care

The general principles outlined already for patients receiving abdominal radiation apply here. With such large fields irradiating the abdomen it is almost inevitable that the patient will experience lethargy, severe nausea, and in some cases vomiting. If the left side is being treated the stomach is irradiated and anorexia and dyspepsia usually occur. For all these reasons unless the travelling distance is short and the home conditions very good, it is probably better to treat these patients in hospital. Those who are treated from home must be admitted if reactions become too severe. During treatment the blood count is kept under review as the white-cell count may fall quite low. Any unusual breathlessness merits a chest X-ray, pulmonary deposits can appear quite shortly after operation despite negative pre-operative reports, and they can then develop rapidly. It is of little use to persist with abdominal radiation in the face of such a development. Persistence in treatment is of little use, but abrupt termination should if possible be avoided. Such a change of plan tests very fully the ability of the team to handle the patient. A reasonable and acceptable explanation must be given to him, an experienced doctor can usually manage this, but at the same time the family must be fully informed of the position.

It is important that patients are not discharged before the symptoms of gastro-intestinal reaction, nausea, vomiting, or diarrhoea have begun to settle. The family may need advice on how to continue the hospital regime, adequate diet, fluids and rest, and how to relax gradually the more irksome restrictions.

Follow-up

At each appointment the patient is questioned about his general health, appetite, weight, and bowel habits. Specific enquiries are made to elicit symptoms of pain, urinary or neurological disturbances. In the latter case symptoms may be no more than transient parasthesiae. X-ray examinations are ordered as indicated but chest X-rays are taken as a routine at intervals. If any urinary disturbance is present an M.S.U. is sent for culture, sensitivity, and cytology, and if the primary tumour was in the renal pelvis or ureter, cystoscopy must be performed to exclude further tumour in the bladder.

Prognosis

Since the disease is so often advanced before medical advice is sought the prognosis is not a good one. However low-grade tumours confined within the kidney have a much better outlook. In operable cases the five-year survival rate is 40% for renal tumours and 50% if the growth is in the renal pelvis. Invasion of the renal vein halves the chance of five year survival in the first case, and there are few survivors if spread is beyond the renal pelvis. No five year survivors are found in the pelvic squamous cell group.

On the other hand adenocarcinoma of the kidney has an unpredictable course. There have been documented cases of spontaneous remission.

CARCINOMA OF THE BLADDER

Aetiology

The same chemical carcinogens are implicated as for tumours of the renal pelvis and ureter. There are however some additional predisposing factors, severe congenital abnormality resulting in the bladder opening on the anterior abdominal wall, certain forms of cystitis, bladder diverticula, and the parasitic disease, schistosomiasis. Leukoplakia although associated with carcinoma of the bladder is not necessarily in this site a pre-malignant condition.

From time to time other substances are suggested as carcinogens, one example is artificial sweeteners. From current research work the concept has arisen that while some substances may be complete carcinogens, i.e. always causing carcinoma in experimental models, others are incomplete and require additional factors to become active, i.e. the presence of urine and stasis. While as yet of little relevance to clinical management, such work may advance our understanding of the process of carcinogenesis.

Age, Sex and Incidence

The incidence of this tumour is increasing, and at present it accounts for 3% of the deaths from malignant disease. The peak incidence is between the ages of 60 and 70, although cases can occur over a wide range. Women less often develop the disease, the ratio male to female being 3:1.

Pathology

Primary

In appearance the tumour is either fronded (papillary) or solid. The second type projects little but grows into the wall while the papillary type may show little or no invasion. The area most commonly affected is the base, particularly the trigone and around the opening of the ureters. Microscopically the growth is of two types, transitional cell with varying degrees of differentiation, and keratinising squamous cell. An uncommon type is the adenocarcinoma. In about a third of cases the growths are multiple, it is generally believed that these are due to multifocal origin rather than to implantation of cells shed from one tumour.

Secondary

The bladder can be involved by extension of tumours arising in neighbouring structures, particularly the large bowel, uterus and ovaries.

Spread

Direct

Tumour spreads initially through the bladder wall and into adjacent structures. Further invasion will result in fixation of the bladder to other pelvic organs.

Lymphatic

In about one-third of fatal cases the disease has spread to the iliac and para-aortic lymph nodes.

Blood

In a similar proportion of patients distant blood-borne deposits are found, occurring late in lungs, bone, liver, skin or other organs.

Implantation

During surgery malignant cells can spill and be implanted. Such recurrences can be found in the urethra, the prostatic bed, and abdominal or bladder scars.

Staging

Tumours of the bladder are staged according to the degree of penetration of the bladder wall.
Stage I.   Tumour confined to the mucosa.
Stage II.   Tumour extending into the muscle.
Stage III. Tissues around the bladder (perivesical) invaded.
Stage IV. Pelvic fixation of the bladder.
    (A Stage 0 has been suggested to include the very superficial carcinoma-in-situ.)
    This staging may be altered after a consideration of findings at operation.
    However, the histology also influences the classification, and there is a tendency to classify tumours as superficial or invasive, and high or low grade. For example superficial high grade tumours can behave in a far more malignant way than low grade ones.

Symptomatology

The symptom which occurs most commonly is painless haematuria. Unlike the bleeding from the kidney or ureter which can be unnoticed by the patient or dismissed as trivial, bleeding from lesions of the bladder is sufficiently marked to cause patients to consult a doctor early. A few patients also complain of pain or frequency. In about 10% of cases the symptoms are more suggestive of an enlarged prostate gland or a urinary infection.

Examination

Since certain carcinogenic factors are known it is important that direct questions are asked about occupation, past and present, or any period spent in an area where schistosomiasis is known to be endemic. The patient should be questioned about the timing of bleeding, if blood only appears in the urine at the beginning of micturition the lesion is most probably in the urethra. The examination must include a general one. A raised blood pressure or changes in the fundus may point to malignant hypertension as the cause.

Investigations

The sequence of investigations will vary according to whether haematuria is still present. If bleeding is still present, after sending an M.S.U. for culture and cytology, checking the blood count and grouping so that transfusion can be given if necessary, cystoscopy is performed. With modern instruments it is possible to wash out the bladder and identify the source of the bleeding, whether it is from the bladder or ureter.

With the patient fully relaxed a bimanual examination can be made. If a bladder lesion is seen it is biopsied, or if it is small resected completely and the base diathermised. If blood clot has been evacuated a drainage catheter is left in place. Investigations described in the next paragraph are then carried out.

When bleeding has stopped the sequence of investigations is reversed, the routine leads up to cystoscopy. The first step is to send urine for culture, sensitivity and cytology. The second voided specimen of the day is the most useful for cytology. It is important to do this before any instrumentation. Pus cells are white cells of a particular type, neutrophil polymorphs. They are important as a defence against bacteria and their numbers are increased in many infections. The finding of numbers of pus cells in the urine, pyuria, without the presence of bacteria is highly suggestive of the presence of tumour or tuberculosis.

Blood Tests

Blood tests will include blood count, blood grouping, electrolytes, and blood urea and creatinine. Any serious anaemia must be corrected before an anaesthetic is given.

X-rays

A routine chest X-ray must be performed both to establish the state of the respiratory system before anaesthesia, and to exclude the presence of metastases. The urinary tract must be investigated by intravenous pyelogram as it is important not only to establish the diagnosis of a bladder tumour, but to exclude the presence of any other lesion. Lymphography has now become a routine investigation and should be performed to show the state of the lymphatics, particularly if spread to the perivesical tissues is suspected.

Other investigations may include liver ultra sound, and X-ray and isotope skeletal surveys.

Cystoscopy

This examination is best performed under general anaesthesia. Many of these patients are elderly men with enlarged prostates and in these cases cystoscopy in the outpatient department may not only be difficult and painful, but lead to complete retention of urine. A further advantage of the inpatient cystoscopy is the opportunity for bimanual examination, catheterisation of the ureters if necessary, and biopsy of any lesion seen. If more than one specimen has been taken these must be listed on the form, and bottles labelled correctly.

Appearance at Cystoscopy

The posterior urethra, the lobes of the prostate, and the mucosa around the bladder neck are first inspected, and then the rest of the bladder is assessed. Notes are made of the condition of the mucosa, the presence of a diverticulum, and the size, shape and appearance of any lesion. A tumour less than half the size of the trigone is considered small.

Treatment

As a result of investigations and findings at cystoscopy a treatment plan is made. Since surgery, radiation, chemotherapy may be used singly, or in combination, it is logical that all specialities should be involved in this planning.

Surgery

Due to the known effect of the tumour histology on prognosis, many centres now adopt a more aggressive surgical approach rather earlier than previously, particularly when superficial tumours are high grade.

Endoscopic Resection

Low grade superficial tumours can be dealt with by transurethral resection. This can be a lengthy process involving several sessions. Routine follow-up cystoscopies must be done, and if biopsy shows a change from low to high grade, more radical surgery must be performed. Lasers have been useful in endoscopic resection.

Total Cystectomy

This involves removal of the bladder and usually part of the urethra and the lower ends of the ureters. The urine is diverted by implanting the ureters in one of three ways: into an isolated loop of ileum which opens on the abdominal well and a bag collects the urine, into the rectum, the faeces being diverted to a colostomy, or directly to an opening in the abdominal wall, again urine collection in a bag.

Patients who are faced with these procedures need the help of a specially trained 'stoma' nurse. If they are able to meet other patients who have had the operation and are coping successfully this also is a great morale booster.

The procedure is used for high grade invasive tumours, when endoscopic resection has failed to control tumour, or when superficial tumour becomes more aggressive.

There must be no evidence of distant metastases or pelvic fixation.

Partial Cystectomy

Only part of the bladder is removed in this procedure. It is only suitable for selected cases such as a small but invasive lesion in the dome of the bladder.

Radiotherapy

On its own as radical therapy radiation has not shown marked success, and is now usually used as a primary treatment when the patient's condition is too poor to permit surgery. As an adjunct to surgery, radiation before cystectomy is held by many centres to reduce the recurrence rate when compared to the results of either method used alone. Studies are also being conducted to assess its post-operative role. Radiation can also control pain and bleeding when the tumour is widespread.

As an alternative to external beam therapy, radiation may be given by radioactive implants, left permanently in the tissues, or left for a short time and then removed, or by putting radioactive colloidal gold in the bladder and then draining it.

If the bladder is being treated by radiation beams careful planning is required. With radio-opaque dye in the bladder and markers on the skin X-rays are taken. These enable the physicist to work out the depth and volume to be treated. It is important to avoid a high dose to the rectum and this can be done either using fixed fields, or rotation through a wide arc.

Preparation of the Patient

A course of radical treatment is a severe strain on the patient and he will tolerate it better if he is well prepared. Very few are able to manage as outpatients, and those who begin in this way usually require admission before the end of the course. The general condition must be improved. Transfusion is given if necessary to correct anaemia, and antibiotics if urinary infection is present. Every effort should be made to keep the patient free of urinary infection as its presence

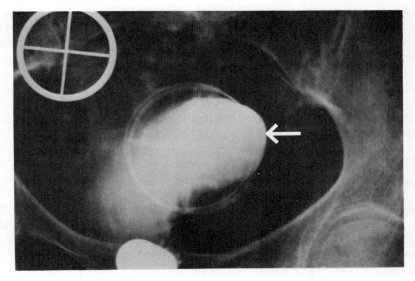

Fig. 18.3.   Cystogram. Radio-opaque solution in the bladder.
Markers in position

will make the radiation reaction in the bladder worse. A urine specimen for culture and sensitivity should be sent weekly as a routine. If the urine flow is obstructed by tumour or an enlarged prostate, resection should be carried out before treatment begins. Radiation produces some oedema and could precipitate complete obstruction.

Some dysuria and frequency will occur inevitably. It is a natural reaction to limit fluid intake but it must be explained that a good urine output will make the urine dilute and less irritating to the bladder. A fluid balance chart should be kept and an intake equivalent to three quart jugs encouraged. Many of these patients are elderly and it may be necessary to supervise and help them at meal times, and also whenever passing persuade them to take some fluid. Radiation of the rectum causes proctitis and some tenesmus (painful straining although the rectum is empty). There may also be some diarrhoea particularly if there has been previous diathermy.

Chemotherapy

Cytotoxic drugs have been found effective in some patients, but no clear advantage of combination over single drug therapy has been found. Some centres have tried intra-arterial perfusion in an attempt to reduce side effects and concentrate the drug in the affected area.

Some progress has been made in treating superficial tumours with cytotoxic solutions in the bladder. Large collaborative studies indicate a reduction in the recurrence rate, and research continues to determine whether this could be a first line treatment, prophylaxis after total endoscopic resection, or whether it should be reserved for recurrences. Drugs so far used have been epodyl, thiotepa, and adriamycin.

Immunotherapy

Attempts have been made to raise immunity by BCG vaccination. Some centres are encouraged but the method is as yet experimental.

Recurrence

Recurrence following radiation is treated by total cystectomy whenever possible. In the reverse situation, or after implantation, radical irradiation is used. No second course of radical radiation can be attempted, nor should it be given, except in rare cases, when there is a leaking suprapubic wound.

Complications of Treatment

All methods carry a risk of late complications. Surgery, even with meticulous care, can result in implantation of tumour, and diathermy after radiation can cause necrosis, contraction of the bladder, pain, frequency, and renal failure due to obstruction. Local necrosis can occur both after interstitial and external radiation. It causes pain, frequency, and some bleeding, but usually heals with symptomatic treatment. A late result can be telangectasia of the mucosa giving rise to haematuria, and fibrosis causing bladder contraction. These conditions are only rarely severe enough to necessitate cystectomy.

Urinary diversion with implantation of the ureters into the colon may result in renal infection and electrolyte imbalance. Patients have to be taught a regime of regular emptying of the bowel and an adequate fluid intake with restriction of salt. They must be warned of the signs of electrolyte imbalance and taught simple measures which they can take immediately, then consulting the doctor.

Follow-up

Apart from the immediate appointment to assess progress after either surgery or radiation, the mainstay of follow-up is regular cystoscopy. At outpatient attendance the patient is asked for details of symptoms and examined, but only regular cystoscopic survey can assess the disease accurately. In the first year the examination should be done at three-month intervals and thereafter six-monthly or earlier if there are symptoms. In advanced cases it may be decided to cystoscope only if symptoms develop. Any suspicion of renal impairment will call for full investigation including I.V.P.

Prognosis

There is a wide range in the survival figures, since both histology and penetration influence the outcome. A figure of 70% five year survival is common for well differentiated papillary tumours, this drops to 30% for solid, undifferentiated tumours. Death is often due to renal failure.

The difference in the behaviour of bladder tumours can best be illustrated by the histories of two of my patients. Mr. – aged 72 had repeated diathermy treatment of an area of papillomata. As he continued to have intermittent haematuria he was referred for radiotherapy. He tolerated this well, the bleeding stopped and he remained free of trouble for six years, and was put on yearly follow-up. By contrast Mr. – 55 had a recurrence-free period of 18 months, then noticed a nodule on the thigh which failed to heal. Others developed on the abdominal wall and the leg. Neither radiation nor chemotherapy controlled them and he died six months later.

CARCINOMA OF THE URETHRA

This is a very rare disease and usually arises only in the patient over 65 years old. It occurs commonly near the external meatus but is also found occasionally along the course of the urethra. Near the meatus it is usually at first papillary, ulcerating later, but in other parts of the urethra it is ulcerative and invasive from the beginning. Most carcinomas are squamous cell with occasional transitional cell areas. Sometimes an adenocarcinoma can arise from one of the adjacent glands. Spread is direct into the surrounding tissues, and to the lymphatic nodes, in the male the inguinal, in the female to both the inguinal and iliac groups.

Symptoms

The initial symptom is discharge or bleeding which does not always accompany micturition. Later pain develops as the lesion ulcerates and sometimes incontinence or retention develops. Women are twice as commonly affected as men.

Treatment

Surgery

To be effective this must be radical. In the male the extent of the operation can range from partial amputation of the penis to removal of the bladder, urethra and prostate. In the female the anterior vaginal wall must also be excised.

Radiation

Early cases can be treated with a radioactive needle implant, and the more extensive growths by megavoltage therapy given in the same way as for treatment of the bladder.

Lymph Nodes

The usual expectant policy is adopted. If nodes remain enlarged after a course of antibiotics, or present following treatment, block dissection is carried out provided they are mobile.

Prognosis is very poor as the disease is often advanced with lymph-node involvement at the time of diagnosis.

CARCINOMA OF THE PENIS

This is an uncommon disease causing at the most 1% of deaths from malignant disease in Europe. It occurs mostly between the ages of 50 and 70. It is never found in those who were circumcised at birth, and usually develops in association with poor standards of hygiene. Certain conditions such as leukoplakia are pre-malignant.

Pathology

Most tumours are well-differentiated squamous cell carcinomas. They can be papillary or ulcerative, and usually arise on the glans or on the inner side of the prepuce. They spread directly along the shaft and are often for some time limited to the penis, eventually spread to the erectile tissues or the inguinal lymph nodes occurs. Blood spread occurs late and is rare.

Investigation

So many of the patients are elderly that a full medical examination and investigation is required. Although syphilis is now less common, serological tests must be carried out. The diagnosis is usually obvious but it must be confirmed by biopsy, and for this a dorsal slit or circumcision may be required.

Treatment

Surgery involves partial or complete amputation, with or without block dissection of the lymph nodes. For the elderly patient in reasonable condition, this is probably the treatment of choice and avoids a long period of discomfort. However, many, and this is certainly true of younger patients, find surgery psychologically unacceptable. Radiation offers a reasonable alternative. The organ during treatment must be enclosed in a mould to stabilise it and the testes protected, treatment lasting four to six weeks. Discomfort is inevitable with erythema and oedema of the skin, and inflammation of the urethra. Non-adhesive dressings and possibly steroid ointment are required and rest should be encouraged. For the elderly patient this should not mean total confinement to bed as so often it is impossible to mobilise him again. For the urinary symptoms the same measures are employed as for reactions in the bladder.

Recurrences after radiation must be treated surgically.

Mr – aged 50 had a full course of radiation for a small carcinoma of the penis. The radiation reaction was severe but settled satisfactorily. He returned for regular follow-up and it was noted 12 months later that there was a recurrence at the edge of the previous site. He had a partial amputation of the penis and remained well. The skin showed marked atrophy and telangectasia and was easily traumatised.

Prognosis

After surgery an overall five-year survival rate of 50-70% can be expected. Radiotherapy can produce equally good results. For early cases many workers claim 100% survival figures.

When all the theories crumble to ashes
The patient and the problem remain,
The doctor also remains
For he must treat,
And in his treatment find his theories.

19 Bone and Cartilage

Skeletal System

This provides the framework of the body. It gives strength and rigidity yet is capable of movement through its joints. The bone of which it is composed looks so solid that it is sometimes easy to forget that like the rest of the body it is in a state of dynamic equilibrium. Even in the adult there is a turnover of tissue, bone destruction being balanced by formation of new bone, one-third of its living groundwork being replaced in three weeks. In the growing child the bone is in a state of even greater activity. Despite appearances bone is a very vascular structure. The tiny canals running through it contain blood vessels, and when a fracture occurs bleeding can be profuse, a pint of blood or more can be lost when the femur is fractured.

Very broadly bones can be divided into two types, the long and short bones of the limbs, and the bones of the axial skeleton. Apart from the upper ends of the femur and humerus, red marrow in the adult is found in the vertebrae and flat bones, yellow marrow in the rest of the skeleton.

Since the position in children is different, we must look at the growing bone, the elements of the bone, and its physiology in the adult.

Growing Bone

Flat bones are formed by new bone, osteoid tissue, being laid down in connective tissue. Long bones have growing ends which are cartilage, the cartilage is replaced and pushed further on by new bone lengthening the shaft.

Long Bones

A growing long bone consists of a shaft with a cap of bone at each end, the epiphysis. Separating the shaft from the cap is a plate of epiphyseal cartilage, this point is known as the epiphyseal line. Activity is greatest at this line. Cells which form new bone tissue, osteoblasts, lay down a framework, matrix, in the cartilage on the shaft side of the epiphyseal cartilage. At the same time new cartilage is formed at the other edge of the plate. Minerals, calcium and phosphates are deposited in the matrix to form bone. It is then remodelled by cells which break down bone, osteoclasts, into cortical and medullary zones. When growth stops the epiphyseal cartilages become calcified and replaced by bone, this is called epiphyseal union. Union in different bones occurs at different ages, the process commences about the age of puberty and is complete by the age of 25. No further growth of bones then normally takes place.

Mature Bone

Flat Bone

The flat bone consists of two plates separated by spongy bone and red marrow. The thin membrane covering it is called the periosteum.

Long Bone

Osteoid tissue is not hard. This only comes from the deposition of mineral salts, calcium and phosphates in the matrix. Osteoid tissue is not opaque to X-rays, but bone due to its mineral content is visible on X-rays.

The dynamic equilibrium of the bone is maintained by the opposing but balanced activities of osteoblasts and osteoclasts, and the constant exchange of minerals in the bone with those in the rest of the body. Any disturbance of this balance results in deformity, e.g. osteoporosis in the elderly, rickets in children.

Tumours of Bone

There are so many elements in bone it is not surprising that a variety of malignancies can occur. We will consider later disease of the blood-forming tissue, leukaemia, polycythaemia, but in this chapter we shall concentrate largely on those that arise from the bone itself or the cartilage.

Aetiology

Little real evidence is available, but a theory is advanced based on the fact that tumours arise more commonly in the areas of high activity in the bone. It is argued that in young people the epiphyseal line is a site of maximum activity and that it is precisely in this area that tumours arise. Older patients may have a disease which is characterised by the formation of very vascular new bone, Paget's disease, and similarly malignant change may occur in these areas.

The one proven cause is the ingestion of radium. This is concentrated in bones and from the earlier chapters it will be remembered that it has a very long half-life. Girls in the watch industry who painted luminous dials with a radium paint licked the paint brushes. They absorbed the radioactive paint which was concentrated in bone and many of them developed tumours of the jaw, the so-called 'fossy jaw'. Theoretically any other radioactive isotope having a long half-life and concentrating in bone could produce the same effect. It has also been noted that several years after the radiation of benign superficial conditions in children they have developed underlying bone tumours.

Terms

These tumours arise from cells which are derived from mesodermal tissue, they are therefore called sarcomas. Mesoderm is the middle of the three embryonic germ layers.

Osteosarcoma (formerly Osteogenic Sarcoma)

This is a tumour characterised by the formation of new bone. The cell of origin is the osteoblast.

Age, Sex and Incidence

The number of patients who develop this disease is small. In England and Wales in 1968 five hundred and fifty-nine deaths were registered as occurring from bone tumours. Most of the cases of osteogenic sarcoma occur in people aged between 10 and 25, with a peak incidence in the two years 18 to 20. It is slightly more common in boys. A few older patients develop the tumour in an area of pre-existing Paget's disease.

Sites

Although any bone can be affected, in young people 75% of these tumours occur around the knee. The point of origin is immediately adjacent to the epiphyseal line, the site of maximum cellular activity.

Pathology

The tumour is bulky and expands the bone, destroying both the cortex and medulla. Within the tumour, areas of haemorrhage and fragments of new bone tissue are found. The periosteum is lifted by the new bone and on X-ray this produces an appearance known as Codman's triangle. This is not however diagnostic of this disease as it can be seen in other conditions. Under the microscope the osteoblasts are seen to be atypical and giant forms can be found. Necrosis, haemorrhage, and small areas of cartilage can be seen, and a careful search often reveals invasion of blood vessels.

The new bone tissues may or may not calcify by the deposition of mineral salts. In the former case the tumour will appear osteosclerotic on X-ray, in the latter osteoporotic.

Spread

Direct

Both up and down the bone, and through the periosteum to involve adjacent soft tissues.

Lymphatic

Rare.

Blood

Occurs commonly and early, the lung is the usual site of the first distant metastases.

Symptomatology

The most constant complaint is pain, very rarely a pathological fracture is the first warning. Patients may sometimes notice a swelling of the painful area and find the skin over the bone red and warm. The pain is unremitting, and when the tumour is in the leg movement is restricted and walking can be difficult.

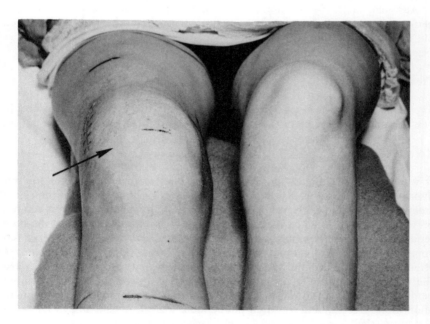

Fig. 19.1.   Osteosarcoma. Note marked difference in size of legs

Examination and Investigation

A full general examination is made followed by the local examination. During the taking of the history details of any exposure to radioactive isotopes is sought, and also of any pain in other areas. The patient's gait is unobtrusively noted when he first enters the clinic. The local examination includes the extent of temperature changes in the skin, the amount of swelling, pain, muscle wasting, and the degree and type of limitation of movement. The limb on the opposite side is also measured for reference. A point is chosen which is a fixed distance from an anatomical land-mark. At the knee this may be x cm above the tibial tubercle.

In the older patient with a tumour arising in an area of Paget's disease, the underlying lesion is so vascular that hypertrophy of the heart can occur, there may even be signs of cardiac failure. Examination of the tibia, clavicle, and femur may well reveal thickening due to other foci of the disease. Cranial or peripheral neurological signs may be present owing to involvement of the skull or vertebrae.

Blood tests include the full-blood picture, and estimation of alkaline phosphatase, this may be raised due to the abnormal osteoblastic activity, and serum calcium and phosphorus. X-rays of the chest and the affected bone are taken, tomograms of the tumour and lungs are required. CAT scans can be very helpful. A skeletal survey with bone scan is necessary to exclude metastases in other bones, and in older patients will reveal the extent of the Paget's disease.

Isotope scans will also include the liver.

Although the X-ray appearances may be virtually diagnostic, biopsy must be performed, particularly to exclude metastases from another site. It is carried out under full anaesthesia.

Treatment

The number of cases is so small, that the best interests of the patients are probably best served if a team of doctors in a specialised centre jointly agrees a policy.

Accessible Sites

It was formerly held that surgery alone was the treatment of choice for this disease. In the limb this involves amputation, and such an operation imposes a tremendous burden, both mental and physical, on a patient. Radiation was not previously employed since the tumour is not very radiosensitive and the dose required jeopardises normal tissue. The frequency with which lung metastases appeared shortly after amputation posed a dilemma. Only surgery could be effective, yet so often the sacrifice of the limb proved to be unjustified, since the early development of metastases showed that spread must have occurred before operation. Megavoltage radiation with its skin-sparing effect made radiation more practical and a revised policy more logical. A high dose of radiation was given, the course lasting six to eight weeks, and the patient observed for the next two to three months. If no pulmonary metastases appeared amputation was then performed. A small proportion of tumours responded to radiation alone.

Following early reports of encouraging results after the use of cytotoxic therapy, adjuvant combined chemotherapy has been widely used, both pre- and post-surgery, and occasionally alone. The side effects are severe, and the value of such treatment is still under evaluation. It seems likely that cytotoxics delay the appearance of the first metastases, but as yet there is not sufficient evidence to conclude that overall survival time is lengthened.

Assessment of results is further complicated by more refined methods of classification of tumours, this makes comparison with past series very difficult. The introduction of CATscans also introduces a new element. Patients may be shown to have lung metastases, when by previous X-ray methods they would have been classified as free of metastases. There is finally the view, held by one centre in the States, that at least among its patients, the natural history of the tumour has changed towards a more benign course.

It is now recognised that in a small proportion of patients one form of the tumour, called juxtacortical osteosarcoma, has a less aggressive tendency. In carefully selected cases some surgeons have taken away the diseased 'bone' with a wide margin, and reconstituted the bone and joint with various prostheses, adjuvant chemotherapy is then given. Such an approach is experimental but may be extended to the more aggressive tumours if the controversy over the results of cytotoxic therapy can be resolved, and if less toxic, more effective drugs can be found.

Immunotherapy, interferon, prophylactic lung irradiation, have all been employed in an attempt to prevent metastases. Interferon is still under trial, the other two methods have so far been disappointing.

Inaccessible Sites and Palliation

The occasional patient has a single lung metastasis only. Surgical removal is then worthwhile as it may be curative. Unfortunately further metastases frequently then appear. Delaying surgery for up to three months will spare patients unneccessary further surgery.

For inoperable tumours, or metastases causing symptoms, a combination of chemotherapy and radiation may be used.

Prognosis

Previously a five year survival figure of 15–27% was given. Centres using adjuvant chemotherapy have claimed 50% in remission at one year, 40% at two years. The prognosis is poor when the tumour is associated with Paget's disease.

The variable course and response of the tumour is probably best illustrated by the histories of two of my patients. In both the histology was proven osteosarcoma and both were treated in the pre-chemotherapy era.

Miss — aged 10 at the time of diagnosis. Two months previously she had developed pain in the upper left thigh, followed one month later by the appearance of swelling. Walking became difficult. On histology the tumour was

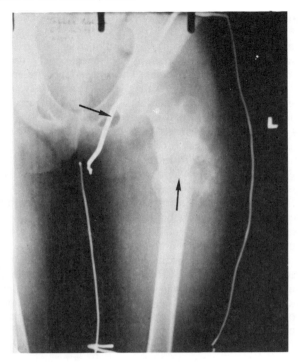

Fig. 19.2.   Osteosarcoma. Lead markers outline field before radiation

considered to be an osteosarcoma of the sclerotic type. Chest X-ray was clear. Hind-quarter amputation was considered but rejected on the grounds of the child's age and the opposition of the parents. She was placed in plaster to relieve pain and facilitate positioning for treatment.

The less usual site of the tumour, upper-third of the femur, posed special problems in addition to the usual ones arising when growing bone is treated. When the epiphysis is radiated growth in length may be arrested, the diameter of the bone may be smaller than normal, and rarefaction or occasionally necrosis can occur. An adequate length of bone must be treated and this meant that in this case the left ovary would inevitably receive radiation.

Megavoltage was not available at this period. A course of therapy using conventional X-rays was given over a period of six weeks. Pain was relieved after a week and at the end of the course she was able to move the leg more freely. The skin showed moderate erythema most marked in the groin. Over the next year or so slight wasting of the thigh became apparent, and on X-ray the diameter of the left femur was less than the right, but no shortening developed. Gait was normal. Menstruation commenced and was regular. At the age of 20 she married, and had two healthy children.

Mrs. — aged 19. Three months previously she had developed pain during labour and subsequently slight numbness of the right knee. Swelling developed

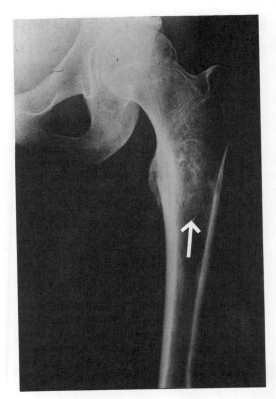

Fig 19.3.   The same osteosarcoma as in Fig. 19.2 after successful treatment

quickly, movement was limited, and she walked with a limp. An X-ray showed an osteolytic lesion at the lower end of the right femur, the chest was clear. The histological report mentioned dense cellular growth, atypical mitoses and malignant cells, an osteosarcoma. When she was first seen at my clinic the knee was hot and tender, and swelling extended below the knee.

Megavoltage therapy was given, the patient was confined to bed to avoid weight bearing on the affected leg. Pain was rapidly relieved. Wasting of the quadriceps developed and although the swelling diminished it never resolved completely. After eight-weeks treatment radiation was stopped as the skin had reached the limit of tolerance. On X-ray some calcification of the tumour was seen. She was discharged on a non-weight bearing regime. She began to walk with a stick, but six months after her first treatment she slipped and fractured the femur just above the tumour site. At follow-up a month previously a suspicious shadow had been noted at the right lung base. During the following months multiple pulmonary deposits developed, and when she died, 14 months after her first visit to the clinic, her doctor reported that metastases were also present in the vagina and bladder.

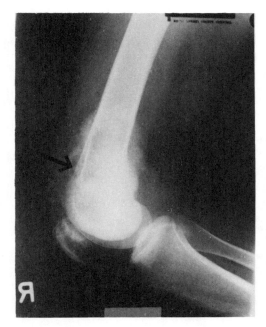

Fig. 19.4.   Osteosarcoma

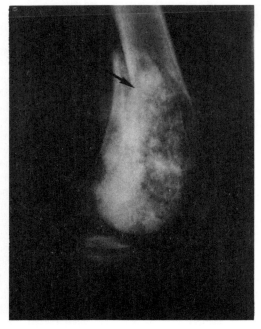

Fig. 19.5.   Fracture just above tumour

The Future

If the results of careful studies show an improvement in survival time, there may then be an attempt to substitute resection for amputation as standard surgical treatment.

Nursing Care

Pain may be severe and adequate analgesia is necessary until radiation produces relief. Immobilisation in plaster may at first be required, this serves several purposes, pain is relieved, the dissemination of malignant cells is minimised, and weight bearing is prevented. Wasting due to disuse and disease will occur. Physiotherapy cannot be too vigorous in the early stages, it will probably be confined to isometric movements (muscle contraction without movement). Later active movement must be re-established.

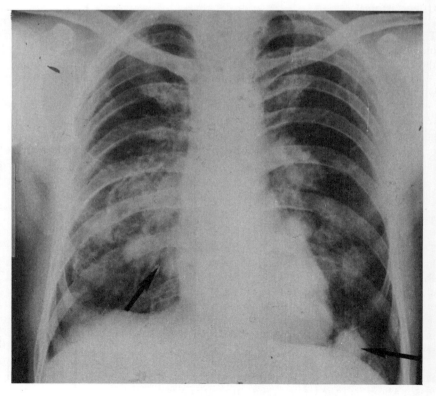

Fig. 19.6.   Osteosarcoma lung metastases

Although megavoltage therapy is used the skin does develop a reaction due to the exit dose or to the presence of plaster. Great care is necessary to prevent traumatisation particularly in the immobile patient. A bed cradle will keep clothes off the leg, and an arm in a sling must be inspected frequently to avoid friction from the bandage. These patients are usually treated in hospital. Analgesic requirements are so high at first that an adequate level can more easily be maintained there, and immobilisation is so important that the supervision of trained staff is necessary. When the patients are children with a natural dislike of restriction constant vigilance is required. Occasionally a very co-operative patient with adequate home facilities can be treated on an outpatient basis.

The prognosis cannot be disguised. Although amputation is not now the immediate treatment it remains a possibility. When apparent recovery has occurred it is more difficult to make the reasons for it seem convincing though they are sound. For the patient the burden of treatment is enough, and only after very careful thought should a procedure which may never take place be discussed.

Osteoclastoma

This is a tumour which occurs far less frequently and is thought to arise from osteoclasts. Usually it is found in the long bones at epiphyseal sites and again there is a predilection for the knee. Most patients are between 20 and 30.

The X-ray appearance is of an expanding osteolytic lesion usually confined within the periosteum. Thinning of the cortex is seen.

If accessible surgery is the treatment of choice, local curettage is often followed by recurrence. Recurrence is treated by wider resection, using bone graft and internal fixation to bridge the gap, this usually gives a stiff joint, or replacing the joint by a prosthesis. When surgery is impossible megavoltage radiation can be used.

Tumours arising from Cartilage

The chondrosarcoma is a growth of cartilage cells. It is most commonly found in the age group 10–30, but there have been reports of its association with Paget's disease in older patients. It is probably due to a secondary malignant change in a pre-existing benign cartilage tumour. Ectopic foci of cartilage can either grow inside a bone or as an outgrowth from it, these are benign chondromas. The pelvis and knee are the usual sites for the primary growth. Increase in size is slow, and spread is local at first but later blood and lymphatic dissemination can occur.

Treatment is by surgery if at all possible. Radiation can produce bone necrosis. Some success has been claimed following the use of one of the newer cytotoxic drugs. About half the treated cases survive five years.

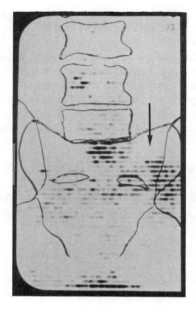

Fig. 19.7.   Chondrosarcoma scan

Tumours Arising in the Fibrous Tissue

The osteoid tissue of bone has a fibrous framework, and it is from cells of this tissue that the fibrosarcoma arises. Spread occurs a little more frequently by the lymphatics than with some of the other bone tumours. It can also be blood borne. The principles of treatment are the same as for chondrosarcoma, the prognosis is slightly less good.

Other Tumours

Ewing's Tumour

Although the cell of origin is not known for certain, it is thought most likely that the tumour arises in the reticulo-endothelial cells within the bone. This is a tumour of childhood and the patient is usually less than 10 years old. The common site is the medulla at the mid-shaft of a long bone.

There is no bone formation by the lesion, but there is a reaction in the surrounding normal bone with new bone being formed next to the tumour. On X-ray the appearance this gives, an osteolytic area with a skin of new bone, is the so-called 'onion skin' appearance.

Other tumours such as neuroblastoma or a lymphoma containing a tumour reticulin (formerly reticulum cell sarcoma), have a histology closely resembling

Ewing's tumour. The diagnosis cannot be therefore regarded as certain until an exhaustive search has failed to reveal any other primary.

There is high radiosensitivity with a rapid response, but unfortunately an often equally rapid local recurrence followed by the appearance of metastases in other bones and the lungs. Megavoltage therapy must be given to the whole bone, and to a high dose, accepting the risk of muscle wasting and bone shortening. For a time prophylactic radiation of the lungs was attempted, but now combination chemotherapy is used over a long period. The previous poor results have improved slightly and a 2 years survival of 50% is claimed in some centres.

Lymphoma (Formerly Reticulum Cell Sarcoma)

Although this is often a secondary from a focus of the disease elsewhere in the body, a solitary bone lesion can occur. Patients are usually young adults. The disease is radiosensitive, the whole bone must be treated.

Rare Tumours

A fascinating but rare tumour is the chordoma. This arises from remnants of the embryonic notochord. This is a structure which in the embryo occupies the position of the adult spine and is replaced by it. In the adult this tissue is represented by the nucleus palposus of the intervertebral discs. The areas most commonly affected are the sacrum and base of the skull. Symptoms are pain and neurological deficits due to the involvement of cranial nerves or the collapse of vertebral bodies. Treatment is by combined surgery and radiotherapy.

The synovial sarcoma (malignant synovioma) is rare. It arises from the synovium and invades bone and local soft tissues. Commonly tumours are anaplastic, producing lung metastases early. Although showing some radiosensitivity surgical excision is the treatment of choice if possible.

Tumours of Muscle

Tumours of muscle are extremely rare. They are of two types arising in smooth or striped muscle. The latter is the rhabdomyosarcoma occurring mostly in young people.

As a rule the tumours are radio-resistant, although radiation can be useful as palliation. Surgery is the treatment of choice.

The prognosis is very poor, but using a combination of surgery, high doses of radiation, and combination chemotherapy for up to 1 year, it has been claimed that children with rhabdomyosarcoma have a 5 year survival rate of 60%.

Secondary Tumours of Bone

In about 20% of patients who die from malignant disease deposits are found in the bones. With a death rate of over 100,000 it is obvious that secondary tumours

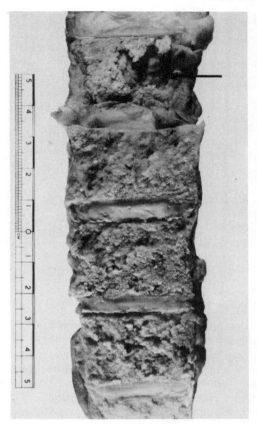

Fig. 19.8.   Spine erosion by metastases

of bone are far more common than primary tumours. Although metastasis to bone can occur from any site, there are five tumours which show a marked predilection for bone. They are breast, bronchus, thyroid, kidney, and prostate.

Treatment

Surgery

Although the bone is often infiltrated quite widely it is usually possible when necessary to stabilise it. A nail can be passed down through the shaft or it may even be feasible to carry out a pin and plate procedure. The advantages are not only relief of pain and achievement of stability, but also the immediate mobilisation which becomes possible. Although only palliative such measures can improve the quality of survival time and are therefore well worth while.

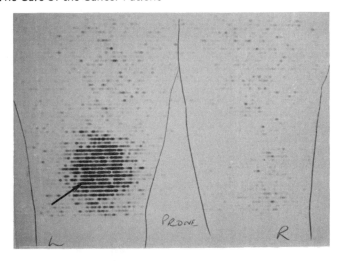

Fig. 19.9. Bone scan. Metastasis in femur

Radiation

Radiation can do much to improve the patient's condition. In some cases healing and calcification can be produced, in others there is marked relief of pain. Metastases from a seminoma are very radiosensitive. Solitary deposits from kidney or thyroid tumours should be treated radically as the results justify such measures. Other procedures which can be adopted for multiple deposits are, hormones for carcinoma of the breast and prostate, and radioactive iodine for certain thyroid tumours, and chemotherapy.

Follow-up

Primary Tumours

At follow-up appointments the aim is to review the progress of the local lesion and search for evidence of secondary deposits. Although careful questioning and examination are important, the mainstay of follow-up is the X-ray and bone scan. Not only the treated lesion must be examined but also sites of possible metastases. The chest X-ray assumes an even greater importance than usual. Special biochemical tests and plasma electrophoresis may also be required.

Secondary Tumours

Unremitting pain in patients with a history of malignant disease should be regarded with suspicion. At first the tumour grows between the trabeculae of bone. There is no destruction of bone or reactive new bone formation so that

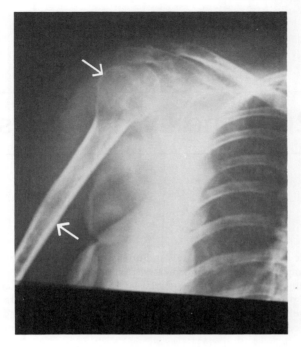

Fig. 19.10. Humerus. Deposits in both head and shaft

X-rays at this stage show nothing. It is then a matter for clinical judgment. While it would be unreasonable to treat every painful area on suspicion, a cautious trial of radiation may be made when justifiable. Relief of pain is regarded as presumptive evidence of metastatic disease. In these cases typical X-ray appearances often follow months after the onset of pain.

To recognise the enemy is not enough,
To defeat him we must know him,
Then we lead rather than pursue,
We can be attackers not defenders.

20   The Lymphomas

The lymphatic system, with its vessels and nodes, is found throughout the whole body. The lymphoid tissue is concentrated particularly in the nodes and in the spleen. Certain cells can take up particles of foreign protein, e.g. bacteria and vital dyes, a process called phagocytosis. Although found in different organs they collectively are called the mononuclear phagocyte system and the lymph nodes which contain such cells form part of this system, the lymphoreticular system.

Before discussing malignant disease of lymphoid tissue it is as well to have a clear idea of the function and anatomy. It will probably be easier to remember the anatomy if some of the physiology is discussed first.

Tissue Fluid

This colourless fluid bathes all the cells of the body, it is constantly being exchanged with the fluid within the cells and the fluid in the blood. It is the means whereby nutriments from the blood and metabolites from the cell are conveyed to and fro. The fluid is formed because of pressure factors within the capillary.

Formation of Tissue Fluid

The walls of the capillary form a semi-permeable membrane, various salts and fluid can pass through, but the plasma proteins are too large and remain within the blood vessel. The capillary itself can be thought of as a loop, one limb being arterial and the other venous. The blood pressure is equal to the pressure exerted by a column of mercury 32 mm high at the arterial end. Pressure gradually falls until at the venous end it is only 12 mm of mercury. This pressure tends to force fluid out, but plasma proteins also exert a pressure which tends to draw fluid into the capillary. In the tissues outside the vessel two pressures are exerted, one holding the fluid in the blood vessel, the other drawing it out. They are both small but they do assist in forming and returning the tissue fluid.

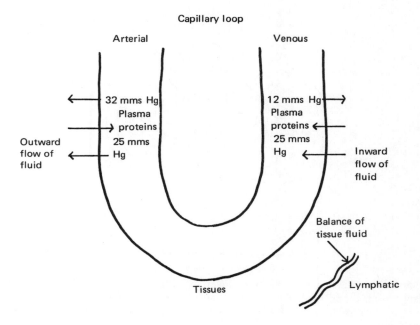

Fig. 20.1.   Formation of lymph

At the arterial end of the capillary the pressures forcing out are greater than those drawing inwards, so fluid passes out to the tissues. Conversely at the venous end the pressure drawing fluid in is the greater of the two, and so the tissue fluid returns to the capillary. However not all returns, and if this were the only drainage system fluid would build up resulting in oedema. Running throughout the tissues of the whole body are vessels which carry this excess. The vessels are colourless and join to form larger vessels and then trunks. They are interrupted by valves and collections of lymphoid tissue, nodes, together the vessels and nodes form the lymphatic system of the body. The trunks open into veins at the root of the neck so returning the fluid, called lymph, to the blood. One of the main lymphatic vessels running up from the abdomen through the thorax to the neck is known as the thoracic duct. To this duct the lymph from the lymphatics throughout the abdomen and part of the thorax drains. After a fatty meal the lymph drained from the small intestine is milky white and is called chyle. Foreign matter molecules are too large to pass into the blood vessels but are taken up by the lymphatics and carried in the lymph.

Lymphoid Tissue

This is widespread throughout the body but is particularly concentrated in the lymph nodes and spleen. The nodes lie along the course of the vessels and in

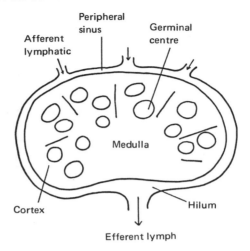

Fig. 20.2.   Lymph node section

specific areas there are many close together. Some are impalpable such as the retroperitoneal and mediastinal, others such as the submental and inguinal may be palpable but normal, while others when enlarged indicate reaction to some disease process.

Each node is bean shaped. When cut across and seen under the microscope the structure is very clear. There is a space, a sinus, lying below a fibrous capsule. Into this the lymph vessels open. Next there is a zone made up of collections of cells, follicles with germinal centres, containing lymphocytes. Sinuses pass between the centres down to the medulla.

Lymph is carried by the afferent vessels to the node, enters the peripheral sinus, drains down through the cortex to the medulla, and leaves in an efferent vessel at the hilum. As fluid passes through, any foreign matter is removed by phagocytic action and destroyed. At the same time lymphocytes are probably stimulated to produce antibody to this foreign chemical and initiate other processes to inactivate it. If the foreign material is in the form of infective bacteria the node will become enlarged, tender, and palpable, this is called reactive hyperplasia. If a finger is septic nodes at the elbow and in the axilla enlarge, and the lymphatics become inflamed and visible as red streaks. If malignant cells are carried to the node this same mechanism can destroy them, but it is possible for large numbers of cells to overwhelm the defences. Also in some way as yet not completely understood a tumour can secrete a substance that prevents this defence mechanism from operating. The malignant cells are trapped but not destroyed. They grow and replace the node which enlarges, but remains mobile until the tumour penetrates the capsule, invades neighbouring tissue, and so fixes the node. This is the secondary deposit, or metastasis. It is not always easy to distinguish between reactive hyperplasia and malignant enlargement when both infection and tumour are present in the primary site, we have already noted this in discussing malignancy of the tongue.

Lymphography

Since deep nodes cannot be palpated means were sought to visualise them and so detect destruction of the normal architecture. Radio-opaque media can be injected and have been used to outline the kidneys, I.V.P., the arteries, arteriogram, and the veins, venogram. Since the molecule of this medium is foreign to the body it was realised that the reticulo-endothelial cells of the nodes would trap this radio-opaque dye and the nodes so become visible on X-ray. If the quantity were kept small it would all be filtered out before it could be carried to the blood vessels in the neck. Because of this reasoning based on normal physiology, the technique of lymphography has been developed. It is used mostly to visualise the pelvic and abdominal nodes by injecting into the lymphatics of the foot, but it is possible, if more difficult, to visualise the axillary and thoracic nodes, also the lymphatic system of individual organs such as the testis.

Technique

Only the procedure for injecting the foot will be described. After skin preparation, a vital dye, methylene blue, is injected subcutaneously in the web of skin between the toes. The dye, being foreign matter, is taken up by the lymphatics which then become visible as greenish streaks. Under local anaesthetic a small incision is made over one of them and it is dissected free of surrounding tissue. Sutures passed round the vessel steady it, and a fine catheter is passed into the lumen. This is tied in place and the catheter connected to a syringe containing the radio-opaque medium. The procedure is repeated on the other foot. A slow steady pressure is applied, so injecting the medium. The pressure should not be too great or the lymphatic vessel will rupture. When the injection is complete the catheters are removed and sutures inserted to close the skin incision. In some centres the first injection made is of water-soluble medium as this is less irritating to the tissues if there is any leak. X-rays are taken at intervals as the medium passes up the lymphatics and is taken up by the nodes. The last picture may be postponed until the day after the injection. The medium remains in the nodes for several months and it is possible therefore to assess both the progress of the disease and of treatment.

The inguinal, pelvic, and sacro-iliac nodes are visualised. The oil can rise higher and on some lymphograms the high para-aortic nodes can be seen. It can be important to assess the relation of the kidneys and ureters to enlarged nodes, both to plan treatment and to see whether the nodes are obstructing the ureters. An I.V.P. performed after the lymphogram will show both nodes and the urinary tract on the same X-ray. If at the same time lead markers are put on the skin to outline proposed radiation fields, both the coverage of enlarged nodes and the relation of the fields can be seen, enabling any necessary adjustments to be made.

Abnormal nodes can be enlarged, deformed, or exhibit a lace-like reticular pattern due to foci obliterating the phagocytic cells, they show up well on CATscan.

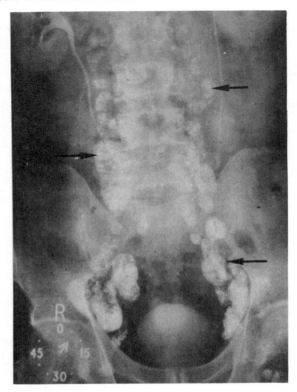

Fig. 20.3.   Lymphogram before treatment. Enlarged nodes in pelvic and
para-aortic groups. Note I.V.P. to check kidneys and ureters

Reactions

The patient usually experiences no reaction and no real discomfort apart from
immobility, but a chest X-ray taken on the following day shows in some patients
transient pulmonary changes due to oil reaching the lungs. Previous radiation,
surgery, or chemotherapy impairs the phagocytic action of the lymphoid tissue
and allows oil to pass through. The maximum reaction occurs in the first 24
hours and is usually asymptomatic. Pulmonary infection and, very rarely, death
have been reported following the examination.

Pathology

Before discussing the types of tumour, a brief reference must be made to the
immune system of the body. This is a defence (protective) mechanism, it involves
the recognition of a 'foreign' chemical called an antigen. Recognition triggers off

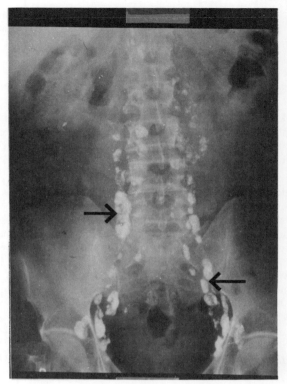

Fig. 20.4.   Lymphogram after treatment. Marked reduction in size of nodes

a defence reaction. Lymphocytes are part of the recognition system. They are formed from stem cells in the bone marrow. T lymphocytes are further differentiated in the thymus, while for B lymphocytes the process takes place in the bone marrow and in the lymph nodes. On meeting an antigen, B lymphocytes divide to form plasma cells which have antibody on their surfaces, while T lymphocytes multiply and initiate cell mediated immune responses.

For more detailed accounts of this fascinating topic specialist literature should be read, this section is meant only to introduce the terms T and B lymphocyte.

Malignant Lymphomas

These are tumours of the lymphoreticular system, which, excluding leukaemias, cause about 2% of deaths from malignant disease. They are divided into two groups, Hodgkin's disease and non-Hodgkin lymphomas. While the first has agreed further subdivisions, the second is still the subject of discussion, and current terms will no doubt be modified further as a result of research. It should be noted that this group includes tumours formerly called follicular lymphoma, lymphosarcoma, reticulum cell sarcoma and, in addition Burkitt's lymphoma.

Hodgkin's Disease

Thomas Hodgkin was the curator of the museum at Guy's Hospital in the first half of the last century. Although the disease had existed before, he was the first to recognise it and describe it as a distinct entity, hence the reason for it bearing his name.

Sites and Appearance

Any tissue of the lymphoreticular system can be affected, but most commonly the lymph nodes are involved. These are usually discrete, firm and enlarged. When cut across they have a rubbery texture and are greyish in colour, this appearance has been likened to that of raw fish. Other sites may be the spleen, liver, or rarely bone. Extremely rarely the brain is involved, this is in contrast to the frequency with which metastases are found there. A curious feature of the disease is the way in which, unlike the pattern of metastatic spread, nodes may be involved in groups which are not adjacent, e.g. cervical and retroperitoneal.

Age, Sex, and Incidence

This is a disease which has two peaks of incidence, young adults between the ages of 15 and 34, and a smaller peak in those over the age of 55. It accounts for about 40% of lymphomas, and males are affected about twice as frequently as females.

Aetiology

No firm evidence as to the cause is yet available. It has been suggested that there may be some element of infection, the clustering of cases and increased risk among relatives of patients might support this. Since the origin is believed to be from the immune system cells, either enhanced response of the system to an antigen challenge, or a failure of the mechanisms which shut down such a response, has been postulated.

Histology

The pattern of the node is destroyed and replaced by various cells. Bands of collagen may divide the node into nodules. The presence of a special type of giant cell called the Reed–Sternberg cell, clinches the diagnosis.

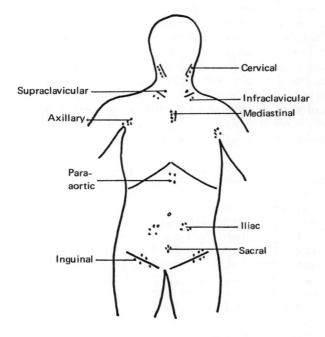

Fig. 20.5. Principal lymph node groups

Four histological types of tumour are recognised, this is known as the Rye classification.

1. Lymphocyte predominance.
2. Nodular sclerosis.
3. Mixed cellularity.
4. Lymphocyte depletion.

These types, taken in conjunction with clinical staging, have prognostic significance, 60% of cases are type 2, and 30% type 3.

Symptomatology

Patients' complaints are varied, but the majority visit the doctor because of painless swelling of lymph nodes, in two-thirds of cases these are in the neck. Often the patient feels quite well. When the enlarged nodes cannot be seen, retroperitoneal, mediastinal, the symptoms may be those caused by pressure. In the chest these can be unexplained cough or dyspnoea, or in extremely rare cases there can be signs of superior vena caval obstruction. There can be abdominal pain from enlarged retroperitoneal nodes, and other organs which can enlarge are the liver and spleen. Bone deposits cause pain. A curious complaint can be of pain in affected areas after drinking alcohol.

Skin irritation may be one of the more generalised systemic symptoms. Patients complain of malaise, lethargy, sweating and loss of weight. They can experience bouts of unexplained fever at intervals of days or weeks, the Pel-Ebstein type of fever, and exhibit all the signs of anaemia. The anaemia can be caused by bone infiltration, but can be due to increased haemolysis (breakdown) of red cells. This can be so marked that prehepatic jaundice can be present.

Investigations

All investigations have two aims, to establish the extent of the disease and to determine its nature. First of the investigations is the taking of a careful history and the physical examination. Particular care must be taken to discover the duration of the symptoms and the presence of any vague complaints which the patient may have dismissed. Apart from palpation of all lymph node areas, the liver and the spleen, the examination must include a full neurological survey. Simple tests which can be done in the clinic are the taking of the temperature and the setting up of an E.S.R. The latter is not diagnostic of the disease but is related to its activity and may be raised although the patient feels quite well. Other blood investigations include, full blood count including platelets, blood urea, uric acid, electrolytes and liver-function tests. If bone-marrow biopsy is carried out, it is most commonly done when intensive chemotherapy is contemplated. It assesses the functional state of the marrow and excludes infiltration, at least in that site.

Of supreme importance is the biopsy, usually of a suspect node. The importance of this cannot be over-emphasised. Although the symptoms may be highly suggestive of disease of the lymphoid tissue, there is always the possibility that the node is the site of metastasis from an unknown primary. Histology is needed to establish to which group the lymphoma belongs and for further classification.

X-rays

A chest X-ray, with tomograms if necessary, is routine. Bearing in mind that retroperitoneal nodes are often involved but produce no symptoms, a lymphogram has now become standard practice. This is followed by an I.V.P., the relation of the nodes and the ureters can then be seen clearly.

Other Investigations

So far the investigations described have been routine, but other tests are available and will be performed when they are indicated. Tests include scintiscanning following the injection of a special radioactive isotope, liver and splenic puncture, laparotomy, with liver and node biopsy to determine the extent of the

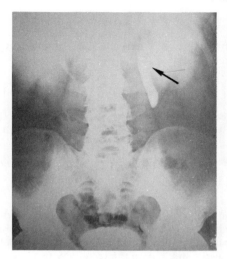

Fig. 20.6.   I.V.P. showing hydronephrosis of the L. kidney due to enlarged
                 nodes obstructing the ureter

abdominal disease (splenectomy may be performed at the same time. N.B. In
view of the efficacy of chemotherapy many centres have abandoned laparotomy).

If there is evidence of widespread disease bone marrow biopsy may be required, also skeletal studies and very rarely, barium meal and follow through.

Staging

Based on clinical findings and the results of investigations a staging is made. This
is the same for both Hodgkin's disease and non-Hodgkin's lymphoma. The
choice of treatment is based on this.
Staging of lymphomas (from Ann Arbor)

E   = Extralymphatic organ or site (i.e. outside node group)
I   = One lymph node region or one E.
II   = Two or more lymph nodes region or E + lymph node region (S). In
        both cases all pathology on the same side of the diaphragm.
III = Lymph node regions on both sides of the diaphragm, +/−E, +/−
        spleen involvement.
IV = Generalised disease of tissues other than lymph nodes +/− lymph
        node regions.

In Hodgkin's disease only, the letters **A** or **B** added to the staging number
indicate the absence or presence of systemic symptoms such as pyrexia, etc.

Treatment

Before any treatment is given anaemia must be corrected by blood transfusion and any obvious infection treated.

Surgery

The part which surgery plays is limited. It is used to establish diagnosis, excision biopsy, laparotomy, splenectomy, and may be required to relieve symptoms due to compression or obstruction. If a young woman is to receive abdominal radiation then the ovaries are moved behind the uterus for protection.

Radiotherapy

Megavoltage radiation is used. It is now the usual practice to treat all the nodes on one side of the diaphragm in one field. Above the diaphragm this is called a mantle field, protection is given to the lungs and larynx. Below the diaphragm an inverted Y field is used, and in men the testes are protected.

Treatment lasts 4–6 weeks. If both mantle and inverted Y fields are to be used, it is then usual for one field to be treated first, and the second after an interval.

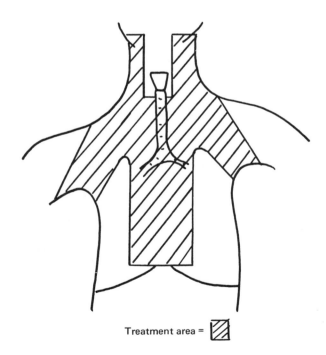

Treatment area =

Fig. 20.7. Mantle treatment

Chemotherapy

In the past various chemicals were used to treat this disease, and although the success achieved was small it was sufficient to encourage workers to look for other agents. Research led to the discovery and use of substances which are called cytotoxics because they are cell poisons. They fall into two broad categories, antimitotics which prevent the cells from dividing (mitosis) or antimetabolites which inhibit the use by the cell of materials vital to its growth and division, for example folic acid necessary for the formation of nucleic acids and hence the nucleus. These cytotoxics act against all rapidly-dividing cells, so that the formation of white cells in the nodes, and red blood cells and platelets in the bone marrow is depressed. However, the malignant cells do not recover as do the normal cells of the body and this is the rationale of treatment.

Aims

The aim of chemotherapy is to relieve systemic symptoms such as fever or pruritus, and to cause regression in affected glands. It is in this setting that it is seen at its best. By introducing the chemical agent directly into the body it can be dispersed throughout the system to reach the scattered malignant cells. To achieve this aim by radiotherapy would involve whole-body irradiation.

Treatment according to Staging

The following plan of treatment is generally accepted, some of the details are still under discussion and studies are being carried out to see whether the present results can be improved.

Adults

IA, IB.	Radiotherapy.
IIA, IIB.	Radiotherapy provided the amount of disease is small, or only two groups of nodes are involved.
IIA, IIB.	Combined chemotherapy followed by radiotherapy to involved areas — used for bulky mediastinal deposits, three or more groups above the diaphragm, older patients.
IIIA.	Combined chemotherapy (or radiotherapy to all nodes) if small volume.
IIIA.	Combined chemotherapy followed by total node irradiation if large volume.
IIIB, IVA.B.	Combined chemotherapy.

Some centres do not use both radiotherapy and chemotherapy since the treatment is prolonged and side effects may be severe, it is therefore particularly in Stages III and IV that efforts are being made to improve chemotherapy, and to assess the benefits and risks of combining the two types of treatment.

Children

Hodgkin's disease is very rare in children, amounting to about 10% of all lymphomas. Treatment must be modified. Radiation must avoid damage to growing bones, and probably splenectomy will be omitted as children are particularly vulnerable to severe infections afterwards. There is a trend towards chemotherapy alone. The optimum regime for children has not yet been defined.

Relapses

Patients who have received only radiation do very well, if given chemotherapy. For those who have been given chemotherapy initially, a different combination can be tried, or if that fails, rotation of single cytotoxic drugs.

Side Effects

The side effects of radiation are the usual ones, and when chemotherapy is given depend upon the drugs used. Patients are more liable to infection particularly when chemotherapy is used, herpes zoster and moniliasis can both be troublesome, occasionally the organism is an unusual one, e.g. Aspergillus. When the spleen is removed infection can be severe, one of my patients had a very severe bout of whooping cough some time after splenectomy.

Two long term effects are infertility and second cancers, the risks appear to be associated with chemotherapy. Infertility is less of a problem with women although some may have an early menopause, it is in men that the more severe effects are seen. A recent suggestion has been that the use of the contraceptive pill while cytotoxics are given may protect ovarian function. There also seems to be a small risk that patients may develop leukaemia or a non-Hodgkin's lymphoma.

It is claimed that the regime known as ABVD (Adriamycin, bleomycin, vinblastine, DTIC) has a lower incidence of both these effects.

Prognosis

According to stage, figures of 5 yrs survival for adults are quoted as, stages I and II with both A and B 80-90%, stages IIA, IIB and IIIA 70%, and stages IIIB, IVA and B 50%. Some would claim even higher figures for Stage I. Children have a good prognosis, 80-90%.

Non-Hodgkin Lymphomas

Aetiology

No factors have been positively identified. A particular virus has been noted in association with Burkitt's lymphoma, but the exact significance of this finding is not clear. Deficiencies in the immune system may prove to be important factors.

Age, Sex

These tumours can occur at any age but are more common between the ages of 50 and 70. They occur slightly more often in men than women.

Histology

There is as yet no clearly agreed classification, but one system is probably a good working basis. It is as follows:

1. Lymphocytic, all degrees of differentiation.
2. Histiocytic.
3. Mixed.

A further subdivision is based upon the presence or absence of a follicular pattern, the former type is called nodular, the latter diffuse.

Use of monoclonal antibodies may provide further clues, particularly on the nature of lymphocytes involved, T or B.

Symptomatology

It is very usual for several node groups to be involved from the beginning, and also for disease to be present in other sites, most commonly gut and bone marrow.

The clinical picture can therefore vary widely, with symptoms related to extra nodal sites being found more often than in Hodgkin's disease.

Investigations

These are as for Hodgkin's disease with the exception that, where indicated, laparoscopy with liver biopsy would replace laparatomy, and a lymphogram and IVP may not be necessary. CATscans are useful in the detection of mediastinal nodes.

Treatment

Very occasionally a patient may have only one node group involved. Radio-therapy will then produce a very long remission, even possibly a cure. For the rest, treatment depends upon staging, and division, by histology, into good and bad prognosis. Most patients are elderly. Cure is unlikely, but very long periods of remission do occur. If patients are well then little or no treatment is required, more vigorous measures being reserved for symptomatic relapse or complications. Good prognosis patients can be managed with the corticosteroid, prednisone, alone.

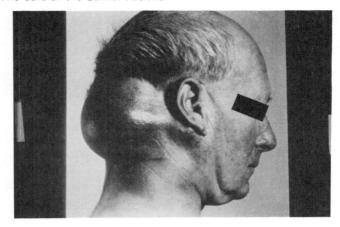

Fig. 20.8.   Non-Hodgkin's lymphoma. Before treatment

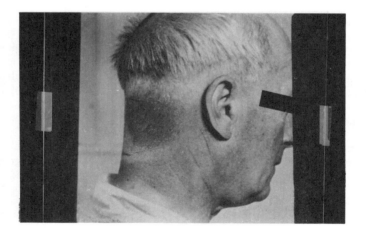

Fig. 20.9.   Non-Hodgkin's lymphoma. After treatment

Radiotherapy

Unlike Hodgkin's disease, it is not necessary to treat adjacent node areas. Radiation is therefore localised to the involved area. It can also be used to relieve symptoms due to deposits, such as pain from bone lesions.

Chemotherapy

Patients with good prognosis lymphomas usually receive a single drug regime, the choice being made from the alkylating group, prednisone may also be given. Combination chemotherapy is used for the bad prognosis group of patients.

Plan of Treatment

Good Prognosis   Stages I and II patients receive local radiation, while stages III and IV, if they require treatment, would be given single drug chemotherapy with or without prednisone.

Bad Prognosis   Stages I and II local radiation, combination chemotherapy is used for stage III and IV and often produces long remissions.

Children

When this lymphoma is found in children it is the bad prognosis type. It is usually treated in the same way as acute lymphatic leukaemia.

One variant is a thymic lymphoma found in the anterior mediastinum. It is large and the disease is either leukaemic from the beginning or becomes so. It usually occurs in adolescent boys.

Prognosis

In adults, good prognosis, stages I and II disease have a 5 yrs survival time of 70-75%, 50% for stages III and IV. The corresponding figures for bad prognosis tumours are stage I 70%, II 50% and III and IV 10-30% according to type. It must be stressed that some good prognosis patients can live much longer, up to 20 years.

In children the prognosis is poor, about 20%.

Burkitt's Lymphoma

This is usually found in tropical E. Africa, but occasional cases have been seen elsewhere. Children between the ages of 5 and 8 are affected. The jaw, gut, ovaries and testes may be involved with single or multiple tumours, the central nervous system may also be the site of disease.

Treatment is by combined chemotherapy. Unfortunately, even when there is a long remission, there is frequent relapse. A survival rate of 30-40% is quoted.

Mycosis Fungoides

This is a chronic skin lymphoma which has a very long course. Radiation and local applications of dilute nitrogen mustard have both been used. More recently a drug called PUVA has been used to sensitise the lesions and a course of ultra-violet light given later, this too has been useful.

Follow-up

The object of follow-up appointments is to assess the response of treatment and detect any extension or recurrence. Obviously the timing of these visits will depend upon the type of treatment given and the severity of the disease.

After careful questioning on general health, appetite, the presence of sweating or pruritus, neurological symptoms such as parasthesiae, the patient is examined for signs of recurrence or involvement of new areas. If the nodes affected have been in the neck or pharyngeal area an E.N.T. examination is required, neuro-logical assessment must not be omitted if the spine has been radiated. A transient myelitis can produce bizarre neurological symptoms such as parasthesiae in the limbs on flexing the neck, and vincristine has neurotoxic effects, already described.

Routine tests at every visit include full blood count, E.S.R., and, at regular intervals, chest X-ray. Bearing in mind that retroperitoneal nodes are seldom palpable, vague malaise can be sufficient reason to justify a further lymphogram if on plain X-ray contrast medium can no longer be seen in them.

In this group of diseases, above all in Hodgkin's disease, real progress has been made in lengthening survival time. It has in fact been so marked that in early cases the word cure is being cautiously used. There is little doubt that as the disease is better understood, treatment can be improved, and further advances expected.

Leukaemia is a volcano.
At times in violent eruption,
At others smouldering quietly,
Yet again silent like a sleeping giant.

21 Leukaemias, Myeloma and Polycythaemia

THE LEUKAEMIAS

A child aged four is taken to the doctor by his mother because she has noticed large bruises appearing on his legs. He looks pale and is described by his mother as being rather quiet and listless lately, the reverse of his usually lively self. The doctor finds the mucous membranes pale and he can feel a few enlarged nodes in the neck and an enlarged spleen. His suspicions are aroused and the results of a blood test confirm them, his diagnosis, acute leukaemia.

Nature of the Disease

The nature of the disease is not fully understood. It is defined as a disturbed proliferation of all the leucocyte-producing (leucopoietic) tissues of the body resulting in changes in both the quantity and the quality of the cells circulating in the blood. While its course is malignant, many hesitate to apply the word to the disease process itself. It can be either acute or chronic, in the acute form the cells are more primitive, 'blast' cells, while the cells in the chronic disease closely resemble normal cells. Before considering in detail the changes produced in the blood and the leucopoietic tissues, the normal development of blood cells must be considered.

Normal Development

The cells of the blood can be considered as a family. Each member is different from the others but it has a common parent. This parent for blood cells is a precursor stem cell which in turn gives rise to a different stem cell for each type of blood cell. As each type of cell develops it goes through a series of changes finally reaching the adult or mature form. The earlier stages are often referred to as the blast cells, this is because the ending blast is attached to type names indicating the more primitive or early forms. To examine either the blood or

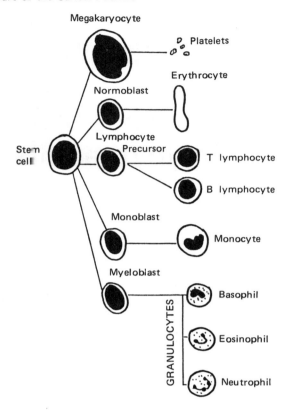

Fig. 21.1.   Formation of blood cells

the blood-forming tissues under the microscope, the material is placed on a slide and stained with a special stain. The different cells will then be coloured and their differences become apparent.

Formation

Red blood cells are formed in the red bone marrow, which in the adult is found in the flat bones such as the ribs and sternum, the skull, pelvis, and upper ends of the humerus and femur. In the early stages of development the cell is known as a normoblast. It gradually becomes smaller, the nucleus becomes condensed and finally lost, and the pigment haemoglobin is acquired. In the last stage before becoming the mature cell it is called a reticulocyte, this is because when stained it has a blue network in the cytoplasm. Mature cells and a few reticulocytes leave the marrow and enter the circulating blood.

Appearance and Function

The adult red blood cell, erythrocyte, is biconcave. The maximum diameter is such that about 3,500 would have to be placed in line to stretch one inch. Its principal function is to carry oxygen and carbon dioxide, it can do this because these gases combine with its pigment haemoglobin. The biconcave shape provides the maximum surface area for the rapid uptake and discharge of these substances. The maximum life of an erythrocyte is 120 days in the body, less when blood is withdrawn and stored in a bank. Ageing cells are destroyed by the lympho-reticular system, notably the spleen.

Blood Tests

There are many tests to measure whether the red cell is being formed normally, and also whether it is normal when formed, only the simplest will be described.

Red-cell Count

First the number of red cells in a cubic millimetre of blood is counted. The blood sample is placed in a tube with a chemical to prevent it clotting and a measured quantity is then put in a special chamber, viewed through a microscope, and the number of red cells counted. The normal range is $4.2-6.1 \times 10^{121}$ ℓ $(4.2-6.1 \text{ million/mm}^3)$. This process has now been mechanised.

Packed Cell Volume

If blood is allowed to stand the cells being heavier will sink to the bottom. The process can be accelerated by spinning the tube of blood in a high-speed centrifuge. The percentage of the total volume formed by the cells is called the packed cell volume. It too has a range, males 40-54%, females 37-47% of the total volume of blood.

Haemoglobin

The haemoglobin content of the blood is determined by chemical means or by light-beam methods. The result is expressed in grams per decilitre (hundred millilitres) of blood, this is sometimes written as g%. In women the normal range is 11.5-16.5 g/dℓ and in men 13-18 g/dℓ. Other tests measure the volume of the erythrocyte, its haemoglobin content, and the relation of these indices to each other.

Anaemia

Anaemia occurs when the erythrocytes are either reduced in number or their quality is changed, for example greatly increased in size. On the results of the tests the anaemia is classified into various types.

White Cells

Mature white cells are divided by their appearance into two classes; if on staining the cells contain granules they are called leucocytes, if they are non-granular then they are either lymphocytes or monocytes.

Formation of White Cells

Leucocytes

These are formed like the erythrocytes in the red bone marrow. They share a common parent but each of the three types develops along different lines. The basic changes consist of decrease in cell size, changes in the nucleus, and the appearance of granules. When mature they are discharged into the circulating blood. One of the earlier more primitive forms is called a myeloblast.

Monocytes and Lymphocytes

Although the primitive lymphocytes are formed in the red bone marrow, further maturation takes place in the thymus and lymph nodes. Monocyte formation is located in the marrow, lymphoid system, and spleen. Primitive cells of the monocyte line are called monoblasts, but it is not now thought that the lymphoblasts found in lymphoblastic leukaemia are the normal lymphocyte precursors. During development, like the erythrocytes, the cells of both types become smaller, the nucleus changing into the adult form.

Adult lymphocytes are mainly of two types, T and B. A few are known as null cells.

Function

The white cells form part of the body defences. They are active in combating infection when their numbers are increased. Many are phagocytic (taking up particles of foreign protein, bacteria, or parasites). Some are a source of the immune gamma globulin. B lymphocytes give rise to plasma cells which also form antibodies.

The life span of the leucocytes within the body is variable, but in stored blood it is a few hours only.

White-cell Count

The white cell count is expressed in a total per litre (previously per cubic millimetre). For leucocytes there is a range in the adult of 4-11 $\times$ $10^9/\ell$ (4,000-11,000/mm^3). A count above 11.0 $\times$ $10^9/\ell$ (above 11,000) is termed leucocytosis, below 4.0 $\times$ $10^9/\ell$ (4,000), leucopenia. A normal lymphocyte count is 1.5 – 4 $\times$ $10^9/\ell$ (1,500 – 4,000/min^3).

Platelets

These are formed in the red bone marrow from megakaryocytes. These are large cells which bud off small processes which become detached and form the platelets. The megakaryocyte is derived ultimately from the same common primitive cell as the other cells of the blood.

The normal adult count is $150-400 \times 10^9/\ell$ ($150,000-400,000$ per mm^3). They are counted both in a counting chamber and on a blood film. If their number is decreased the condition is described as thrombocytopenia. Platelets play an important part in the formation of a blood clot (thrombus). If their number is deficient abnormal bruising and bleeding occur on minor trauma.

Examination of Bone Marrow

When abnormalities of the circulating blood cells are found the blood-forming tissues are examined, either by biopsy of a lymph node or by aspirating red bone marrow. The two most accessible sites for marrow biopsy are the sternum and the iliac crest. The aspirated marrow is spread as a film on a slide, dried and stained, and viewed under the microscope. The early stages of cells of all series are seen and the haematologist by experience can detect any abnormal increase or decrease of one element, in aplasia there is a complete absence of all cells.

Acute Leukaemia. Incidence

Deaths from leukaemia in England and Wales accounted for less than 1% of all registered deaths. Although the condition is world-wide it is more common in countries with a high standard of living. It is popularly believed that this is a disease of young people but it is also found in adults in whom there is a peak incidence in the age group 40-60 years. Among children there is a peak incidence in the under fives, while young people between the ages of 15 and 25 are the least often affected. There is a very slightly larger proportion of males among patients. Certain conditions may terminate in an acute leukaemia.

Aetiology

The cause of leukaemia is unknown, and though certain factors have been incriminated the links in the chain of proof are incomplete. Much research has been done in animals for the disease is widespread among them, but there are often differences between the animal and human forms and caution must be used in applying the results to man.

Genetic

Research has shown chromosome abnormalities in the cells of some patients with leukaemia, and patients with Down's syndrome (mongolism) have a higher than normal chance of developing the disease. It is suggested that when cells are dividing small parts of a chromosome may be accidentally attached to another, this is called translocation. Such translocations are usually of no advantage to the cell or result in its death. However the theory is advanced that, if, by chance, a part of a chromosome containing genes which govern the working of the cell is translocated, so that it is close to 'promoter' genes which it normally never approaches, then unrestrained division takes place. This division results in a large number of this abnormal cell.

Virus

It is known that viruses can induce leukaemia in animals, this not unnaturally led to the search for a similar agent in man. Although viruses and virus-like particles have been found in the blood of leukaemia patients, they have also been found in association with other conditions. Injection of patients' serum has not so far induced the disease in animals. However a very rare type of tumour found in Japan and the West Indies may, on the early evidence, be caused by a specific virus. It is also suggested that viruses may potentiate or maintain these 'leukaemic translocations'.

Pathology

The leukaemia is defined according to the cell type which predominates, this cell type is characterised by its appearance (morphology), staining characteristics, enzyme content, and immunological reactions. The two main types are acute lymphoblastic leukaemia (ALL) and acute myeloblastic leukaemia (AML). Further subdivision can be made. This is important as more precise identification of the leukaemic cell not only enables better estimates of prognosis to be made, but also improvements in the nature and timing of treatment. Other names used sometimes are acute lymphocytic, or acute myeloid leukaemia, and for AML, acute non-lymphoblastic leukaemia (ANLL).

In children 85% of cases are lymphoblastic (ALL) while in adults acute myeloblastic leukaemia (AML) predominates.

It is important to grasp that the finding of abnormal white cells or of an increased number in the circulating blood is not sufficient for the diagnosis to be made. It must be supported by the presence in the bone marrow of leukaemic cells. Without this the blood changes are spoken of as leukaemoid, but not true leukaemia. This type of picture can be found in some acute infections, in tuberculosis, and sometimes in patients with carcinoma of the colon and stomach.

Changes in the Body

If we look at the body tissues in a patient with this disease certain changes are obvious. A study of these will make it easier to understand the variety of symptoms with which such a patient can present.

Bone Marrow

The marrow is crowded with cells, leukaemic and immature cells. The tissue producing erythrocytes and megakaryocytes is reduced.

Blood

As a consequence of the reduction in normal haemopoietic tissue there is an anaemia. The red-blood cell count and the haemoglobin level are reduced, but cells are usually normal in shape and size. The white cell count is usually raised, there is a range from normal up to $200 \times 10^9/\ell$ ($200,000/mm^3$).

Some cells are normal, but most are leukaemic or early primitive forms of the development line. The platelet count is decreased.

Spleen and Lymph Nodes

There is some enlargement, the degree varies with the type of leukaemia. In children a greater degree of enlargement is found. The spleen shows loss of pattern and infiltration by leukaemic cells, while the nodes although generally showing similar infiltration may occasionally contain masses which are like tumours.

Other Tissues

Deposits of leukaemic cells can be found in almost any organ. Some which are affected are the central nervous system, the tissues around the eyes, and the skin.

Clinical Presentation

In the younger age group there is often a sudden onset but in older patients symptoms may appear slowly.

Symptoms due to Blood and Marrow Changes

Due to anaemia there is lethargy, pallor, and dyspnoea on exertion. The skin is often waxen. With platelet depletion there is a tendency to bleeding, large bruises can appear with slight or no trauma at all, and small wounds tend to bleed for longer than normal. In many adults the diagnosis has been made on investigation following prolonged haemorrhage after tooth extraction.

Although the number of white cells is increased, the cells are immature and abnormal, they can no longer play an effective part in the body's defence against infection. Accordingly patients are liable to become infected and many have mouth ulcers with associated enlarged cervical glands.

Toxic Symptoms

Even in the absence of infection, similar symptoms may be present. There is a fever and rigors may occur.

Spleen and Lymph Nodes

When the leucopoietic tissues of the spleen and lymph nodes are involved there is enlargement. The degree is variable but can be very marked. In the case of the spleen there may be associated pain.

Bones

The infiltrated bone can be tender, this is particularly true of the sternum. In children joints may be swollen and painful and there may be changes visible on the X-ray.

Central Nervous System and the Eye

Deposits on the meninges or in the brain or spinal cord can cause convulsions and neurological signs. It is often difficult to determine clinically whether these are due to leukaemic foci or to a small haemorrhage caused by the lack of platelets. Infiltration of the tissues around the eye may produce bulging of the eye, proptosis, and severe bruising, 'a black eye' can also be present.

Review of the Opening Case History

Armed with these facts it is now possible to explain the symptoms and signs described at the beginning of the chapter. The lethargy and pallor are due to anaemia, while the bruising is caused by the low level of platelets. The enlarged cervical glands may well be the result of infection in the throat, and leukaemic infiltration is responsible for the increased size of the spleen.

Examination

A full history must be taken and this must include any exposure to the known carcinogenic factors. The mother of a child must be questioned about any diagnostic X-rays which she may have had during the pregnancy. A full clinical examination is necessary and this must include the neurological system.

Investigations

Blood Tests

A full blood count including platelets, together with bone marrow biopsy, provides the evidence on which a diagnosis is based. Chemical tests can be made on the white cells, the enzyme content determined, and, using mono-clonal antibodies, their antigens typed.

Blood grouping in preparation for transfusion, and the determination of the histocompatibility profile in case a bone marrow transplant is required, are both part of early testing. Other investigations, X-rays, ultrasound, etc., are carried out as clinically indicated.

Treatment

The aims of treatment are threefold:

1. Supportive.	Measures to combat initial conditions consequent on normal bone marrow depletion, and complications of treatment.	
2. Induction	of complete remission. In practice this means reducing leukaemic cells to a count below 1×10^9. At this level they are not detectable in the marrow.	
3. Maintenance.	This is designed to prevent relapse.	

The treatment of acute lymphoblastic leukaemia in children is described first. The regime for adults is similar, any differences will be noted at the end of the section.

Supportive

Anaemia and thrombocytopenia are treated by transfusion of packed red cells or platelet concentrates. Since repeated transfusion may lead to reaction, and also since large quantities of blood may be required, it is essential that there is easy access to a transfusion service with adequate facilities. It is usual not to raise the haemoglobin above 10 g/dcℓ (10 g/100 mℓ) until the white cell count begins to fall, this avoids the complication of intra-cranial haemorrhage due to stasis of leucocytes.

Infection may already be present, or develop during intensive chemotherapy. Adequate anti-bacterials, anti-fungals, and in some cases the antiviral drug acyclovir, may all be necessary. Reverse barrier nursing reduces the risk of infection from other sources (extrinsic), but not from the patient's own com-mensals, skin, gut organisms. It is therefore usual to take swabs before intensive chemotherapy begins, to enable identification and sensitivity of these com-mensals to be made. It is not possible to wait the routine 48 hours for a culture and sensitivity report, treatment must begin at once. It is based on the known sensitivities of the likely extrinsic organisms, or the patient's commensals. Non-absorbable antibiotics are given by mouth to sterilise the patient's gut. If there is severe neutropenia (too few neutrophils) concentrated granulocyte trans-fusion will be given.

Children, and non-immune adults, are at risk from infections such as varicella and measles. Antibody levels, particularly in children, should be measured at the beginning of treatment. In hospital contacts can be avoided, but when out-patient treatment is given, parents and adult patients must be warned of the risk. If there is contact, the appropriate immunoglobulin should be given within 48 hours. Children should not receive live vaccines, e.g. measles, poliomyelitis, but toxoids, e.g. tetanus, diphtheria are permissible.

The diagnosis of leukaemia is a severe shock to the parents, and the treatment, with perhaps isolation, to the child. It is necessary to give all the psychological support possible to both family and child. The social services may need to be mobilised, particularly if the demands of hospital visiting put a financial strain on family resources. The medical social worker is a vital member of the team, not only can she contact the official bodies, but also those in the community who can organise the good will of voluntary helpers in supporting family life, shopping, meals for working husbands, care of any other children, etc. However, the most important factor is the time given to explain not once, but many times, what is happening, what can be expected, and what the family can do to help. The initial shock and the continuing tension mean that explanations must be made over and over again, and time given for patient and family to work out the feelings of frustration, despair, and anger which are very natural.

Induction

This is carried out in hospital, preferably at a specialised centre.

Combination chemotherapy with oral prednisone or prednisolone and weekly injections of vincristine, together with either L-asparaginase or an anthracycline (daunorubicin or doxorubicin) is used. In about four to six weeks about 90% of children will be in remission. It may be possible in future to define a good prognosis group who only need the oral steroid and vincristine.

It is known that relapse can occur owing to the leukaemic cells finding sanctuary in the C.N.S., and in boys, in the testes. It is therefore usual to give prophylactic intrathecal methotrexate at intervals and also radiation to the C.N.S. In view of the known complications of this treatment attempts are being made to substitute additional methotrexate given intravenously for radiation, but it may be that only good prognosis patients are suitable for this regime. Children under 2 years of age are given only methotrexate, radiation is withheld until they have reached the age of 2.

There is less agreement on prevention of testicular disease. Prophylactic radiation after intensive chemotherapy will cause sterility, but without prophylaxis 30% of boys will have a relapse following the end of maintenance chemotherapy due to testicular involvement, and if tumour is actually present when radiation is given, systemic or C.N.S. relapse will occur in the majority. Again it may be that supplemental intravenous methotrexate may prove to be the answer. It is possible that routine biopsy at the end of systemic chemotherapy may detect early infiltration and indicate those requiring treatment.

Complications During Induction

Apart from bone marrow depletion and infection, there is an initial hazard due to the accumulation of three products of the breakdown of leukaemic cells, uric acid, calcium, and phosphates. These products may precipitate in the kidneys and cause renal failure. The problem can be prevented by adequate hydration, alkalinisation of the urine, and use of the drug allopurinol.

C.N.S. prophylaxis has both short term and long term sequelae. A temporary sleepiness may occur 4–6 weeks after radiation, and more severe neurological symptoms with fits occasionally follow combined radiation and methotrexate.

Slightly lower performance in mathematics and reasoning may occur as a long term effect, more commonly if radiation is given to a child under two years old.

Watch must be kept for the late development of second malignancies, particularly well-differentiated thyroid carcinoma which is treatable, the main risk of malignant damage from chemotherapy appears to be associated with the alkylating drugs which are not used in these regimes.

Preliminary evidence from long term survivors does not seem to confirm fears of malignancy or malformation in children of successfully treated patients.

Maintenance

This can be carried out on an outpatient basis. With due attention to the risk of infection, normal life can be resumed. This is particularly important for children as they can go back to school and join their friends in other activities.

The mainstay of treatment is daily 6-mercaptopurine and weekly oral methotrexate. The doses may need to be adjusted to keep the total and differential WBC at a steady level. In addition many centres give a mini-induction course of vincristine and oral prednisone at monthly intervals. Most centres continue treatment for three years but some consider five years give better survival figures.

This phase of treatment can often be supervised jointly with the local hospital and the family doctor.

Relapse

Patients who relapse while on chemotherapy or after maintenance treatment has been stopped, may obtain remission by a regime either of the same drugs at higher dosage, or a different drug combination. Some centres are trying to identify poor risk patients and give them more intensive induction and maintenance therapy. Improved methods of treating bone marrow depletion and intercurrent infection make this possible. Relapse is suspected if there is a return of bone pain or an unexpected drop in the blood count.

Testicular leukaemia is treated with local radiation, C.N.S. prophylaxis, and systemic chemotherapy. The symptom is a painless swelling of the testicle.

The development of signs of increasing pressure, headache, vomiting, papilloedema, or abnormal weight gain (through infiltration of the hypothalamus) are indicative of C.N.S. relapse which must be confirmed by examination of the C.S.F. Intrathecal methotrexate at weekly intervals, and then at longer intervals will control this. The insertion of a reservoir within a ventricle enables this to be given more easily. Further radiation can be given, but is more liable to produce reactions.

Bone marrow transplant using a histocompatible donor, usually a sibling, is considered in the second remission, and possibly for poor risk patients in the first. The patient must be immunosuppressed by the use of cytotoxics and whole body irradiation. This of course brings the risk of infection and the consequences of marrow depletion, both are dealt with as outlined previously. A poor appetite promotes poor resistance to infection, and intravenous feeding including additional vitamins may be required.

Rejection of the graft by the host is unlikely owing to prior conditioning, but graft versus host disease (GvHD) was until recently the usual cause of failure. Various steps have been advocated including the use of cyclosporin-A and removal of incompatible red blood cells and T lymphocytes from the donor marrow. However the latter may also remove some anti-leukaemic effect of the graft marrow. It is also interesting that patients who survive moderate or slight GvHD have a lower relapse rate. About 25% of patients develop chronic GvHD which can be treated with low doses of steroids and a drug called azathioprine, but they will probably have a lowered immunity for life, while survivors of the acute disease recover full immunity in about two years.

Adults

Treatment is similar, but the results, for reasons as yet unknown, are worse. Patients who are identified as having T-cell or B-cell ALL, may be considered for bone marrow transplant earlier, soon after the achievement of the first remission.

Immunotherapy

As in other malignancies attempts have been made to improve the patient's immune defences. The method used may be passive by transferring antibodies against the leukaemic antigens, adoptive as in the transfer of immunologically competent cells in marrow transplants, or active by the use of BCG vaccine or irradiated leukaemic cells.

BCG has probably been the most widely used method. During the time that it has been used chemotherapy and supportive measures have both improved, and results are therefore difficult to interpret. BCG is not now used alone to maintain remission.

Discussion of further development in marrow transplants, and the use of monoclonal antibodies, is reserved for the section on research.

Acute Myeloblastic Leukaemia (AML or ANLL)

Here the situation is reversed, it is more common in adults. Their treatment will be described first, any modifications in children noted later.

Supportive

All the measures outlined for patients with ALL are needed with particular emphasis on infection risks. For some patients daily granulocyte transfusions may be required.

Induction

Combined chemotherapy using cytarabine, 6-thioguanine, and an anthracycline (daunorubicin or doxorubicin) will induce remission in most patients in 4-6 weeks.

Maintenance

The average survival time after diagnosis is three years, so the same statements cannot be made about maintenance treatment as in ALL, namely that continuous maintenance therapy lengthens survival time. There is at present no obvious policy, but agreement that treatment must be more aggressive than for ALL. Either the induction drugs are given at monthly intervals, or combined with others including methotrexate, 6-mercaptopurine, and prednisolone.

Immunotherapy

The use of treated leukaemic cells and BCG have been shown to prolong survival time in this disease. However the actual length of remission remained unaltered, the therapy was therefore only palliative, not curative.

Bone Marrow Transplants

Since chemotherapy and immunotherapy failed to make a marked impact on the disease, bone marrow transplantation was an attractive additional measure.

The procedure and precautions have already been outlined. Patients who achieve a first complete remission and are under 20 years of age appear to respond better. Long term results are awaited.

CNS Treatment

One quarter of patients develop CNS involvement, but this differs from that seen in ALL. Symptoms are frequently focal because of pressure on the cord, or cranial nerves. As there is no evidence of an effect on survival time, prophylactic CNS treatment is not used.

Children

Treatment is identical but intrathecal methotrexate or cytarabine is given as CNS prophylaxis. Bone marrow transplantation complications are better tolerated.

Prognostic Factors

Attempts have been made to identify factors which influence prognosis and may therefore affect the choice and intensity of treatment. Some are noted at the time of diagnosis, some as response to treatment. Some caution is required with regard to the latter since they may be influenced by subtle differences in treatment regimes. The one common indicator for both types of acute leukaemia is age, results become less good with increasing age.

In children with ALL there are certain features which indicate a high probability of relapse. They are age, less than 2 years or more than 12, a high WBC, early involvement of the CNS, a mass in the mediastinum, enlargement of organs other than the marrow, and finally male sex.

Results

Acute Lymphoblastic Leukaemia

About 50% of children may currently remain in complete remission after maintenance therapy has stopped. Most relapses occur within 18 months of this, and while late relapses are known, a patient who continues disease free for four years is probably 'cured'.

On the other hand children who relapse during treatment have a poor prognosis, 80% die within a year of relapse.

The figures for adults are less good. While 78% achieve complete remission, the median survival time is just over 3 years. Current studies using intensive maintenance regimes have not yet reached the point at which conclusions can be drawn, but the preliminary figures look encouraging.

Acute Myeloblastic Leukaemia

There are as yet no firm figures since no real advances have been made, also in different series the age groups were markedly different thereby influencing results. Some centres have patients who have survived almost 5 years, but as an average only 10-20% of adults are long term survivors. With successful marrow transplantation up to 50% of patients remain in remission, again age has an important effect.

Research

Much of the success in the treatment of leukaemia has stemmed from a better understanding of the administration of the cytotoxic drugs, improved transplantation techniques, and better treatment of the complications both of the disease and the treatment.

Current research is looking at new cytotoxic drugs and their incorporation into various regimes. Of equal importance as efficacy is a decrease in toxicity. So far none of the drugs is specific for leukaemia cells alone, and normal cells of the body are also attacked but recover more quickly than the abnormal cells which are the real target.

Various methods have been suggested, mostly they have centred on methods of carrying the drug to the leukaemic cell in such a way that the drug only becomes comes active when it is split from its carrier. Cytotoxics have been coupled with fragments of DNA, the low density lipoprotein (LDL) and lysosomes are being explored, but theoretically the most promising is the monoclonal antibody. Each antibody will only combine with the corresponding specific antigen on the leukaemic cell. If the cytotoxic could be linked with it without destroying its antibody activity, the cytotoxic could be homed in on the target cells and released exactly where it is wanted, without exposing unduly normal cells.

Monoclonal antibodies can also be used to determine the specific sub-groups of leukaemia, each antibody reacting only with one antigen. They are also able to deplete donor marrow of unwanted cells. This research, leading hopefully to clinical usage, is only possible because these antibodies can now be produced more easily.

The greatest barriers to more widespread use of marrow transplantation are the lack of suitable donors, and the risk of GvHD even when the donor and recipient are compatible. Here again monoclonal antibodies by ridding the marrow of unwanted cells may not only reduce the risk of GvHD, but also enable donors who are not completely matched to be used. A further advance would be the ability to pre-treat the patient's own marrow with monoclonal antibodies and complement before whole body radiation or intensive chemotherapy. The marrow could then be stored and used as a 'graft' after treatment.

Further work will continue to look at the role of viruses particularly in relation to translocation of chromosome fragments, and also the special factors which enable the leukaemia cells to leave the marrow and settle in other sites.

Nursing Care

Nurses who are attached to special units receive a full training in all the aseptic and barrier nursing techniques, but for those who never see such a unit, or who may be briefly involved in the care of a patient prior to transfer, it may be helpful to describe some of the principles, techniques and problems.

Special Units

Every member of staff, nursing, medical or auxiliary, must practise and maintain a discipline which can become very irksome. For personnel such as cleaners or orderlies with no medical knowledge, the rules may seem unduly restrictive. Every effort must be made to explain and maintain understanding, for the kind-hearted orderly who slips into a cubicle to give a child a sweet or pick up a newspaper, is not only sabotaging the system, but endangering the patient.

It would be impossible here to describe in detail such a unit. Only the principles of its operation can be stated and some of the consequent problems.

Aim of the Unit

The primary aim is to place the patient in a sterile environment. Everything with which he comes in contact must be sterile, the air, the room, and its contents, must be sterilised. Having achieved this it must be maintained and controlled by periodic bacteriological checks. To maintain sterility nothing contaminated, either human or inanimate, must enter this environment. The staff must have their carrier sites, nose, etc. swabbed, and if staphylococci are found, vigorous efforts to eradicate them are made. All food, dishes, medicines, must be sterile and so special preparation units must be set up. In the unit itself the patient's sluice must be separate from his room, and a chute for dirty articles situated well away from the hatch through which sterile articles enter.

As already described steps must be taken to prevent the patient's own commensal organisms from becoming a source of infection.

The Cubicle

The number of staff entering the cubicle is kept to a minimum. Before entering the unit everyone leaves outdoor clothing in lockers and puts on clean over-shoes. At the entrance to the cubicle, the nurse or doctor may go into a preparation room, and after removing all clothing, take a shower and then put on special sterile clothing and mask. On leaving the unit the procedure is reversed. Before touching the patient, hands are scrubbed as for a surgical procedure. This has been found to be the most important single action. As far as possible disposable articles are used, cutlery, plates, syringes, towels, a long list could be made. Any infection among the staff, however minor, must be reported. The patient himself must be put into sterile clothing after a bath before entering his room, and nothing that cannot be sterilised, not even a well-loved toy, can be taken in with him.

Psychological Effects

Although an adult usually has sufficient mental resources to cope with this situation, it is the effect on the child in fact which may be more damaging. Long separation from the mother has been shown to have adverse effects, and prolonged visiting by parents is now encouraged in hospitals. The nature of the treatment and of the barrier unit makes it impossible for a mother to nurse her child. Close physical contact is an important part of the mother/child relationship, and cannot be entirely replaced by telephone and visual communication. The number of nurses handling a child is kept to a minimum for reasons of bacterial sterility, but it does enable a nurse to build up a closer relationship with her patient. She must be prepared to spend time playing with the child and becoming in some ways a foster mother.

The Family

At least the patient is the focus of activity but the family is confined to a spectator role. Visitors often play a quite unconscious part in a patient's treatment. They bring news of the outside world, small attentions, picking up a paper, giving a drink, maintain physical contact and the sense of belonging together. The deprivation the patient may suffer in the unit has been discussed, but it must be realised that the relatives can be even more deprived and emotionally disturbed. A mother may want to spend all day with her child, but because she has other children and family responsibilities, cannot do so. It is important to regard the other members of the family as also being in some sense patients.

As much care and attention may be required for them. Time for explanations and for just listening must be found. Patient repetition of the treatment planned, of the meaning of changes, discussion of progress, all these are part of total patient care. From the very outset the medical social worker must be in close contact with the patient's relatives. She needs to be experienced in the special problems involved and will probably need an office for her own use in the unit. The responsibility for the care of patient and family involves the whole team, and that team includes all ancillary staff. Every member should be briefed according to his role, to understand his part and the general policy, and the task must be regarded as a joint one.

Staff

The ratio of staff to patients is very high. The bacteriological and laboratory control of a large unit will require the full time services of doctors and technicians. The training of staff and the maintenance of sterility routines requires unremitting vigilance. Many departments of the hospital will be involved and if the purpose of the unit is explained clearly and simply, co-operation will be maximal. If the filtration plant develops a fault, the duty engineer who gets up at night will then understand the urgency of his job and be better reconciled to a lost night's sleep.

Chronic Leukaemia

This disease presents many contrasts with the acute form, it rarely affects children, the onset is slow and insidious, and it is possible to state clearly to which group of white cells the leukaemic cells belong. The two commonest types are granulocytic and lymphocytic, the latter occurs more often. For convenience a comparison between the two is given in a table below.

	Lymphocytic	**Granulocytic**
White Blood Cells	Lymphocytes up to $300 \times 10^9/\ell$, 99% of them are B-lymphocytes	Leucocytes up to $100-250 \times 10^9/\ell$ or more, mostly neutrophil granulocytes and their precursors
Platelet Count	Falls only in terminal stages	Normal or slightly raised
Anaemia	Slight	Moderate
Marrow	Hypercellular, increase in lymphoid series	Hypercellular, very high increase in myeloid series
Spleen	Moderate enlargement	Gross enlargement, often painful
Lymph Nodes	Painless enlargement	Enlargement not often found. Develops into acute leukaemia

Enlarged tissues

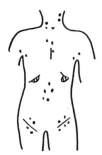

Lymphatic. Mainly lymph nodes

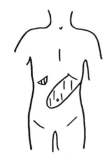

Myeloid. Mainly spleen and liver

Fig. 21.2.   Chronic leukaemia

Chronic Lymphocytic Leukaemia

Incidence

This is the more common disease of the two chronic types and accounts for about one-quarter of the deaths from leukaemia. It is rare to find it in a patient under 35 for it is a disease of the older age groups, its rate of incidence increasing with age. Males form two-thirds of the affected group. In certain countries, notably Japan, the incidence is very low.

Aetiology

This is one form of leukaemia which does not seem to be caused by radiation.

Symptomatology

There is a gradual decline in health. The patient complains of loss of energy, but usually only consults a doctor when he notices enlarged lymph nodes, these are often in the neck. A small proportion of patients are symptomless and only discovered when a routine blood test is performed as part of some other investigation. Occasionally patients consult the doctor because they have noticed a lump in the abdomen due to an enlarged spleen, or because they have skin nodules, leukaemic deposits, or skin rashes.

Course of the Disease

Patients with this disease have shown considerable variation in clinical behaviour. Some have had few or no symptoms and survived 20 years, while others have had progressive deterioration and have died within a year. Research work has now shown that the clinical condition mirrors pathological findings. In addition to the findings already tabulated, some patients have a positive direct antiglobulin test (Coombs') due to a haemolytic anaemia, and others may have a reduced platelet count due to platelet antibodies rather than marrow failure. About half the patients have a reduction of the immunoglobulins. Infection, bacterial, viral, or fungal is found and is often a terminal event.

The disease can be staged 0 to IV, the range being from symptomless lymphocytosis to lymphocytosis with reduced platelets +/− lymph node or liver or spleen enlargement.

Examination

A full history and examination is made as for the acute leukaemic patient. It is important that the site of enlarged nodes is carefully described and the size recorded. If the spleen is palpable, then the degree of enlargement is noted.

Investigations

Since the condition is variable and hence the treatment, it is important to establish the nature of the disease. As with the acute condition, a full blood count, including platelets, is necessary, and also bone-marrow examination. A chest X-ray is routine and possibly tomograms will be required if mediastinal involvement is suspected. The full extent of abdominal lymph-node enlargement is assessed by a lymphogram. The presence of haemolytic anaemia is determined by performing a direct antiglobulin test. It is important not to omit this estimation as a positive result indicates a less favourable prognosis and influences the choice of treatment.

Treatment

The choice of treatment depends upon the clinical state and the blood picture. Patients who are symptom free and not anaemic, can reasonably be left untreated but kept under observation with regular blood counts, this stage may last for years. For the rest treatment consists of a judicious use of chemotherapy or radiotherapy combined with supportive measures, transfusion and antibiotics.

Chemotherapy

This is used when there are systemic symptoms or impending bone marrow failure. The drugs are oral chlorambucil or cyclophosphamide. Both are immunosuppressive, and it is probably best to give the drug in short courses, assessing the patient's condition afterwards during a rest period. The majority respond with a fall in lymphocyte count, smaller numbers of patients experience a reduction in the size of lymph nodes or spleen.

Prednisone

A positive antiglobulin test or a rapidly falling haemoglobin indicating active haemolysis, requires the urgent administration of prednisone. Usually the response is dose dependent, 40 mg daily are given, gradually tailing off the dose. The risk of infection is increased with the use of steroids.

Supportive Therapy

Blood transfusion is given where necessary and antibiotics if infection is found. Gamma globulin can also be given.

Radiation

Radiotherapy is usually given to relieve troublesome symptoms due to leukaemic deposits or enlarged nodes. When the spleen is treated, white-cell counts and haemoglobin levels must be charted daily. The dose of radiation is small, it is often given on alternate days, and adjusted according to the blood picture.

Prognosis

Since the disease shows a gradation of severity, the prognosis shows a similar variation. The average survival time is given as three to five years but many patients have survived 20 years and died of some other condition.

Chronic Granulocytic Leukaemia

Incidence

The disease is found equally in men and women, can occur at any age, but usually in patients over 40 years of age.

Aetiology

Radiation is definitely linked to this form of leukaemia. It occurred in patients who received high irradiation for the treatment of ankylosing spondylitis, and in Japanese survivors of the atomic bombs. Nearly all patients have an abnormal

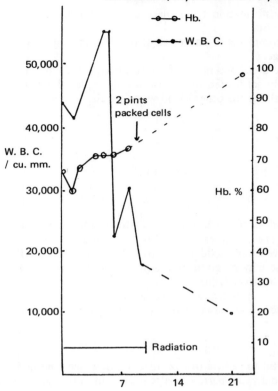

Fig. 21.3.   Effect of splenic radiation on W.B.C. chronic lymphatic leukaemia

chromosome, the Philadelphia Chromosome, material from chromosome 22 is translocated to another chromosome, usually 9.

Clinical Picture

Like chronic lymphatic leukaemia, the onset is slow. Complaints are of general ill-health with weight loss and loss of appetite. Later there may be breathlessness and oedema of the legs due to anaemia. Due to gross enlargement of the spleen some patients consult the doctor because of an enlarging abdomen which is often quite painful. Pain is due to thrombosis of a vessel in the spleen causing an infarct.

Progress of the Disease

The initial chronic phase of the disease progresses eventually into a transformed 'acute' phase, this may take place between three and ten years after the diagnosis.

Occasionally transformation takes place in a matter of days, this is sometimes called a 'blastic crisis'.

The patient complains of any or all of these symptoms, fever, sweating, bone pain, haemorrhage.

The blood picture shows mainly primitive blast cells, simultaneously the bone marrow is heavily infiltrated or almost wholly replaced by myeloblastic cells. Primitive blast cells of the other blood series are also sometimes seen.

Treatment

Chronic Phase

Chemotherapy

Busulphan is the drug of choice, it is given daily until the WBC reaches $20 \times 10^9/\ell$ (20,000/mm^3). The count must be plotted daily as some patients are unduly sensitive and have a very sudden, abrupt fall. After reaching the desired level a maintenance dose may be given, but count plots must be continued as a severe, potentially fatal, marrow failure may occur.

Hydroxyurea is an alternative drug. Recently a combination of bulsulphan and 6-thioguanine has been used as this may give better control with less toxicity.

Radiotherapy

This may be useful to reduce the size of a spleen which does not regress. Counts must be charted daily and particular attention paid to the rate of fall.

Marrow Transplantation

If a suitable donor is available bone marrow transplant is considered early in the chronic phase. This procedure is relatively new but early results are promising. Current research may enable slightly mismatched donors to be used so making transplantation available to more patients.

Transformation Phase

Chemotherapy

When the onset of this change is slow, a switch from busulphan to another drug such as hydroxyurea may cause regression to the chronic phase, but more often combination therapy used for AML is required. If a lymphoblastic picture predominates then an acute lymphoblastic leukaemia regime may be tried first. Remission is less frequent than in the acute leukaemia condition.

Auto Transfusion

The blood of patients often contains pluripotential stem cells, these can be harvested and stored in liquid nitrogen. After intensive chemotherapy, these stored cells can be reconstituted and transfused back into the patient. However the chronic phase which may then ensue usually only lasts a few months.

Children

Treatment is the same as for adults. Splenectomy is beneficial in some patients.

Prognosis

Survival time is variable ranging from 3 to 10 years. Children and Philadelphia negative patients have a poor prognosis.

The almost certain biphasic nature of the condition means that the life span of the patient is inevitably shortened. For the young or the middle aged patient this may be crucial to his plans for himself and his family. The expectation of a period of reasonable health may make it possible for him to make changes in his life style if he wishes.

PLASMA CELL MALIGNANCY (MULTIPLE MYELOMA)

Plasma Cell Tumours

Plasma cells are derived from B-lymphocytes, and the tumours may be found in bone, usually multiple but occasionally single, and extra-skeletal sites such as skin, cervical lymph nodes, gut, and upper respiratory passages. The majority of patients have multiple bony lesions, multiple myeloma, and are usually in the older age groups.

Symptomatology

The patient with this disease is often first seen in the casualty department. The story is that nothing wrong was noticed until a spontaneous fracture occurred. The following case history is typical.

Mrs. – a woman in her late fifties was doing her housework. She reached into a cupboard to bring out her vacuum cleaner and felt a sudden sharp pain in her upper right arm. She noticed some change in its shape and went to her local hospital. On X-ray she was found to have a pathological fracture of the upper humerus. She was kept in hospital for a few days and during this time developed retention of urine and paralysis of the lower limbs. A further X-ray showed a collapsed vertebra, at laminectomy biopsy confirmed this to be a myelomatous deposit.

The retention of urine and lower limb paralysis illustrate another form of presentation, neurological symptoms due to pressure on the spinal cord or peripheral nerves.

All these patients are at risk of hypercalcaemia consequent on bone destruction and may have symptoms of thirst, nausea, vomiting, constipation, mental confusion. About half the patients will have signs of renal failure.

Many patients state that they were perfectly well before the sudden onset of symptoms, but close questioning often reveals vague malaise, lethargy or repeated infection during the preceding weeks.

Examination

After a careful history a full examination is made. This must include the nervous system. When moving painful limbs care must to be taken as fracture occurs so easily. Signs of weight loss are sought. A pyrexia may occasionally be found.

Investigations

These are designed to discover the extent of the disease, and to make a firm diagnosis since other conditions can also show the abnormal M protein (paraprotein) in blood and urine.

Blood Count and Marrow Examination

Anaemia is usually found, initially not severe. Occasionally immature forms of all the blood cell types are found, or a few plasma cells. The sedimentation rate is high. Marrow findings are variable, usually a general increase in plasma cells is found, but by contrast the marrow is abnormal only in the site of a solitary lesion, not outside it.

Proteins

Plasma cells form immunoglobulins, and in this disease an abnormal paraprotein, M-protein is found in blood and urine. On electrophoresis the serum shows a characteristic pattern. Normal globulin levels may be present, but albumin is often low, thereby changing the normal albumin globulin ratio.

There may be proteinuria. This is usually due to some loss of albumin, but mostly to a particular fraction of an immunoglobulin molecule, this is called the Bence-Jones protein. On heating the urine it precipitates out at about 60°C, disappears at boiling point, reappearing on cooling again at about 60°C. Tubular damage to the kidneys allows the protein to pass into the urine, and electrophoresis of concentrated urine gives a characteristic pattern.

Electrophoresis is used to identify and quantitate the serum M-protein.

Biochemistry

Serum calcium, blood urea or creatinine, uric acid, and alkaline phosphatase must be measured. The level of urea or creatinine is used to add A or B to the staging number of the disease.

X-rays

A skeletal survey is needed to establish the extent of the bony lesions. If there are neurological signs and symptoms, or evidence of a paraspinal mass, a myelogram is needed, a CATscan may be helpful. The cerebrospinal fluid should be sent for examination.

It used to be held that an I.V.P. was dangerous in these patients, but it is now believed that the preliminary dehydration caused the problems. If needed the examination can be carried out, provided precautions are observed.

Other Investigations

Special tests may be needed. Some of these are the viscosity of the blood, biopsy for amyloid deposits, and aspiration of joint effusions.

Staging

Based on all these findings the disease can be graded stages I to III. If the blood urea is below 60 mg/100 mℓ, or creatinine below 2.0 mg/100 mℓ it is also designated A, the converse B.

Treatment

Surgery

This is usually palliative and will be designed to relieve obstruction, to prevent pressure on the cord, laminectomy, or to stabilise a fracture by the insertion of a pin.

Occasionally operation is required to remove a residual extra-skeletal tumour after radiation.

Radiotherapy

Radiation will relieve bone pain. Solitary bone lesions and extra-skeletal tumours can also be controlled. Large bone lesions should be treated either prophylactically before fracture, or after surgical stabilisation.

Chemotherapy

Intermittent courses of melphalan and prednisolone are given. Weekly blood counts are made. Therapy is continued as long as the M-protein decreases, the dose of melphalan being increased until this point is reached, or a decrease in neutrophils or platelets occurs.

Some patients may be able to discontinue therapy.

New bone lesions appearing despite successful chemotherapy are irradiated.

If the platelets decrease, there is no response to melphalan, or there is relapse, treatment is changed to intermittent cyclophosphamide and prednisolone, if there is still no response, chlorambucil or carmustine may be tried.

General Measures

Patients should wear supporting corsets or collars where necessary to enable them to be mobile. These relieve pain until radiation or chemotherapy can take effect and also prevent sudden strain causing small fractures. Immobilisation increases bone demineralisation and the risk of hypercalcaemia.

Patients should be encouraged to take 2–3 litres of fluid a day (4 or more pints) to enable them to excrete the abnormal load of proteins, calcium and uric acid, etc. If hypercalcaemia is present, intravenous infusion may be needed, and prednisolone until the serum calcium is normal. Infections require prompt treatment. Occasionally allopurinol is used to control uric acid levels.

While the disease is controlled, regular checks of urea/creatine and serum calcium are made. Once stabilised, blood counts are repeated at each visit, M-protein every 1–2 months, and X-rays as clinically indicated.

Eventually all patients enter terminal acute marrow failure, some develop an acute leukaemia.

Nursing Care

Although some patients can remain at home most will require admission. The nursing care can be very demanding, patients are often in poor condition and may have multiple fractures. They require the skills applied to medical, orthopaedic, and neurosurgical nursing. At the same time the physiotherapist and occupational therapist need to exercise all their expertise and ingenuity to rehabilitate the patient if at all possible. Simple measures such as a comfortable bedrest, a mirror for the patient who cannot sit up, and tongs for retrieving articles which may have slipped out of reach, may raise morale greatly.

From the earlier description of the disease the complications to be expected are pathological fractures, spinal-cord compression, and renal failure. The first two conditions have already been discussed previously. Signs of renal failure are sometimes very slight and the onset is insidious. Often the first abnormality to be noticed is the passage of large quantities of dilute urine particularly at night. The blood urea or creatinine may then be found to be raised. Acute onset with the passage of little or no urine is rare and usually associated with an I.V.P. preceded by dehydration. Since renal failure does occur an adequate fluid intake must be maintained and a fluid balance chart should be kept. Signs of any of these complications should be reported at once. Infection may be masked by the steroids given. Particular watch must be kept for signs and symptoms which may be quite slight.

Supportive therapy includes blood transfusion and adequate analgesia. Many patients are afraid of making a fuss and put off asking for analgesics. Established pain is more difficult to treat, by intelligent anticipation a nurse can not only spare the patient but make it possible to sustain analgesia at a lower dose level.

Pain relief is important in its own right, but in these patients it has the additional benefit of enabling them to be mobile thereby diminishing bone demineralisation. It should not be forgotten that supervision of the proper fitting of supports is in itself a form of analgesia.

Prognosis

Patients with extra-skeletal lesions do best, followed by those with solitary bony lesions, and finally multiple myeloma. Survival time in solitary as opposed to multiple lesions is longer by about five years, but the solitary deposit is held to be merely an early form of multiple myeloma.

Figures are given as stage I 46 months, II 32 months, III 23 months. Patients whose disease is graded B have shorter survival times. About 15% of patients treated with melphalan and prednisolone are alive at 5 years.

POLYCYTHAEMIA

Although not a leukaemia, this interesting condition is included in this chapter because it is a proliferative disease of the blood. The total red-cell mass is increased and the level of haemoglobin, the red-cell count, and the haematocrit are raised. This blood picture is called polycythaemia.

Physiological Increase

At first the infant has raised values due to the massive intake of blood from the placenta. The figures quickly fall to normal. If the environment has a lowered oxygen tension, as at high altitudes, then the oxygen saturation of arterial blood is lowered. To compensate for this, in those people who live permanently at such a height, the red-cell mass is increased so making more cells available to carry oxygen.

Secondary Increase

Diseases which produce reduced oxygen saturation in arterial blood, induce a secondary polycythaemia. Examples are certain congenital heart diseases, and pulmonary disease. Some conditions of the kidney and lesions of the brain are also associated with this blood change. It can also occur in association with an erythropoietin producing tumour.

Polycythaemia Rubra Vera

Polycythaemia rubra vera develops independently, and no cause, as in the other cases quoted can be found. It is a rare disease, men being slightly more often affected than women. The usual age of presentation is between 40 and 70.

Clinical Appearance

The increased red-cell mass causes a variety of symptoms. Headache and vertigo relate to the effect on the brain. Normal people may occasionally see a few spots before the eyes, but this is very common in these patients. Other complaints are of lassitude, dyspnoea, and epigastric discomfort. A few patients have gout, and others peptic ulcers. Both thrombosis and haemorrhage can occur and patients can experience symptoms due to these vascular accidents in vital organs, brain, lung, in coronary vessels, or in peripheral vessels.

On examination, these patients have a dusky blue tinge to the skin and mucous membranes. The spleen is often enlarged, the liver less frequently, and half of the patients have hypertension.

Diagnosis

This is made on the result of the blood investigations and the absence of any predisposing cause. Not only are all the red-cell values raised, but the leucocytes and platelet counts are also increased. In the marrow there is hyperplasia and an increase of all the precursors of the blood cells.

The red cell mass is estimated by the use of radioisotope labelled red cells.

Other investigations include chest X-ray, and in biochemistry plasma uric acid and estimation of the alkaline phosphatase content of the neutrophils.

Treatment

The aim of treatment is to reduce the red-cell mass.

Venesection

This is useful to relieve symptoms, but if it is the only measure taken, it has to be repeated frequently. The haemoglobin is raised relatively less than other elements of the blood and repeated venesection can lead to quite severe anaemia. If the platelet count rises or there are ischaemic symptoms it may be necessary to give a plasma volume expander to reduce the risk of thrombosis.

Chemotherapy

Cytotoxic drugs such as busulphan have been used successfully but the platelet count may fall rapidly. Melphalan and chlorambucil are alternatives, but the risk of leukaemia is greater.

Radiation

Irradiation of the bone marrow by external means has been replaced by the use of radioactive phosphorus. Bone has a high turnover of this mineral and so the radioactive isotope is concentrated more in the bones than in other tissues. The maximum effect on granulocytes and platelets is seen within three weeks.

The injection can be repeated 8 weeks later if the response is not adequate.

Administration

Although administration can be oral, there is always the risk of the patient being sick and it is more often administered intravenously. There is little risk to the doctor and nurse as the radiation emitted is in the form of beta rays which only travel a short distance. If venesection is to be performed before injection, it is probably best to admit the patient overnight, otherwise the treatment can be given on an outpatient basis. The couch and the floor around are covered with absorbent paper laid over polythene. The doctor and nurse don gowns, gloves, masks and overshoes. The patient is covered except for the injection site with a paper and polythene protection. After the usual checking of the dose and the patient's name, the liquid isotope is drawn up into the syringe and injected into a convenient vein. Firm pressure is applied over the injection site to prevent any bleeding and leak. The contaminated syringe and swab are discarded, together with the gloves and patient's covering, into a specially labelled waste bin. The patient, doctor, nurse and room are monitored with a radiation counter. Since the range of beta rays is so small, patients can go home at once with no risk to their families.

Results

When remission is produced it can last several years, untreated patients survive about 2–5 years. Some patients develop leukaemia, others may have a fatal thrombosis or develop myelosclerosis which destroys the bone marrow.

Summary

It will be obvious that many different branches of medicine are involved in the treatment of these conditions. In many cases investigation and treatment will be carried out in specialised centres, but the later follow-up stages and also the treatment of the chronic disorders may well be undertaken in peripheral hospitals. It is for this reason that so much detail has been included, without it a nurse may find it hard to understand the treatment policies.

Observing man from the cradle to the grave,
It becomes clear that his life
Is but one event in the continuing cycle of human affairs.
When a child is born,
One cannot but wonder what link he will forge
In the unending chain of human progression.

22 Malignant Disease in Children

Chromosomes and Genes

When a cell reproduces itself normally by mitosis, the daughter cells have the same structure, and carry out exactly the same functions as the parent. A cell's activity is governed by the chromosomes in the nucleus. Each chromosome is formed of a special nucleic acid called deoxyribonucleic acid, D.N.A., and along its length lie concentrations of organic chemicals, bases. These are different from each other, are called genes, and the total combination of them is the plan of a cell's activities. At division the genetic blueprint is passed unchanged to the daughter cells, so a skin cell will not produce daughter stomach mucosa cells.

Chromosome Number

Chromosomes are found in pairs. Both the total number of chromosomes and the number of pairs varies with the animal or plant. The potato has 48 chromosomes, the crayfish 300, and man 46. A pair of chromosomes is joined at one point called a centromere. It is possible with the aid of the microscope to sort the pairs into groups according to their size and the point along the chromosomes at which they are joined. These pairs are then numbered. A pair usually consists of chromosomes similar in form, but in man the sex chromosomes are distinct from each other in appearance. Man therefore has 22 pairs of chromosomes, each pair composed of two similar chromosomes, and one pair of sex chromosomes. In the female the sex chromosome is X and all her cells contain an X pair of chromosomes, XX, while in the male a Y sex chromosome is paired with an X chromosome, XY, and Y determines the sex as male.

Dominant and Recessive Genes

In pairs of chromosomes certain genes may be dominant, the characteristics they carry will always appear. Conversely the characteristics of a recessive gene will only be expressed if the corresponding gene on the other chromosome is

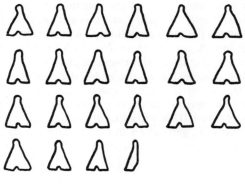

All
causes

_____

All
malignancy

Fig. 22.1.   Comparison of deaths under the age of fifteen

also recessive or is absent. A non-recessive gene can suppress a recessive gene, but the organism will be a carrier for the recessive factor. If two recessives are paired in a succeeding generation the condition then becomes clinically apparent.

Inheritance

Gregor Mendel formulated the laws of inheritance. These explain inherited traits which may skip one or two generations and then reappear. An example is blue eye colour. The eye colour gene is recessive, if both father and mother have received recessive blue eye genses, then the child can have blue eyes through neither of his parents has. Certain rare diseases are both sex linked and recessive.

Each individual inherits two sets of genes, one from each parent. When we consider that the pairing of these sets is random, that each parent possesses in turn two sets similarly acquired, we begin to have some idea of the vast genetic pool from which each individual draws. It is no longer surprising to us that brothers and sisters have different genetic constitutions. Furthermore genes cannot be considered in isolation, they are modified by the presence of others, and so, though two individuals may possess the same gene, due to a differing genetic constitution the expression of that gene can vary. Only identical twins have the same genetic blueprint. They result from the splitting of a fertilised ovum before it begins to develop into the embryo and they therefore share a common genetic constitution.

The interaction of genes blurs the simple lines of Mendelian inheritance, as does also the interaction between the genes and the environment. A condition may therefore be in some measure genetically determined and for this reason be more common in a family than in the general population, but at the same time occur sporadically only. We often call this a familial tendency in contrast to the situation in which the mere possession of a gene causes inevitable development of the condition. A clinical example of the latter situation is a disease of the central nervous sytem called Huntington's chorea.

Mendel based his laws on the results of hundreds of plant breeding experiments. Even the largest human family cannot reproduce these experimental conditions, and so in one generation all the possible combinations of the parental genes will not be expressed. This will account not only for characteristics which fail to appear in the next generation but often also for cases of genetically-determined disease in which there is apparently no family history.

Abnormalities

These can consist of either an irregular number of chromosomes, a major irregularity in one of them or in a single abnormal gene. Such a change is called a mutation. Of the non-sexual chromosomal abnormalities Down's Syndrome (mongolism) is the most common form. There are three chromosomes, number 21, present.

Major Irregularity in Chromosome Shape

Chromosomes can be broken and recombine incorrectly, or fragments can join other chromosomes. This is most likely to happen during division. The resultant abnormality may appear in all cells or only in certain cells. A partial or complete loss of chromosome 5 shown in all cells is associated with mental retardation and certain physical characteristics. Many patients with chronic myeloid leukaemia show the loss of part of chromosome 21 or 22 producing the so-called Philadelphia chromosome. This loss is shown in myeloid cells and megakaryocytes only, not in lymphocytes.

Abnormal Genes

A chromosome may look normal but carry an abnormal gene. This gene is the result of a mutation. We call the gene abnormal because it produces disease or abnormality in the individual. Certain diseases are genetically determined and their clinical occurrence is governed by whether the gene is dominant or recessive. A disease carried by a recessive gene will only be clinically apparent if the individual receives such a gene from each parent. It will thus seem that the disease has arisen by chance. Nurses are familiar with the procedure of testing a newborn baby's napkin for the presence of an abnormal metabolite in the urine. Untreated this condition of phenylketonuria, which is an error of metabolism, results in mental retardation. Both parents carry the gene and are normal, only the child receiving two genes develops the disease.

Sex-linked Disease

This is one of the most fascinating aspects of genetic inheritance and probably the most well-known example is the disease of haemophilia. This is a condition characterised by abnormal haemorrhage following minor trauma. It is due to a recessive gene carried on the X chromosome and is therefore said to be sex linked. Caution must be exercised in applying Mendelian laws to actual families. In the usual small family it is chance which genetic pairings occur.

Causes of Mutation

Some of the factors causing abnormalities of the chromosome are known. Experimentally radiation has been shown to cause failure of the normal division of the chromosome and of pairing after division. Certain infections, particularly those caused by viruses such as measles, can break-up the chromosomes, and the occurrence of an extra chromosome, as in Down's syndrome, is more frequent among children of older mothers.

The causation of point mutations, changes affecting single genes, is less well understood. Again radiation is known to produce this type of damage, but unless the change becomes inherited or affects the life of the organism it is not easy to detect. Some mutations may be lost or their effect may be so damaging that the cell dies or is unable to divide.

Mutations and the Germ Cells

The reason for the care exercised by those who handle radiation devices and for the advice in family planning offered to patients now becomes clear. Radiation can cause a mutation in a cell of one line, for example a skin cell, so that all the daughter cells inherit this change, or it can affect a germ cell and so potentially the whole of a future organism. It must be remembered that while a germ cell contains half the blueprint for the new organism, the genes of the fertilised ovum will contain all the genetic code for the whole development and future function of the new organism. As the embryo develops so cells become more and more specialised until eventually a cell performs only certain functions and reproduces only itself. Certain cells however retain the primitive characteristic of developing in several possible ways. A child can receive radiation from background cosmic sources, from fall-out incorporated into food such as milk, and from diagnostic X-rays of the abdomen of the pregnant woman.

It must also be remembered that cytotoxic drugs are mutagenic, and for this reason the rules for handling them must always be observed.

Teratogenesis

During the first three months of intra-uterine life the embryo's organs are formed. Viruses, such as rubella (German measles), certain drugs like thalidomide, and radiation or cytotoxics can disrupt this process producing malformations.

We call this teratogenesis. As yet we do not understand how the damage is caused.

Malignant Disease and Genetics

We can now see a little more clearly the possible role of inheritance in malignant disease. So far a dominant gene which causes malignant disease in every individual who inherits it has not been identified in man. This could be because such people might be unlikely to survive and have offspring. We do however have certain genetically-determined conditions which predispose to the development of malignancy, the most well-known example is polyposis coli discussed in Chapter 14, and we have seen that an abnormal chromosome in certain cells is associated with leukaemia. While the existence of a definite 'malignant' gene has not been proven, its existence may be suspected. When discussing tumours of the retina we mentioned that over half the children of parents who have had a retinoblastoma successfully treated will in turn develop the disease.

It is also possible to postulate that several genes interacting between themselves and with the environment may cause malignant change. In such a case the mere possession of these genes would not of itself be carcinogenic, but it would mean that the same disease would be more likely to occur in members of a family. This is what we mean by a familial tendency or a strong family history, and it is possible to find this when surveying for example the female relations of a patient with carcinoma of the breast.

Future Study

The common tumours occurring in childhood differ quite markedly from the adult types. They are usually solid and frequently the tissue is embryonic or sarcomatous. Sarcomas arise from structures represented in the embryo by the middle germ layer, mesoderm, osteogenic sarcoma is one example of this type.

Malignant disease in children represents a change occurring comparatively early in the life span of the organism. Many workers therefore feel that a genetic basis for such disease is a strong possibility. As we understand more about the mechanism of teratogenesis and the biology of chromosome damage, and as the science of genetics expands it is probable that more will be learned of the role of the gene in carcinogenesis.

Radiation and Cytotoxic Drugs

In children the tolerance to these types of treatment is the reverse of the situation in the adult. The total dose of radiation which can be given is lower and roughly matched to the age. The whole body is growing and the cells are very active. When considering the dosage of cytotoxic drugs it is often found that children tolerate comparatively higher doses weight for weight than adults. When the dose is related to surface area this difference is less marked.

It would be unwise to believe that our explanations are complete. Until we understand more fully the mode of action of both radiation and cytotoxics we can only formulate theories. Indeed we can only base our treatment on observed reactions and the cumulative experience of ourselves and others.

Tolerance of Tissues in Children

The reactions in specialised tumours to high doses are on the whole the same as in adults, pneumonitis in the lungs, nephritis following high renal dosage. There are two exceptions, the lens of the eye and the bones, both are more sensitive than in adults. In children under one year old the lens is very sensitive. Submitted to the same dose ratio as adults a higher proportion of them develop cataract. Growth in bone may be slowed, and in the spine this may result in uneven growth of the two halves of vertebrae resulting in permanent lateral curve, scoliosis. In the long bones length may be affected because of arrested or slowed growth.

Of particular concern is damage to the gonads. Effects may not be seen until the child reaches the sexual maturity, and there is always the possibility of mutations which could be passed on to future generations. In one follow-up study eight out of ten men receiving radiation during childhood for abdominal nephroblastoma, despite shielding of the testes, had reduced or absent spermatogenesis. Similarly girls receiving radiation can have primary ovarian failure.

Radiation of the hypothalamic-pituitary axis can cause growth hormone deficiency, which may not become apparent until several years after treatment despite repeated testing. Hormone supplements can be given but the response is variable. Clearly long term follow-up studies are required, particularly when new cytotoxics are introduced into regimes.

Tumours Following Radiation

It should not be forgotten that radiation in childhood has been followed by the development of malignancy later. I have already described thyroid carcinoma following successful spinal radiation for medulloblastoma, other examples are radiation of the thymus producing thyroid carcinoma, and X-ray epilation of the scalp for ringworm followed years later by multiple basal cell carcinomata.

Chemotherapy

Many of the cytotoxic drugs produce similar effects to radiation in children. However much depends on dosage. For example a dose which produces gonadal damage in adults affects pre-pubertal children far less frequently.

For successful treatment radiation and chemotherapy are often combined, and this may enhance the risk of damage.

Tumours of the Central Nervous System

Although these tumours have already been described in Chapter 9, in children they display certain characteristics worth noting. About one-third of childhood

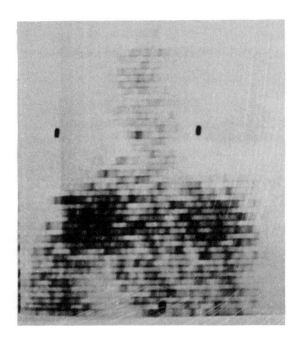

Fig. 22.2.   Scan showing metastases in the upper pelvis, medulloblastoma

tumours occur in the central nervous system and many workers would describe this as the most common tumour. Whereas in adults the majority are astrocytomas and arise in the cerebrum above the tentorium, in children the astrocytoma is less common, usually occurs in the cerebellum, is often Grade I or II and has a better prognosis than in adults. In children the commonest tumour is the medulloblastoma and indeed it is exclusively a childhood phenomenon. Secondary tumours in the brain are found but are far less common than in adults.

Other Childhood Tumours

Neuroblastoma

Though rare this is one of the commoner tumours occurring in children. It is occasionally found in adults but as a rule most patients are under the age of five. *Sites*   Sympathetic nervous tissue is found in all parts of the body. In the foetus this tissue contains primitive cells called neuroblasts and it is from residual cells of this type that this tumour is developed. The primary growth will be found in the same sites as the sympathetic system but most commonly in the adrenal medulla, the posterior part of the mediastinum in the chest, and in the abdomen in close relation to this special nervous tissue. It can also lie partly within and partly without the vertebral canal forming a dumb-bell shaped tumour.

Pathology

In appearance the neuroblastoma is greyish-white and may grow to quite a large size. Seen under the microscope the cells are small, have deeply-staining nuclei, and are often arranged in rosettes.

Spread

Direct

This occurs early. Adjacent structures are infiltrated and the tumour becomes fixed to them.

Blood

Metastases can occur anywhere in the body but are found most frequently in the bones, the liver, and the adrenals. This type of spread also occurs early in the course of the disease.

Lymphatics

Nodes are often invaded, usually the regional groups.

Symptomatology

The child is usually so young that specific symptoms are hard to elicit. There is a vague malaise, and the mother may notice signs due to pressure, this will be especially likely if the tumour is in the chest and causes respiratory embarrassment. Other symptoms due to pressure on nerves or the spinal cord may be varying degrees of paralysis or sensory loss. If the tumour develops in the adrenal gland a lump in the abdomen may be the first sign of trouble. The spread of the disease from each adrenal gland differs, from the left deposits seem to occur more often in the skull and orbit, while liver secondaries are more commonly associated with right-sided tumours.

Since spread occurs so early in the course of disease the first symptoms may well be caused by the secondary deposits and may for a time obscure the diagnosis. Bruising round the eye due to metastases can lead to an initial suspicion that the child has leukaemia.

Examination and Investigations

Since the patient is *usually* a very young child the story must be obtained from the mother. Often there is little that is diagnostic but it may be possible to get some idea of the length of history. Since leukaemia will enter into the differential diagnosis questions about abnormal bruising must be put. The examination though gentle must be thorough, palpation of a mass in the abdomen or of an enlarged liver may be the first clue to the nature of the disease.

A blood count if normal will virtually eliminate leukaemia. A chest X-ray may show metastatic deposits or a tumour in the posterior mediastinum, in the latter case tomograms will be required. If an abdominal tumour is found and it is thought to lie in the region of the kidney it is important to try and determine whether this is within the kidney or not.

X-rays

Chest and abdomen X-rays are required, with tomography if necessary. In at least half the cases flecks of calcification are seen.

I.V.P.   This will distinguish the tumour from a Wilms' tumour which lies within the kidney. It is likely to show displacement, but not distortion of the kidney substance.

Arteriogram   In some cases this may be necessary.

Myelogram   Any suspicion of a dumb-bell tumour may requre a myelogram, and the studies described under brain tumours, if there is any question of a brain deposit.

Skeletal Survey   This is needed because of the tumour's tendency to metastasise early.

Lymphangiography   This will be done to examine the abdominal lymph nodes.

Blood

In addition to the routine haematology and biochemistry, the urine must be screened for high quantities of metabolites of substances produced by the tumour (e.g. homovanilic acid). As some foods and drugs interfere with the test, the child has to be put on a special diet.

The test is not positive in all patients, but if it is, it is repeated during follow-up as a marker of possible recurrence.

Bone Marrow

Histology of an aspirate may show spread to the bone marrow.

Biopsy

Though the diagnosis may be almost certain, histological confirmation is still required, particularly in the case of the adrenal tumour to differentiate it from Wilms' tumour.

Treatment

It is now usual to combine surgery, radiation and chemotherapy to achieve radical therapy.

Surgery

Total surgical removal is usually impossible as the tumour invades neighbouring tissue early and becomes fixed. Nevertheless, apart from obtaining biopsy material, surgery by removing as much tumour as possible may relieve pressure symptoms. It is also possible in certain sites for the surgeon to insert clips at the naked-eye limits of the tumour so providing useful guides for the radiotherapist planning post-operative treatment.

Radiation

Treatment will last three to four weeks, and for the adrenal tumour include both sides of the spine and the other kidney. This opposite kidney will be shielded after part of the dose has been given to avoid total permanent damage. As much lung as possible is shielded when a mediastinal tumour is treated.

Chemotherapy

A combination of drugs is used, usually initially, and thereafter at intervals during the following year. Since the haemopoietic system is receiving a double assault when radiation is also given, an even closer watch than usual must be kept on the white cell count.

Secondary Deposits   A decision to treat these will depend on whether the secondaries are widespread and on the general condition of the patient. A solitary metastasis in lung or bone causing symptoms can often be irradiated with good results.

Anaemia

Due to bone-marrow involvement some patients have a severe anaemia. This must be corrected before treatment begins. Earlier we discussed the effect of lack of oxygen, anoxia, on the radiosensitivity of cells. With the present means of radiation available this can cause a serious decrease in response. Radiation with other particles of the atom, at present experimental, is less affected by anoxia. The constant emphasis on the correction of anaemia will have been noticed and at this point it is probably worth while repeating the reasons for such treatment. They are, improvement in general condition, lessened systemic effects of radiation, and improved radiosensitivity.

Spontaneous Transformation

A benign tumour of sympathetic nervous tissue is the ganglioneuroma. The cells of which it s composed are the mature type into which the neuroblast can develop. It has been shown that a neuroblastoma can be transformed into a benign ganglioneuroma.

Prognosis

The results of treatment depend upon the degree of spread and the age, children under two years of age do better. The assessment of treatment is difficult. The disease is rare and it is usually necessary to look at the results in several series, these may be difficult to compare as the method of treatment and the clinical state of the patients are very variable. Figures quoted are 80% for localised disease, 40% over-all, but only 20% in the older child. Spontaneous regression occurs in about 8%. The case history of one of my patients will illustrate the favourable response that can be obtained. It will be obvious that it is impossible to say which element of therapy was responsible, or even whether this is an example of spontaneous maturation, particularly since he was treated before the advent of the currently available cytotoxic drugs.

Master — . After a normal delivery and pregnancy, apart from the mother's involvement in a slight car accident at seven months, the baby was discharged home. The parents believed the legs were then moving normally. He failed to thrive, became fretful, and it was noted that the left leg hung down and movement was poor on the right. He was found to be febrile, the right leg was paralysed and failed to respond to stimuli. An X-ray of the spine showed widening of the intervertebral foramen at the level of L1-2. On I.V.P. the left kidney, though functioning normally, was found to be displaced downwards.

At laminectomy a dumb-bell shaped tumour was found. Only partial removal was possible. Histology showed it to be an undifferentiated neuroblastoma.

He was started on injections of Vitamin B_{12} and received a four-week course of radiation to the area of spine involved. As the haemoglobin was low he was given an intraperitoneal blood transfusion before treatment began. Intravenous injections of Vincristine were begun and maintained for four months, then both this and Vitamin B_{12} were discontinued.

Control of the sphincters was difficult to obtain. The left leg regained good power but no movement or sensation was regained in the right.

He is now a normal adolescent walking with the aid of a caliper. Sphincter control has been difficult, and ulceration due to slight trauma has also been a problem. However he is very determined and joins in as many activities as possible, even a cross country run.

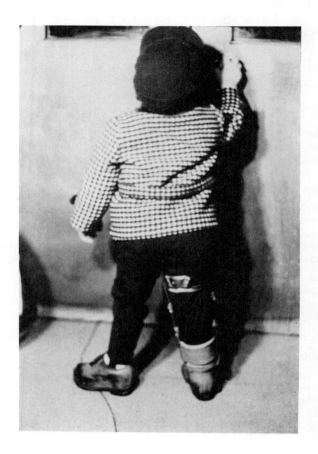

Fig. 22.3. Three years after irradiation of a paravertebral neuroblastoma.
Now a teenager

Wilms' Tumour

One-fifth of the tumours occurring in childhood are of this type. It is thought
to arise from embryonal tissue and often contains both primitive renal and
connective tissue. The alternative names are embryoma and nephroblastoma.
Both sexes are equally affected and it is rare after the age of seven. Most commonly the children are about three years old. Usually one kidney is affected,
but in a very small proportion of cases tumour is present in both.

Aetiology

No known factors have been found, but it is more common in children who have abnormalities of the urinary system, complete or partial absence of the iris in the eye, and overgrowth of half of the body.

Spread

Blood

This is common and deposits can be found in the lungs, liver, and brain. Apart from the usual spread of cells which reach the blood stream, solid growth can be seen extending into the renal vein and the inferior vena cava. This is very fragile and fragments can easily be detached and form tumour emboli which can be carried away by the blood.

Direct

The tumour spreads through the kidney, into the blood vessels, and outwards to involve adjacent structures.

Lymphatic

At the time of diagnosis the regional nodes are often already invaded.

Symptomatology

Usually the increasing size of the abdomen or the presence of a large mass is the presenting symptom. Closer questioning may reveal symptoms related to anaemia, lethargy, lack of appetite. Once the diagnosis is suspected the child must be admitted at once to hospital.

Examination and Investigations

One very important fact that must be borne in mind by all who handle the child is the danger of tumour emboli. After the initial examination the abdomen should be palpated or handled as little as possible to minimise the risk of these occurring.

Investigations

Apart from the usual haematology and biochemistry, X-rays are used to confirm the presence of the mass, to define it, and to look for metastases. They will include chest, plain abdomen, IVP possibly with tomography, skeletal survey and possibly also radio-isotope scan, ultra sound of the abdomen and liver, and possibly isotope scan for the latter, abdominal and lung CATscans. Arteriography and venography may also be necessary.

Treatment

It is now usual to use chemotherapy, radiation and surgery. The staging of the disease is based upon the results of investigations and findings at operation. Chemotherapy may be given for a few days prior to surgery, nephrectomy is then performed. Post-operative abdominal radiation follows, the opposite kidney being shielded as for neuroblastomas.

Combination chemotherapy is given finally in cycles, usually for a period of eighteen months.

Metastases

The treatment of metastases following prolonged radical treatment calls for judgment. There may be occasions when it may be decided that no treatment should be given, but reliance for the control of symptoms be placed on other drugs such as analgesics, sedatives, etc. Radiation can be useful in palliation.

Treatment of the lungs for multiple secondaries has been advocated, but there is a risk of pneumonitis and consequent fibrosis. Much will depend on the age of the child. It is well known that the prognosis is best for babies under one year old and worst for those of five years old and more. A solitary metastasis is probably well worth treating particularly if it appears some time after the original tumour, but in these circumstances lobectomy if at all possible should be the treatment of choice.

Prognosis

The findings at operation and the age of the child are probably the best guides to prognosis. Children below the age of two do best, particularly if the nodes and renal vein are free from tumour and the adjacent tissues are not infiltrated. Survival rates of 80% are now quoted for patients with localised disease, and 60% is possible for more widespread disease.

Follow-up

Apart from the history and examination of the local condition it is obvious from the behaviour of these two tumours that a chest X-ray at regular intervals must be a routine procedure. The blood count, and if necessary estimation of blood levels of urea, creatinine, and electrolytes, are also standard tests. The blood count is a sensitive indicator of bone-marrow infiltration and may also point to a radiation nephritis. In this latter case the other blood tests may be helpful but an I.V.P. is certainly needed in addition.

Other Tumours

Two other rare conditions should be mentioned, histiocytosis X and rhabdomyosarcoma. The former exhibits a range of malignancy and is treated with radiation for bone deposits, and chemotherapy. Rhabdomyosarcoma has now been quoted as having a two year survival rate of 75% if treated with a combination of surgery and chemotherapy.

Nursing Care of Children with Malignant Disease

Children suffer the same reactions as adults during radiation and chemotherapy but due to their natural resilience they often tolerate them better. The blood count is particularly vulnerable and a careful watch must be kept on this. It should not be forgotten that vomiting can rapidly lead to dehydration and shock in young babies and young children. Anti-emetics and adequate hydration measures should be instituted early.

Changes in a child's condition can be swift, whether it be deterioration or improvement. The latter is gratifying, but it is the former which can be disconcerting, though to the trained observer usually not unexpected. Unless very ill a child is usually reasonably active, any unusual quietness, refusal of food, or irritability should alert those in charge. A mother rarely needs to be told to look for these signs, she is acutely aware of them and may in her anxiety find them when they are not there.

Hospital or Home

In the initial stages most children are acutely ill and need to be in hospital. There is no question that intensive chemotherapy can only be given there, but it is more difficult to decide when only palliative treatment is given. Much will depend on distance and on the mother. If she is able to cope both with her child and her other responsibilities there is probably much to be said for outpatient treatment, but such an arrangement will only work if there is close co-operation and understanding between the parents and the radiotherapy team.

Preparation for Treatment

Most toddlers and older children are co-operative and will remain still during treatment, but babies and very young children require sedation. It is important that there should be full understanding between the nurses in the ward and the radiographer treating the child. If sedation is administered on an empty stomach treatment can be given first thing in the morning. A time should be fixed and proper arrangements made for moving the child.

If the nurse understands that a moving target cannot be treated and that the child becomes increasingly upset with each failure, she will find it easier to co-operate in getting the timing right. Equally the radiographer must ensure that the appointment time is kept and that other treatments which might be difficult to set up and overlap should be fitted in later. To avoid disturbance the child is moved in the cot or bed. During treatment sandbags or inflatable holders are sufficient to keep the child in position, it should not be necessary to tie the limbs down.

Older Children

Probably the most important factor in securing the co-operation of a child is the attitude of the parents. There are very few who do not want the child treated, and those few have usually based their refusal on mistaken ideas of the disease and the treatment. The inevitable question 'how long?' cannot be answered. The attitude to be cultivated is rather 'what can we do at the moment?' When the condition is a recurrence further treatment can only be given with the full agreement of the parents. At all stages this willing co-operation, this sense that parents and staff together form a team, is vital, for the attitude which the parents develop inevitably affects the child. A tense, fearful atmosphere will produce a fretful, unco-operative child. If possible the nurse should be present at this vital interview, she can then be certain of the aim of treatment and the way in which the parents have been handled.

Gaining a Child's Confidence

It is probably best if someone familiar, the mother or a nurse, accompanies the child to the department. The presence of a well-loved toy is often helpful. Experience enables the staff to handle a child, a gentle, kind, but firm attitude is usually best. When skin marks have to be used some children like to see the toy marked first and will happily lie still for treatment if the toy is there too. Few machines are noiseless, so that on the first day it is probably better that they should just hear these, feel the treatment couch being moved, and get used to the radiographer. If a mother can watch this she can both be reassured herself and in turn reassure the child. Sedation is rarely necessary in the older child but there are exceptions to every rule, and in extreme cases anaesthesia may be necessary. In my experience this has only happened once.

Mother in the Hospital

Nowadays unrestricted visiting in children's wards is the usual practice. There is more understanding of the psychological damage that separation from the mother can cause. It must not be forgotten that the mother also has needs. She may be exhausted by the emotional tension of discovering her child has a malignant disease and be unable to stand the strain of prolonged visiting. She may have family responsibilities that make it impossible for her to spend long periods at the hospital. It is important in these circumstances that she should not be made to feel guilty because she is not conforming to the present pattern. Equally she must not be banned from her child. If the needs of any treatment are explained she can usually be relied on for co-operation.

Children often cry when parents leave, only to turn happily a few minutes later to play. It is often hard for a mother to realise this, but if she can, she will feel less guilty if she is unable to stay. Very rarely her absence may be beneficial, for she can be so emotionally disturbed that she can affect the child adversely. The doctor and staff of the department, the nurses, the medical social worker must all unite to include the parents in the therapy team. In this way the best interests of the child will be served.

Whatever articles appear in journals, the child being treated and his family are individuals, and the conclusions and theories expounded by researchers are only guidelines. It is fatally easy to rely on them as dogma and apply them unthinkingly, far harder to spend time and thought applying them, even breaking them, if necessary. Each family must be treated individually, there are no unchanging golden rules.

Close co-operation with the general practitioner is desirable. As far as possible the child needs to be treated as normally as possible. If of school age he should attend school where he can play with his friends and not be 'spoiled'. The latter in particular is a mistaken kindness, the relaxation of familiar routine makes the young child uneasy. The older child, often aware that he is ill and may die, then has to cope with the burden of being set apart. The support of the family doctor who knows the whole family is often its sheet anchor, particularly since it may not be the child who is disturbed but the parents or other members of the family.

Emotional Attitudes

In an earlier chapter I discussed the impact which patients with malignant disease can have on those treating them. This is probably most marked when the patient is a child. Death is the inevitable end for us all but for children it is not expected so early, and the realisation that the child's disease is incurable can be a profound shock.

At the same time we must not lose hope. To win time and make survival comfortable is a gain, and few parents would feel the effort to achieve it is not worth while. Always there is the chance that during this respite research may yet produce some advance making a further treatment possible.

These children have such a resilience and often a gaiety that we feel the losers when they die. If the whole family has become part of the radiotherapy team it is inevitable that we should have this sense of loss. Yet in a subtle way we also gain, the memory of the relief we have been able to give, and the courage of the child, these enable us to begin again with the next patient.

The depth of human suffering cannot be measured,
It is matched only by our human response,
The response which achieves victory despite defeat.

23   The Auxiliary Services

The Patient and the Problem

A diagnosis of malignant disease means an upheaval in life, nothing will ever be quite the same again. Whether the patient suspects the nature of the complaint or not, his life will be narrowed down to the disease. After an intense period of activity when the diagnosis is made and therapeutic decisions are taken, there follows the comparative tedium of treatment. The mind is empty and there is time to doubt and despair, to withdraw from life. From the very nature of their work doctors and nurses regard these people as patients, and they in turn expect this attitude. To return to normal life they require rehabilitation, to be regarded as people not patients, and it is here that so many of the auxiliary workers play their part. We can none of us be all things to all men, and patients require contact with many people at many different levels both within and outside hospital if they are to rebuild their lives.

At various times in this book I have mentioned the help that auxiliary workers can give and the expression 'The Team' has been used. In the radiotherapy department the doctors, nurses, and radiographers are very much in evidence and their work is vital, but they represent the apex of the pyramid. Their work would be far less efficient without a large number of others who make up the base, and who, because they may be unseen, may be forgotten. It is time to look at their work and see how they help us, and how we can make it easier for them to do so.

The Medical Social Worker

It is a very rare patient who has no problems. When illness is short and acute the family and friends can usually help and find the solution, but when the condition is chronic or incurable then very special difficulties and strains arise. The medical social worker is not just there to arrange convalescence or a home help, she is the point at which needs are identified and if possible met. She is the ready listener, and that is often her most valuable function for many problems are solved merely by talking them out, and others shrink when discussed. Her influence extends far beyond the hospital, for not only is she in touch with official and voluntary bodies, local authorities, Red Cross, health visitors, terminal-care organisations, but often she can tap other resources in special cases, local church organisations, youth clubs, women's institutes. She should be given as much information as possible before meeting a patient, and in return she may quite often glean facts which can make contacts easier between the patient and the department staff.

To the patient the medical social worker becomes a friend. Although associated with a hospital her concern is with all aspects of the patient's life and her influence extends to his life outside. The trivia of day-to-day family affairs can be discussed and the implications of illness set aside. Yet at times of need problems can be raised, with the relief of leaning on a familiar shoulder. Above all the patient feels that to this member of the team he is a person whose human and social needs are more important than his disease.

One history is given to stand for the many which could be quoted to illustrate the help this worker gives.

A young woman of 38 was referred by a surgeon to the department with a diagnosis of inoperable breast carcinoma. She had three young children and her husband was doing two jobs to bring in a reasonable weekly wage. The medical social worker met her and soon learned all about her family, the finances, and most important of all something of the patient's temperament. After radiation and an oophorectomy a convalescent holiday was arranged and the patient returned home.

Unfortunately the course of the disease was rapid and quite soon she developed skeletal metastases. These caused pain and difficulty in walking. She was reluctant to enter hospital as this meant that her children had to live some distance away with relatives as her husband was unable to stay at home. Financial assistance was given to enable a neighbour to care for them and a further short convalescence was arranged. The nursing home was chosen with great care by the medical social worker, it was close to the patient's home and suitable for her age group.

During the next few months at home the patient gradually deteriorated. With great skill and sympathy the medical social worker, in close co-operation with the patient's doctor, reacted to her changing mood and sensed her fear that she would be sent away to die. The local Young Wives' Group was contacted and a roster organised so that she always had someone with her. The community nurse cared for her physical needs. Arrangements were made for the children to spend part of the day with neighbours so that they were not overburdened with their mother's illness, but yet were with her often enough to make her feel still part of a family. That this woman was able to remain with her family and die at home was directly due to the sustained efforts of the medical social worker.

Occupational Therapist, Physiotherapist

These two workers are discussed together because, although their skills and training differ, their work is so often complementary. Both aim at the mental and physical rehabilitation of the patient. The physical exercises taught by the one can be continued by the other through the choice of occupation. Despite understanding the importance of their work nurses sometimes find their presence on the ward inconvenient. There are times in the day's routine when it is awkward to have extra workers around, but with goodwill on both sides it is usually possible to make arrangements convenient to both. The ward is in some ways a nurse's special kingdom, she must be on guard that she does not treat all other workers as intruders.

The physiotherapist has a direct physical contact with the patient and this can be very reassuring. She can note and comment on small improvements in movement and her encouragement gives the patient an incentive to continue. Simple breathing exercises alone can not only produce physical benefits but often psychological improvements as there is a feeling of active participation in treatment. The occupational therapist can choose some form of handwork which will continue physiotherapy. It provides interest for other patients and a topic of conversation divorced from hospital affairs. There is a sense of achievement in making something, however simple, and quite often patients turn themselves into miniature production lines and indulge in friendly rivalry. Both workers not only rehabilitate the physical condition, they also provide invaluable food for the mind and occupation to fill the long hospital day. The help given by both of them need not stop with discharge, if necessary the patient can return as an outpatient to continue these activities, ideally in a day hospital.

A patient who had a left hemiplegia benefited very greatly from these combined efforts. When first admitted he was on a stretcher, unable to use the left arm and leg, nor raise his head from the pillow. He was very withdrawn and silent. Intensive physiotherapy was started and he began to respond. Every improvement was commented on and the patient soon began to register these himself and became determined to make some gain each day. The occupational therapist had been judging her time, and as soon as appropriate introduced him to simple weaving of a stool seat which required the use of both hands. As soon as he could walk, his work was taken to a table so that he had to walk to it from his bed. All this time both of them were discussing day-to-day affairs of the outside world with him. He became more animated and confident, left hospital walking with only slight help from a stick and was eagerly looking forward to returning to work.

Dietician

Patients rarely need this member of the team, but at times her special skill can affect a patient's progress very markedly. This was obvious when discussing the treatment of carcinoma of the post-cricoid and oesophageal areas, and good co-operation between nurse and dietician will make the feeding of an ill or difficult patient more successful. It is possible that not enough use is made of this specialised worker. When discussing after-care at home many families would be glad to have skilled guidance on how to meet dietary requirements without too much extra expense. This is the type of problem which can face a dietician. One of my patients was a diabetic who had a post-cricoid carcinoma. She was responding to treatment but had severe dysphagia due to radiation reaction. Not only was she anorexic but she also had decided food likes and dislikes. She needed a high-calorie diet which was within her diabetic allowance and which would also suit her taste. After the sister of the ward and I had discussed the situation with the dietician, she saw the patient and eventually produced a diet which not only met all these requirements, but was easy for the patient's relatives to prepare when she went home.

Prostheses

Some patients need surgical supports, wigs, or prostheses and the services of a skilled fitter are required. If a nurse can give this worker the background of the patient and the reason for the request it will make his task easier. If she then introduces him to the patient he can work more quickly and easily. Despite all his care the appliance may not always fit exactly or be completely comfortable. The nurse who takes the trouble to talk to the patient can often help the fitter by being able to tell him exactly what the problem is.

Some patients will require colostomy belts or urinary bags. Unless they can feel completely comfortable and confident they will be unable to go out and mix freely with their friends at home and at work. The special skills of the fitter consist not only in measuring and fitting an appliance, but in helping the patient to use it correctly. From his experience and his knowledge of how other patients have overcome difficulties he can help, encourage, and advise. This knowledge can also be of use to the doctor in his preparation of another patient.

Speech Therapist

While not often called in to help, there are occasions when the speech therapist's very special skill is most valuable. Patients with cerebral tumours who have speech disorders become very frustrated at their inability to communicate. Their emotion makes the defect more pronounced and a self-perpetuating destructive process begins. Patiently by encouraging writing, card games, memory work, and in many other ways, he is helped to overcome his disability. Because something active is being done his tension is relieved and that alone may produce marked improvement.

Medical Illustrator

Adequate records are important, not only to preserve details of treatment but also as a means to follow its progress. An illustrator or photographer can be invaluable in providing pictorial information. He can either work in a hospital studio or visit the wards. It is not always easy for him to know exactly what is required. He makes great efforts to do so, but it will be much better for him if either the doctor or nurse can explain not only what the purpose of the present request is, but also how the lesion will progress. The illustrator can then plan his work so that each picture will form part of a smooth series, thereby recording as much information as possible.

Other Helpers

There are many people who have contact with a hospital patient, cleaners, receptionists, orderlies. They all contribute to the comfort of the patient and can in turn be affected by him. The workers so far described have prolonged contact with patients and are prepared for the fact that some of them can be demanding and difficult. These other workers see them less often and it is only fair that they should be told of any special difficulty with a particular patient. Their good humour and cheerfulness are often a tonic to a ward or department, and many patients enquire after them when they return to the hospital.

Other Departments

A little thought produces a long list of workers and departments forming part of a therapy team. The physicist and technicians preparing moulds and treatment plans, the theatre and diagnostic X-ray staff, the laboratory, the pharmacist, the kitchens, the engineers, the community nurse, the health visitor, ambulance personnel, it becomes a long catalogue. To many, work is a routine and there is little to remind them that they too share in the care of a patient. Every order for work to be done should not be turned into a live-saving drama, but due acknowledgement of their services can be made, and a little time should be spent explaining the reason for 'out of office hours' requests.

Voluntary Workers

In this country we are fortunate that many people devote both time and money to helping hospitals. The Red Cross provides invaluable help, equipment on loan, wheelchairs, bed pans, bed rests, escorts for patients returning home long distances, and libraries for hospitals. The W.V.S. often brings a mobile shop round the wards, runs a canteen for visitors and outpatients, and will do individual shopping for ward patients. Many a centre would be hard put to it to organise the transport of patients on treatment were it not for the voluntary car drivers. Very few of these workers have any nursing or medical experience and do not understand the inevitable delays which can occur. Hospital workers have to be patient and try to explain as far as possible both the patient's condition and the hospital working.

Clergy

Some hospitals are large enough to have a full-time chaplain, others are served by the ministers of the neighbouring parishes. Patients with strong religious convictions welcome visits from the clergy and gain much help and strength. To other patients the minister is just another of those friendly people who pop in and out of the ward and bring a breath of the outside world. In moments of crisis both patients and relatives may need to turn to him, and at such a time and indeed always, he can only help completely if he is told all the relevant facts.

Outside Hospital

The needs of the out-patient differ and many of the auxiliary workers will have no contact with him. It is the medical social worker who will probably meet him most often, but at any time he may need other services and help. While less easy to organise these for the patient at home, a little ingenuity often enables most complex situations to be resolved.

Human Contact

The term auxiliary workers is an awkward one and includes both medical, nursing, and paramedical staff. It does not express the significance of their work and is such a dry phrase that there is a danger of forgetting their importance in the therapy team. If a patient is to return to a normal or near-normal life, he must be kept anchored to the outside world. By their contact with him, by reacting to him as a person so that he is not constantly reminded of his disease, the auxiliary workers make this return easier. They also ensure that the hospital is a place of friends, so that when, as so often happens, he has to return, he will not be with strangers.

The Place of the Nurse

How does the nurse fit into this picture? She stands at the very centre of affairs. In close contact with patient, doctor, and relatives, it is usually she who conveys and receives information. She is usually there when auxiliary workers are called in and through her many requests are relayed. She must be diplomat, information officer, listener, and occasionally activator. She should value and use the services at her disposal. If she is doing her job well her reward will be the instinctive cry 'Nurse!'.

I fear Life more than I fear Death.
No death is feared more than a Life with Death
And during life I have suffered death too long.

24 The Care of the Patient and Family

This is one of the most difficult and yet rewarding parts of our work. It taxes all our resources. Each new patient is both a fresh challenge and an opportunity, and we not only give, but also receive. Above all we require humility, we must be on guard that we never regard ourselves as infallible or as the only and best judges of a patient's needs.

When a nurse first begins work in an oncology centre she may find it hard to appreciate the reasons for either the continuation or cessation of treatment. She may search for the rules only to find that in fact each patient must be treated and managed as an individual. Decisions will depend not only on the experience and convictions of the doctor, but also on his assessment of the real wishes of both the patient and his relatives.

The Decision to Tell

There is much discussion on the right of an individual to be told he has cancer or that he is dying. Here we must beware of theories. A patient can resent being treated like a child or being overprotected, but at the same time he can over-estimate his courage. We in turn can fall into the error of telling him what we or the theorists believe he should be told, rather than what he actually wants to know. We can be trapped by our own successes or failures in the past. We can seek to take what we have learned and use it as an infallible guide to our handling of the next patient, forgetting that this patient and his family are individuals and cannot be treated in exactly the same way. Many very well-intentioned people stung by the experience of others, or themselves, cry out that 'We were badly treated, they should do this or that', making the fatal mistake of believing that what is right for them is right for everyone else.

If there is any rule it is that at no time should a deliberate lie be told. On the other hand it is rarely necessary to tell the whole truth in detail and at length at one time. How much is said, and when it is said, will vary according to the mental and psychological status of the patient, to his financial and family responsibilities, and to the type and stage of the disease. It is important that whatever he is told, all in contact with him, both staff and relatives, should know and therefore be ready for questions which may arise.

At first the staff are strangers to a patient, yet it is essential that very speedily he learns to trust. Such trust only comes through confidence which in turn depends upon how quickly the doctor can establish mental contact with him. A nurse in her casual conversations may gain information which will give a clue to the patient's personality, to his hopes and fears, and so make the doctor's task easier.

It will be noticed that although the doctor's personality remains unchanged, his method of approach and his language will be tailored not only to the individual patient, but to his needs at that particular time. Only when rapport has been established can treatment really begin, and while it is essential that this condition is reached at the first interview, paradoxically its full development can only be gradual and take time. It is impossible to describe how this mutual trust and respect is achieved, one can only recognise it. It is established when a patient feels that the doctor and centre can help him, can take over the responsibility and burden of the disease, and above all that there is a sincere interest in him. It is as if he has come in from the cold and at last is warm and able to relax.

When the patient has reached this frame of mind, the doctor can begin to feel his way on answering questions. Because this is so intensely personal, it is impossible to say in advance how the question 'Is it cancer?' will be answered. To some a confirmation would be a sentence to fear and despair, to others it would be welcome as a first step to a mental reassessment. Between are all stages, and not only do the patients vary in their needs, but the same patient will change from day to day. The doctor through his understanding will know and judge the right time and the right answer. Often this question which seemed so important in the waiting room becomes less urgent and even irrelevant after the first interview. It may no longer be asked because the reassurance which the patient was seeking from a denial has been given in other ways. When confirmation is given it must always be coupled with constructive suggestions. They must be told that pain and unpleasant sequaelae are not inevitable, but that if they do come they can be controlled, that nobody will think the patient slow, weak or tiresome because he asks questions. It is his body, and mind, and, some also believe, soul. We must give him time, and the assurance that someone cares.

The reaction of the patient and his relatives to the diagnosis is infinitely variable. There are certain common patterns, fear, resentment, anger, guilt. Often the question is 'Why, what have I done to get cancer?' Everyone in the team must be prepared to accept the anger and resentment, realising it's not personal. Anodynes have no place in the discussions. Telling a patient not to worry, that there are far worse diseases to get, that he will upset his family, is making the burden he carries even heavier. He has good reason to worry, he is afraid of treatment, afraid it won't work, is not interested in other diseases, only the one he's got, and worried about letting himself and his family down. His world has fallen round his ears and he must make a new one. Some can only cope by burying the knowledge so deep in themselves that they deny ever being told, others will swing to the other extreme and assert their 'independence', coming later or missing appointments, arguing for some unfounded major variation in treatment, or trying to get intervals between appointments lengthened to show they don't really need treatment.

Although this close relation between doctor, staff, and patient has been stressed, it must not be allowed to become completely absorbing. If this happens emotion can cloud judgment, and mental reserves can be so exhausted that there is nothing left to give either to this or any other patient, or to one's own family and friends.

The Family

The patient cannot be treated in isolation. He is a member of a family, he has a job and a place in society, and his situation in regard to each must be considered. Closest to him and the most intimately affected is his family. From the very beginning time must be given to discussion and explanation of both the patient's condition and his treatment. Such time is never wasted, for not only will the patient benefit from the resultant greater understanding of his family, relatives are often able to give information which he has forgotten, or to discuss fears which he has been unable to voice. They will thus give a more complete picture of his personality. At these interviews misconceptions can be removed. Many relatives have interpreted incorrectly what they have already been told, or have been distressed by accounts of the effects of treatment given by those who are unfamiliar with modern techniques. A father of a six-weeks-old baby was adamant that he did not wish his child to be treated. Gradually it became clear that he had gained the impression that treatment was useless and that the child would be badly burned. He felt such additional suffering was unjustified. In the end he agreed to radiotherapy, and the child is alive and is now a teenager. These interviews and enquiries must be dealt with personally. Discussion over the telephone or by letter is not only far less effective, but may be mischievous because misunderstandings so easily arise. One discussion is never enough. The doctor must see relatives during and at the end of treatment, at follow-up appointments, or at any time they are worried. In this way the family becomes part of the team and plays an active role in the patient's treatment.

During treatment and the continuing follow-up the alert members of the team may uncover many problems, some patients are either too shy to raise, or they fail to voice them because the right questions have not been asked. Any aspect of family life can be a problem, finances, social attitudes, how to handle the other children, 'are the rows we're having normal', or most intimate of all, the attitude and behaviour of the sexual partner. These queries must be passed to the whole team and a decision made on how to handle them, contact by a medical social worker, telling the doctor the analgesic isn't working and the patient doesn't like to say so, referral for psychiatric help, a call to one of the voluntary mutual help organisations. Often the action needed is quite small, but the benefit to patient and family is out of all proportion.

The Questions

Prognosis

The first enquiry is invariably 'What are the chances?' It is posed in many forms, but basically the family want to know whether the disease is malignant, how far advanced it is and the chances of treatment, whether the patient will suffer, and whether he can be cured. Answering these fundamental questions must be a gradual process, the bald truth will almost certainly be such a shock that the fact that treatment can be offered would not be appreciated nor even accepted. It is often helpful to trace the history, the investigations, and any treatment such as surgery already given, and during this discussion to give the relevant facts slowly. Then it is possible to move on to the proposed treatment and the patient's likely reaction, and only at this point to reach the possible prognosis. To give this will tax the most experienced doctor. Setting a definite period of time is seldom justified and so often it turns out to be a wrong forecast. It is common hearsay that a patient given six months to live has been alive and well years later. With malignant disease it is impossible to be completely certain how it will progress, nor how it will respond to treatment.

Statistically the average survival for patients with carcinoma of the lung is six months from the time of diagnosis, and in the majority of cases this is a correct figure. However I have in my care patients who have had proven lung cancer, who received minimal radiation, and who are alive and well years later. Had I given the statistical figure as a prognosis I would have induced unjustifiable despair in the relatives. On the other hand I cannot use these exceptions to engender unwarranted optimism in all the other cases. A forecast of survival time can colour and limit the thinking of both doctor and relatives. Unless family or business affairs must be settled it is usually better to discuss the stage of the disease and stress that the important consideration is the immediate possibility of treatment.

From this the nurse will realise that giving a prognosis on a new patient is almost an impossible task and so far we have only considered the proven cases of malignancy. It is even more difficult when clinically the disease is considered to be cancer but histological proof cannot be obtained. Symptoms are often so severe that treatment is given despite lack of evidence. Favourable response is regarded as proof but this is not complete. In these cases to give any forecast of survival would be mere guess work.

Progress

On Treatment

These questions on prognosis having been dealt with adequately the relatives will now want to ask about the treatment. It is unfamiliar to them and as we have already noted they may have heard inaccurate stories about it. They will want to know whether it is to be given in the hospital or on an outpatient basis, how long it will last, and what the patient will feel. Not all patients have to be admitted, skin lesions can often be treated while the patient is still at work. The doctor will be able to tell them how many treatments are planned and how long each treatment lasts. Reactions to treatment are less definite. They can vary for radiation both with the patient and the site of treatment. Relatives can be reassured that the patient is under constant review and that local changes can be dealt with as they arise. Some patients experience no untoward effects. Others may be tired, some become depressed to a variable degree. Adequate rest will minimise or even prevent these general effects. If the relatives have been told of this they can see that the outpatient takes sufficient rest. In the ward this is easy to ensure, but the patient at home may feel so well at first that he is tempted to overdo things. This is particularly so in the case of a woman with a family.

Chemotherapy may need the patient's admission for a few nights or not at all. The same precautions as for outpatient radiotherapy are needed. Some feel so well that they are able to return to work between sessions, others may be more debilitated by disease and have to stay at home. Every effort must be made to avoid nausea and vomiting by the use of anti-emetics and anxiolytics. Reported symptoms must be treated seriously, even if they are so delayed after treatment that the link seems tenuous. If unpleasant toxic effects are not controlled. patients, or the relatives, may lose heart. A little imagination will enable us to understand. What must be the apprehension when each appointment comes round with the inevitable prospect of another bout of sickness to follow? Advice on meals, adequate rest, must of course be given too.

On Discharge and Follow-up

Many patients require little in the way of special care after their treatment but not unnaturally their relatives will have questions to ask. If there has been a reaction of any kind during therapy they will want to know how long it will last, how it will progress, and what special care is required. For example a patient who has had a radiation field including the buccal mucosa may have lost his taste and his family will ask for advice. Although during therapy diet will already have been discussed and the need for oral hygiene explained, these points will need covering again for reassurance. Arrangements for dressings, visits by the community nurse, or the provision of special aids will have already been made, and any convalescence planned. The rearrangement of the home to enable easier management of a disabled or bedridden patient is made by the medical social worker in conjunction with the community services. In fact all these provisions for the patient's welfare are complete before his discharge, but so often relatives require to discuss them again in order to be reassured that they will be able to look after him adequately and maintain his comfort. The question of further treatment if there is a recurrence may be raised. An assurance can always be given that the patient will be cared for, but the situation is at that time theoretical, and discussion as to the nature of further active treatment must wait on events. In addition a question on a return to work may be asked, whether this will ever be possible, if so when, or whether a change or modification of occupation is necessary. This discussion enables the family to assume a more active role in the care and treatment of the patient. This is not only beneficial to him but also gives those around him an easier mind.

At follow-up appointments a relative may accompany the patient and wish to see the doctor to discuss progress. This can yield extra information and is always a means of maintaining contact and continuity. Occasionally questions are asked on the subject of any symptoms which should be sought. Advice will vary according to the individual case. While it is unwise to burden families with the task of watching daily for a long list of signs, it is sometimes advisable to suggest a key symptom which should be an alert. For a patient with a cerebral tumour this could be a fit, severe headache, or vomiting.

Liaison with the General Practitioner

Although close relations with the staff are established, a patient and his family are usually known best by the family doctor. It is therefore exceedingly important that at all times he is kept fully informed, not only of treatment and progress, but also of any discussions which have taken place. In this way there will be two sources of help and advice. He will be able to give reassurance quickly, or alternatively ask for an early appointment if he is concerned about a patient's progress. Additionally from his close knowledge of the family he may be able to alert the centre to problems, or supply background information. Many doctors visit their patients in hospital. This close contact should be welcomed by all members of the staff, for the family doctor completes the team responsible for the total care of the patient.

Enquiries by Employers

The confidence of a patient is always respected. No enquiries from employers should be answered without written consent. When the question concerns fitness for work or the likelihood of work ever being resumed, agreement must be specifically given. It is not always possible to discuss with the patient the implications of such a report. He may not realise the full nature of his disease, but the family must be adequately informed of the report made. It must be both fair and complete. In some cases employers may decide, after reading it, that they cannot keep the patient on, and the relatives must be warned of this possibility. In my experience this happens infrequently, most employers are very sympathetic and helpful, and when it has happened, in most cases the patient would have been unable to work again. It must be appreciated that when the work involves the safety of others, as for instance with an airline pilot, or a bus driver, the employer is not only entitled, but has an obligation to ascertain his fitness for work. Usually attempts are made to find some other duties.

Parents and Children

Children although seriously ill are often surprisingly cheerful and active. Their reaction is usually a reflection of the parents' attitude. If they show openly their distress and are full of doubts about treatment, this tension is transmitted to the child, he becomes fretful, restless, and difficult to handle.

It is therefore even more important than usual that in these cases the parents should not only be fully informed, but also be in complete agreement with any proposed treatment. This state is only achieved if time has been spent establishing their confidence in the doctor and the department. To do this at the first interview the history of the illness, past illnesses, and the family health are discussed. The doctor usually has already received the full details and rarely learns anything new, but it enables both parents, particularly the mother, to unburden and to feel that this new doctor fully understands their child.

Next there is a need to discuss the disease itself. Parents seek desperately for some reason for this to have happened to their child. They may quite irrationally think that they are in some way responsible, and so feel guilty. If they can accept that in most cases the cause is quite unknown and they are blameless, they will be relieved of some of their tension, and be free to turn all their attention on the question of therapy.

The treatment is discussed in detail and any misconceptions gathered from uninformed sources firmly dispelled. The most common is that radiation inevitably involves severe burning and sickness. Parents also fear that the child will experience suffering because of radiotherapy. They can be completely reassured. I have tended to stress the question of what relatives have heard about radiation as misunderstandings are so common and can cause much distress. In fact children usually tolerate treatment far better than adults. This may well be because if wisely handled they do not experience fear, and they also lack an adult's apprehension for the future.

The same cannot be said for chemotherapy. There is no way that the unpleasantness of injections can be avoided. With skill they can be virtually painless but the experience is strange, and trying to hit a moving target is traumatic to both child and staff. A calm, informed parent can make all the difference, but if this is impossible, sedation may be needed. Parents in these circumstances must not be allowed to feel guilty.

Whatever the treatment plan, reassurance must be given that no major changes in treatment will be made without the parents' knowledge and consent.

The next step, if radiation is involved, is for the radiographer to be introduced and for the parents to see, if possible, the first treatment given. In this way they meet the whole therapy team and are reassured about the handling of their child. They feel that they know what is happening. If the first interview has been successful, they will leave, confident that their child is not only in competent hands, but in the understanding care of the entire staff, doctors, radiographers, and nurses.

Throughout treatment the doctor will see the parents at regular intervals to discuss progress. Certainly whenever major decisions must be taken, he will see them, discuss the situation, and so obtain their willing consent and co-operation. On discharge future care, the handling of the child, and schooling will be talked over and advice given.

Recurrences

As will be appreciated from some of our discussions all too frequently the problem of recurrence must be faced. The question of further treatment, whether radiation or chemotherapy, has then to be discussed with the parents. Inevitably they will wish to know the immediate effect on the child and the prospects of a remission and its likely duration. In many cases it is impossible to predict the outcome, and the treatment, particularly when chemotherapy is involved, may cause the child discomfort and some suffering. This must be stated and the whole topic discussed fully. Before the final decision is taken, parents must be led to consider what their feelings will be at the end, so that when the decision is taken together, they will believe that they have done all they could, and not feel in the future that they have failed in some part of their duty. In fact most parents feel such confidence in their doctor that they are willing to be guided. They seize any chance however slim, for they feel any time gained is worth while and hope that some other treatment may in the interval become available. Even when disappointed, the comment is 'We tried. He had his chance, it was worth while'.

Management of the Later Disease

Treatment is always designed to be in the patient's best interests, and this will mean that the emphasis will vary with the stage of the disease. In the early condition there is an all out onslaught on the disease. But when palliation only is possible, the balance shifts. The patient's comfort becomes all important and treatment of the disease is secondary. This is not to say that active therapy is not worth while, but its aim is different. It is designed to maintain the patient's comfort. It is of little use to prolong life if its quality is unacceptable. This is true rehabilitation, enabling the patient to cope with his present condition and maintain his dignity. In fact even when a patient is dying, the proper use of analgesics and sedation, the patience and understanding of the staff, should be regarded as active treatment which only ceases with death.

General Considerations

There are certain general questions which must be considered and discussed with the family and patient. There is more and more a willingness to discuss treatment with patient and family, particularly when there are alternatives. It avoids a 'them and us' situation, and the feeling of being part of the team restores the sense of control so often lost in the hurly burly of referral and diagnosis. It may seem that discussion has been overemphasised in this chapter, but unless its importance is realised, nurses may feel that the time spent on it delays a clinic unnecessarily. Relatives feel that when they have been able to spend time with the doctor they are fully considered. More important still they will be able to know later, in their grief, that together they and the department have done all they could for the patient.

Examples of topics to be talked over are the place of treatment, home or hospital, the provision of help, financial or nursing, and care if the patient becomes too ill for relatives to continue home nursing. This last question is so important that it is dealt with in a separate section later in this chapter.

It would be easy, if boring, to catalogue procedures and treatments, but a description of four lines of therapy will probably best illustrate the principles of patient care.

Radiation

A patient who has had a carcinoma of the bronchus treated and who develops severe and persistent headache due to cerebral metastases, has very little likelihood of cure. To control his symptoms with analgesics is difficult, and will almost certainly involve heavy sedation. Radiation can give good relief for certain tumour types, and even if survival is only a few weeks may be regarded as worth while since it makes this period pain free.

A frail elderly woman who has severe vaginal bleeding due to advanced carcinoma of the cervix, should not be regarded as being beyond help. Despite her frailty the risk of an anaesthetic should be taken. It enables the insertion of radioactive boxes which will control the haemorrhage and make her remaining life more comfortable.

Surgery

The procedure of pinning and plating a pathological fracture of the femur is a major one and the operation may take an hour or more. When a patient has wide-spread skeletal metastases and has a short-life expectancy, a superficial consideration will condemn surgery as over-zealous. The patient will think differently. To be able to stand and walk again, instead of being confined to bed for the rest of his life, will be regarded as very worth while. In certain cases even amputation may be justifiable.

When intestinal obstruction occurs and the patient has exhausted all possible therapy, to fashion a colostomy is still justifiable unless death is regarded as being only a few days away. A prolonged period of nausea and vomiting, or of continuous suction, is a burden to the patient and distressing to the family, and therefore should be avoided.

Spinal Injection

It is also possible that procedures carrying some risk may be beneficial. A special intrathecal injection of phenol destroys pain fibres, and so blocks appreciation of pain in the relevant area. When the pain is bilateral there is a risk that control of the sphincters may be impaired by the injection. One young woman who died two months after such an injection was in no doubt about its value. She had widespread pelvic secondaries from a carcinoma of the cervix and was in severe pain. Due to its severity she was confined to bed and one leg was completely flexed. Not only was she relieved of her symptoms, she was able to walk and to enjoy a holiday before her death.

On the other hand there are times when to do nothing is in fact the best treatment of all. If a patient has a very advanced lesion, perhaps in the tongue, he may have a severe haemorrhage. To transfuse him or to try and tie off the vessel would be meddlesome. Only heavy sedation and analgesics should be given. One patient had a rodent ulcer which he neglected until it penetrated bone. He had exhausted every mode of therapy, and when the external carotid artery was eroded no steps were taken to resuscitate him.

Pain

It is still believed by many that patients with cancer must suffer prolonged and severe pain. This is not so. When pain does occur, there is available an armoury of drugs and procedures which should ensure comfort. It is most important that the family should be assured of this. It is equally important that drugs should be given in adequate dosage and frequently enough. A wise nurse will learn to judge for herself, rather than to rely on the patient's often spartan estimate of his requirements. The precautions on respiratory depression, addiction or liver toxicity, should not cause a valuable drug to be withheld. If a patient has widespread lung metastases and pain severe enough to require morphia, its respiratory depressive effects should be disregarded. Other useful drugs are various tranquilisers and anti-emetics, chlorpromazine (Largactil) is useful since it combines both properties, analgesics, pethidine, omnopon, mist. aspirin nepenthe, heroin, the non-steroidal anti-inflammatory drugs, and the various hypnotics. Prednisone is often very useful in improving the appetite and the sense of well being, this contributes to the relief of pain.

Surgical procedures are all designed to interrupt the pain pathways. Formerly cordotomy by blind cutting, cautery, or sclerosing injection, was the most commonly practised. This cut the tract of fibres in the cord conveying the sensation of pain to the brain. A later development has been the injection of phenol into the spinal intrathecal space. This chemical destroys the fine pain fibres leaving other sensory and motor fibres intact. The level of the injection is determined by the site of the pain.

Alternative Medicine

Such, unfortunately, is the dread mystique surrounding cancer that many patients and their families have sought with desperation any method which promises 'cure'. This has led to many being attracted by costly 'quack' remedies, and experiencing the despair of disappointed hope. It cannot be denied that 'orthodox' treatments for cancer are not pleasant. The intensive chemotherapy used by some for tumours that are not responsive, has caused a revulsion against cytotoxic therapy among many lay people, quite blotting out the very real gains it has achieved in certain malignancies. The so-called 'alternative medicine', 'the gentle method' has gained prominence as a consequence. Much that is advised is sound, a patient's co-operative positive attitude of mind is always a joy to a doctor, we have all seen patients who turned their faces to the wall. A sensible well balanced diet is an asset to anyone, healthy or sick, and moderation in all things has been a sound philosophy since the days of the Ancient Greeks.

The problem arises in the use of the word alternative. It implies that a choice must be made to reject all orthodox methods in favour of unproven regimes. In cancer therapy we all know that patients can have long, and sometimes unexpected remissions, it is then tempting to ascribe these to the last treatment given, orthodox or alternative. Without long and painstaking research it is not possible to be sure. That is not to say that there may not be very valuable lessons to be learnt from some of these other treatments, but they will only be learned if they are carefully investigated in an impartial way. A better title would be complementary medicine.

What do we then say to our patients who remain with us but sample other treatments, or leave the oncology centres? There is no place for hurt pride. We can offer a great deal in the way of palliation and some cures, but in many cases only the former. Provided that the alternative is not harmful we should welcome the evidence of a patient's healthy determination. If we think that the new regime is toxic we should say so with reasons. If the patient persists and events go well, we must be philosophical, if not there must be no suggestion that the patient should have listened to us. If they leave us, or fail to consult us until late on in the disease, we must still be there ready to help when they come, no patient should be made to feel abandoned. It is the patient who matters, not our self esteem.

Terminal Care

Frequently it has been suggested that this section should have been longer, with precise details of pain control, psychological counselling, etc. The subject could be the theme of a whole book, and there are many excellent ones available, written by those who have worked in the hospice movement. However for me merely to give lists of techniques or drugs without emphasising basic attitudes, would be to deny my strong belief, which is shared by many others, that this care is an individual matter, and depends upon the patient, the family, and the doctor.

Whether he is in a special hospital or at home depends not only on the wishes of the patient and those of his family, but also on the available facilities and their physical capacity. It is always wise to look ahead and make contingency arrangements. It is very distressing if a family has come to the end of its physical, mental, and spiritual resources, only to find that there is a delay of several days or weeks before admission can be arranged.

Each patient will need to be treated differently and with compassion. Those who care for the dying must consider their own attitude to death. They must evolve a personal philosophy which will enable them to sustain the very real mental and spiritual pressures of the situation. However surrounded by love and care, in the end each man dies alone. We may believe that for some death is a beginning, and that for them there are moments when the next world has already begun. For others death may be regarded as a finality, the end of all things, while others may think of it as an uncertainty, a hovering on the brink of the unknown. We can only guess, we do not know what a man truly thinks.

The only certainty is that he has the right to expect that he should be able to die in dignity and peace.

Those who frequently see patients in the last stage of their illness, often detect a withdrawal and gradual loosening of ties. Matters which were judged of vital importance only a short time before are now accorded only a passing interest. This can be very distressing to relatives who can interpret this as a rejection of their love and concern. Many patients are well aware of their condition and it is insulting to engage in false cheerful discussion of what they will do when they improve. If they really wish to discuss the fact that they are dying then the doctor and staff must be prepared to do this. Those patients who find consolation in religious faith should have every opportunity to receive frequent visits from the minister of their choice. Care should be taken however not to press this service too strongly on those who are reluctant or frightened, nor should it be assumed that a strong religious faith necessarily banishes fear and worry.

Patients often feel the need to be useful. The sharing of some cherished hint or skill, listening to the hopes and ambitions of their attendants, helping other patients, these and many other actions give them a dignity, a value as human beings.

If patients are being nursed at home every effort must be made to help the family to cope and to avoid the patient feeling himself to be a burden. Here the close co-operation of the family doctor, the community services, and voluntary organisations can achieve wonders. The home nurses provided by some of these organisations can mean that patients can be at home where they want to be, without intolerable strain on the family.

If patients prefer to be in some form of unit then the family must be involved as far as possible, this avoids the feeling that it has been cut off from the patient. For the patient there must be the assurance that whatever the problem, pain, offensive discharge, depression, somebody will help and go on helping until there is relief. There is a need for time for someone to listen, and it may be anyone, voluntary worker, nurse, physiotherapist, each patient selects his own anchor. The great fear is of loneliness, we all die and go forward alone through that gate, but to have the assurance that someone will be there at that moment is a great comfort.

It must be realised that knowing that cancer has reached its final stage is a matter both of heart and mind. Many patients discuss their condition with great frankness, but it is a knowledge of the mind only, and often it is only shortly before death that they remark with surprise that they are really very ill. Similarly relatives can refuse to accept the prognosis and will not discuss it with the patient although he knows the situation, the 'anchor' then becomes very important.

The decision as to whether a child is told he is dying is one for the parents to make. Doctors and nurses can discuss this with them, but the matter is too intimate for any outsider to interfere. Some of the factors to be considered are the parents and their relationship with each other, other siblings, and the likely time span of the illness. Many children know intuitively, and seem to accept the situation more readily than adults. In a way they have less to relinquish and are perhaps more clear sighted than we are, what matters most to them is that they are secure in a loving, caring atmosphere. It is usually the parents who have to make far more adjustments.

After the patient has died the family has to go on with ordinary life. The help that can be offered by the acute oncology unit is limited, but if relatives come to see staff afterwards it is most helpful if they are allowed to talk, even if most of the time it is repetitive. Mourning has its own pattern, and only if we follow it can we return to normal life. Many mutual help associations have been formed by relatives and patients with cancer. They are a support not only during the illness, but also afterwards when the activity is over and the recovery must begin.

Because I feel it so important to stress that individuals vary so much in their reaction to what they are told, I shall talk of two women, both with a strong religious faith, one with cancer, the other with severe heart disease. The first was proving a sore trial to her family. She was a widow with several loving children. She had advanced cancer of the large bowel and palliative surgery only postponed further symptoms. She was very angry with her doctors and her family since she felt nobody took her condition seriously. When she was told her diagnosis, she relaxed completely, since she felt that shortly she would be with her husband. The second woman, also a widow and confident that she too would eventually be reunited with her husband, was very independent, and often did more than her cardiac condition allowed. In an effort to restrain her the family doctor explained the risk she ran of a sudden fatal heart attack. The effect was quite other than intended. She became depressed, and eventually told her daughter that she was haunted by wondering each night whether she would wake up in the morning, and whether she would see her roses again next year when she sat in her garden.

To care for the dying is a privilege. We are often permitted at this time to know a human being completely stripped of all pretence, so we must be humble and know that while we give, we also receive. Many patients unconsciously enrich us, we remember them and turn renewed to fresh tasks.

Proportion

All that has been said so far should not lead a nurse to adopt a hushed voice, tiptoe attitude towards the patient with cancer. He is no different from anyone else who is ill. He is not marked out in some special way, nor is his disease more tragic than many others. Patients with multiple sclerosis, chronic pyelonephritis, or severe psychosis, have conditions which can be just as refractory. Cancer is still a forbidden word and so those with the disease may be regarded with a morbid fascination. There is a real place for gaiety, for cheerful gossip, and even occasionally healthy impatience.

Despite the fact that this book has concerned itself entirely with the care of these patients, it must be remembered that in a death rate of half a million there are many causes of death, and not all of us die from cancer.

I think of Life as a complex,
An intertwining of all human experience,

From the microscopic biological
To the intangible spiritual.
I have never thought of Death
As other than an episode
In the march of human existence.

Life is danger.
Yet danger makes Life.
We do not choose to live,
We choose how to live.
For what is Life but a flirtation with Death.

25 Protection

A geiger counter registers radiation not only on a dial but also by an audible click. If we put a counter on a table we hear only a few clicks, this is the register of the natural background radiation. As the wearer of a watch with a particular type of luminous dial brings it close to the instrument, the audible count rate increases and dies down as he moves it away. A dummy radioactive needle has no effect, but if we ask a technician to bring in a lead pot containing live needles, there is a change. As he comes through the door we can see that he is carrying the container on a long handle. If the lid is taken off and the counter held over the pot the rate again increases. Using long-handled forceps a needle is lifted out, the count now sounds like a staccato volley, and if the needle is changed for another the same size but containing more radioactive material, the volley becomes a rapid machine-gun fire.

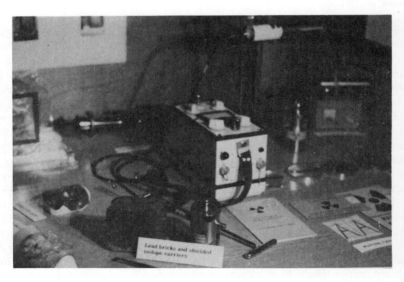

Fig. 25.1. Monitoring and protection equipment

This simple demonstration teaches us something of radiation sources and safe working methods. Background radiation comes from minerals in the earth, and outer space. Man has always been exposed to it and its amount has varied little. Radium represents both a natural and an earlier medical form of radiation, while the luminous watch is an example of a man-made addition to the background type. The geiger counter shows us that the further we are from the source the less radiation we receive, and it is obvious therefore that the radioactive materials should never be touched, but should be manipulated with long-handled instruments. Speed will also lessen the dose received. All lined containers with their sources should be placed in a safe place as soon as possible. Radiation should be respected but not feared.

Why Protection?

If Man has always been exposed to radiation, why then do we need protection measures? To answer this question it is necessary first to consider the effects on the human body. These have only been investigated since the medical use of X-rays and radioactive isotopes, and there are still many problems to be resolved.

We have in our earlier chapters stressed that time is needed for the long-term results to become apparent. The short-term effects are quickly appreciated, locally moist desquamation of the skin, and if whole body exposure, severe often fatal bone-marrow depletion. The development of skin carcinomas by some pioneer radiologists led to the investigation of radiation damage to other tissues, and it was realised that certain organs were more vulnerable, among them the lens of the eye, the gonads, the kidney, the skin of the palms and soles.

Atomic Radiation

Since the advent of the atomic bomb with its fall-out of radioactive materials attention has been focused on the dangers of genetic damage and the effects on children who are still growing. Not only were those in the area exposed to immediate radiation, but airborne radioactive dust was carried away and deposited at some distance. While it was insufficient to kill vegetation, it could contaminate it, and if animals which yielded milk or meat for humans ate it, the radioactive traces would enter the human body. If the half-life (the period taken for the radioactivity to fall to half its original value) was a long one, then there would be considerable exposure to radiation. We have already learned that leukaemia is a disease affecting the bone marrow and the white cells of the blood. One of the fall-out products of the atomic bomb was strontium and this is concentrated in bone. Since activity in the growing bone of children is high it was feared that strontium would be accumulated at this site and thereby the incidence of leukaemia be increased. This led to international efforts to limit or ban atomic-bomb tests, and the setting up of devices to measure background radiation. It is also known that radiation can cause sterility by damaging the gonads, or at a lower dose a change in the genes of the chromosomes, mutation. Such a mutation might be the cause of an abnormality in a subsequent embryo.

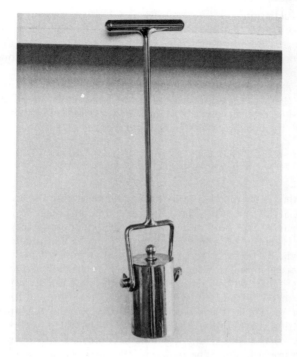

Fig. 25.2.   Long handled protective carrier

As yet the incidence of such mutations and their effects on the following generations are not clear. It is obvious that a long period of time is necessary to
evaluate them, and that we must be certain that radiation could have been the
only cause.

Natural Radiation

Since Man has been exposed to natural radiation during the whole of his evolution,
mutation has occurred, some bodily changes may have been beneficial and
have been retained, while the processes of natural selection have probably
eliminated those that were too damaging. Over this long period it is likely that
an equilibrium between Man and his background has been reached. Protection
is designed to deal with the additional burden from the industrial and medical
uses of radiation.

Unnecessary Radiation

Since the dangers are now appreciated, the first step is to remove all unnecessary radiation. X-ray machines to check the fittings of shoes are no longer in use in shops. Radium is not now painted on luminous dials. New machines and processes must be checked. Cooking by microwave is being developed and it has been realised that there is a small radiation hazard which must be eliminated. When colour television receivers were first operated it was found that radiation was being emitted, by a change in design this was reduced and screened off.

Monitoring

Monitoring, that is the process of detecting and measuring the level of radiation, requires special instruments. The geiger counter, although it has caught the public fancy, is in fact only one of a range of detection devices. These can be mounted permanently on a machine incorporating an alarm device if levels become too high, be portable for moving around an area for periodic checks, or be designed for personnel to wear. They must all be specially designed to respond to the type of radiation being measured. Hospital staff usually wear film badges. These are changed fortnightly. When developed the film will be blackened by the radiation to which it has been exposed. By varying the thickness of the plastic, or putting in a thin filter, the 'windows' of the holder will permit differing energies to reach the film. The blackening is compared with a standard, and the level of exposure recorded. The radiation exposure for each person is recorded and summated for a given period.

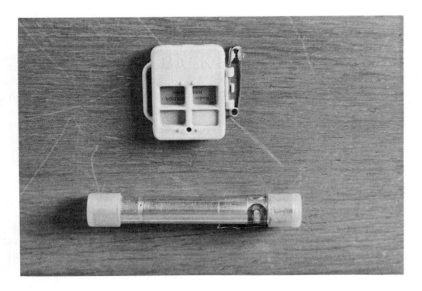

Fig. 25.3.   Radiation staff monitoring badges

Protection and Permissible Doses

After considering all the evidence, regulations have been drawn up governing the levels of exposure which can be permitted. In practice, not only are these well below danger levels, they are also seldom reached. It was realised that it was impractical to use the same figure for the whole population and so slightly higher levels were set for those whose work was with radiation. The radiation incurred during medical investigations is excluded as it is regarded as an acceptable and necessary risk, therefore it is important that only necessary X-rays should be ordered.

International agreements have been made about the signs warning of radiation areas, and the storage and carriage of radioactive materials. These agreements are on minimal protection measures, and national regulations are usually more strict and made by special regulatory committees. In Great Britain there is a code of practice on protection measures for each of a number of situations, industry, research, hospitals. Wherever there is a source of radiation one person is responsible for safety. He checks radiation levels and maintains safe methods of machine operation and personnel working. In a radiotherapy department he is usually the physicist. Among his duties is the instruction of nurses and radiographers in safe working methods, and his advice should always be sought when any doubt on custody of sources or procedures arises. He cannot however be everywhere at once. Each individual must maintain standards and must not become careless because radiation is an unseen hazard.

Protection and Machines

In a radiotherapy department, machines are protected by thick walls or a maze device. This keeps scattered radiation within the machine room. When not in use the window of an X-ray tube is closed by a shutter; a radioactive source is stored in a heavily screened compartment and the machine will not operate unless the doors or barriers are closed. Control is from a panel outside the room. Periodic monitoring checks are made on the efficiency of the machine, the scattered radiation within the room, and the level outside it. If a nurse visits the department, she should not enter treatment rooms without the permission of the radiographer who is responsible for the safe working of the machine. If she works in the department she should also keep a wary eye open for the lay person accompanying a patient and straying into working areas.

Protection in the Wards and Theatre

Patients who are receiving external radiation are not radioactive, but those who have implants or gynaecological sources and others who are given radioactive isotopes are sources of radiation. A nurse will see hanging on the bed or door the international sign carrying the safe working times, both with and without protection in place. These have been drawn up as if one person were solely attending the patient, but in fact it is better if the nursing duties are shared and

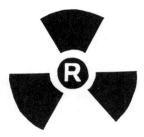

Fig. 25.4.   Radiation warning sign

the exposure of each person thereby reduced. The rules of safe custody of sources and disposal of radioactive waste must be followed strictly. It is most important that eating or drinking should not be done in the same room as storage, this is a commonsense caution, but may be neglected. In the theatre the basis of safe working is speed and distance. Sources should not be removed from containers until actually required. Long-handled instruments should be used and the same nurse should not assist at more than one procedure in the same list. The advent of powerful modern machines has considerably reduced the numbers of implants and insertions required and hence the exposure of staff.

Radiological Department

The energy at which the radiodiagnostic machines work is lower than that of most therapy machines and therefore less penetrating. It is possible for the radiographer to remain in the room but to stand behind a protective screen when the machine is operating. If she has to move about the room during screening procedures, she wears a lead and rubber apron, and the radiologist will wear an apron and stand behind a portable screen. If he thinks he will need to put his hands in the X-ray beam to manipulate a patient, he puts on protective lead and rubber gloves. A nurse who accompanies a patient to the X-ray department will be in no danger if she follows the instructions of the radiographer. Radiation to the patient is minimised by better techniques, such as the use of screens to watch the progress of a meal and by recording on tape. It must be appreciated that if the annual dose of radiation which is genetically significant is calculated for the whole population, diagnostic medical radiation is responsible for only 32% of the total figure. Natural background radiation contributes almost 67% of the total.

During pregnancy X-rays are kept to the minimum. Ultra sound is now used routinely to check the lie of the foetus and the position of the placenta.

Discharge of Patients, Visitors

The nurse should be familiar with the instructions given to patients leaving hospital after permanent implants or after receiving a radioactive isotope. She should be certain that they are understood. When patients are in the ward it is usual to exclude children and pregnant women from visiting when sources are in position. Care should be taken to place visitors to neighbouring beds correctly. If radioactive isotopes have been administered, the rules governing visitors will vary with the type of isotope. If in any doubt, advice on protection should be sought, particularly if the substance is being used for the first time.

Death of a Patient

Occasionally a patient dies shortly after one of these procedures. Advice will be given when radioactive isotopes have been given. It may be necessary to keep the body in special conditions for a time, or to forbid cremation. This can be very distressing for the relatives and the nurse will need all her tact and sympathy at these times.

Accidents

Radiation accidents are very rare. It is impossible to lay down rules for every emergency, but there is a certain drill which a nurse should know. The emergency service is alerted, entry to the area by unauthorised people is prevented, contaminated staff are held in a safe area, and steps taken to prevent a spread of contamination.

Relative Risks

Those who are new to the world of radiation may well at this point decide the work is too hazardous and the risks to the patients and staff too great. Many nurses harbour a secret fear that such work may render them sterile or liable to have abnormal children. The radiographers who have a greater exposure, do not seem to suffer this fate, they marry and often revisit their friends in the department to show off their healthy beautiful babies. Nor do the families of the doctors seem to suffer. There is a risk, but it is small and minimised by good protection measures.

To be alive at all is a risk. A man can stay in one room from which all hazards are excluded, yet he may still be killed by lightning striking the room or a lorry demolishing the wall. We are constantly choosing the degree of risk to which we will expose ourselves. We decide that in view of the benefits or the pleasure, we can accept the danger. The action of governments regulates the risks which we cannot choose, pollution of the atmosphere, dangerous machines, and it must be admitted that sometimes that action is slow. In our pressure for national measures we must beware of rejecting some process of which the risks have been over dramatised, while ignoring those from less-publicised and more insidious sources. Radiation may well be an example of this illogical approach, while we concentrate on this we may neglect the pollution of the environment by man-made waste, or the destruction of the soil by greedy or ignorant farming.

Balancing the Risks

Let us then try to balance the risks. In England and Wales in 1965 over 1,300 new cases of acute leukaemia, cause unknown, were recorded. Yet in the same period more people died either from renal disease, committed suicide, or were killed in road accidents. It has been calculated that to survey the population of men at risk for carcinoma of the lung by an annual chest X-ray would be 100 times more likely to detect a lung carcinoma than to induce a case of leukaemia.

For the nurse and all others working with radiation, the lesson is clear. There are risks, but they are no more, and very probably less, than those we accept as part of the normal pattern of life, and they are far outweighed by the benefits. We are no longer ignorant and so do not incur the penalties suffered by early workers who did not realise the potentiality of this new therapeutic

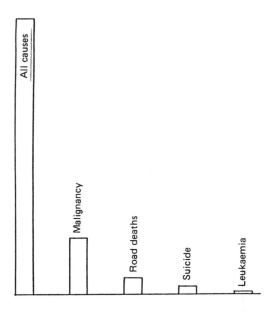

Fig. 25.5.   Comparison of death rates all ages

weapon. Within the hospital the methods of working and of protection are constantly under review and nurses are fully represented on all the relevant committees. The assurances given can be accepted, and sensible behaviour together with the vigilance of the authorities will keep any risk at the lowest possible level.

What is fact?
It is surely nothing
But an evolution of ever changing truth.

26   Radiation of Benign Conditions

The previous chapters have dealt entirely with the treatment of malignant disease, but there are a few benign conditions which can benefit from radiotherapy. When X-rays and radium were first discovered it was believed that this field of use was a large one. The realisation of the carcinogenic nature of radiation caused the early workers to reconsider. The policy which was then formulated is still followed today, this is that all other treatments should be tried or considered first, and that total dosage and area should be restricted. The wisdom of this policy is evident when it is remembered that intractable dermatitis, skin carcinomas, and leukaemia have all resulted from excessive radiation of vulnerable healthy tissues.

Principles of Treatment

For all benign conditions certain principles govern treatment. They should never be abandoned and the nurse will notice that they vary quite markedly from those followed in the radiation of malignant disease.

1. The smallest dose and the energy with the minimum penetration for the condition are used.
2. The area is carefully demarcated and no margin included.
3. The dose is less for sensitive areas, groins, axillae, soles, palms.
4. Watch is kept for individual variation in tolerance.
5. Accurate records must be kept and no more than a fixed dose given to one area in a lifetime.

This last point is a very important one and the records should carry not only notes of the anatomical area, but also a drawing or photograph. Patients must be told that they must always remember that they have had treatment and must tell the doctor if they are ever referred for any reason to another radiotherapy department. Parents have a particular responsibility to see that this knowledge is given to children as they grow up. That this policy is not easy to follow is illustrated by a patient referred to me from a dermatologist for treatment to eczema of one hand. She was asked the routine question 'Have you had treatment like this before?' She said that she had, that she could not remember when, at what centre, or to which part of her body! We had no record of a previous attendance by her. Since radiation of a benign skin condition is never urgent nor life saving, I referred her back to the dermatologist, who in turn made enquiries of her doctor. She arrived back in the clinic six weeks later with a letter to say that she had received treatment three years previously before her marriage. This time our records registered under her maiden name were traced, the hand had not been radiated, and she received a full course. Though amusing, this is a cautionary tale, and all staff should be on the alert for this forgetful type of patient.

The conditions treated mainly affect two tissues, skin and joints. For the former low-voltage radiation with little penetration is used, but the latter needs a better depth dose and requires more penetrating radiation.

Skin Conditions

Depending upon the thickness of the lesion and the area involved, the energy used ranges from 5 to 140 kV. At the lower end of this scale (5-15 kV), the rays are soft or Grenz rays. At 1 mm depth in tissue only 20% of the dose remains, so that the sebaceous glands and hair follicles which lie deeper than this are not damaged. Intractable eczema often responds. A small dose is usually given three to six times at weekly intervals. The area is carefully marked with a skin pencil. As it is usually irregular and the applicators are of a regular shape, a tracing is taken of the skin mark and a cut-out made in lead, this protects adjacent areas not being treated. Rings must be taken off or moved out of the field.

Keloid Scars

These conditions involve a greater thickness of the skin and for this reason require a more penetrating type of radiation. Keloid scars are a thickened fibrous reddening of the skin and can arise spontaneously, this is more common in the negroid races, or as a result of trauma. The latter type particularly if treated within one year of occurrence usually responds better. The policy adopted by centres varies slightly, but usually 100 kV is used and a dose of 6 Gy (600 rads) is given, with a careful lead cut-out in position. After six to eight weeks the dose is repeated if necessary. Great care must be exercised when treating children and due consideration given to the underlying tissues. Treatment to the neck has in the past resulted in the development of thyroid carcinoma in a few cases.

Vascular Naevi

If the decision is made to treat a cautious approach is used. Small doses up to 4 Gy (400 rads) are given and repeated only after observation for periods of three months or more. An alternative is the use of radioactive isotopes such as phosphorus which emit beta rays. Plaques of the isotope to fit the area are made from a careful tracing and are bandaged into position. They are removed when the correct dose has been given. This is usually after about 45 minutes. The eyes and lips must be carefully protected whatever form of treatment is given.

Joint Conditions

The condition which was most commonly treated is ankylosing spondylitis. This is a disease process which causes stiffening of the spine due to bony tissue replacing joint spaces and ligaments. At first the joints are inflamed, then fibrous tissue joins the bones obliterating the joint space, ankylosis, and finally the new tissue is ossified. On X-ray at a late stage the spine has a characteristic 'bamboo spine' appearance with squaring off and thickening of the vertebral bodies. The costo-vertebral and sacro-iliac joints are usually also affected, and in addition the hips, knees, and ankles can be involved. The cause is unknown but it is thought by many to be a form of rheumatoid arthritis.

Men in the second to third decade most commonly are affected, but the occasional woman patient is seen. It is a fairly rare disease.

The condition is painful and the patient complains also of stiffness. Inflammation of the iris, iritis, can develop, and sufferers from this disease are warned to consult a doctor for reference to an ophthalmologist as soon as it occurs. Considerable deformity can follow, the spine becomes very bowed, kyphotic, and in extreme cases the patient is bent almost double and is completely unable to look up or forward. Stiffening of the costo-vertebral joints limits expansion of the chest and restricts breathing, consequently respiratory infections can be

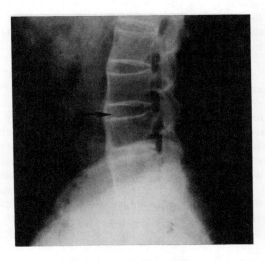

Fig. 26.1.   X-ray of the spine. 'Bamboo' appearance of the vertebrae. Calcification of the ligaments

difficult to eliminate. While a brace may improve pain and prevent deformity, the harness restricts breathing, and it is often difficult to decide which requirement is the more important.

The disease was frequently arrested and pain relieved by radiation. The whole spine and the sacro-iliac joints in men were treated, but in women these joints are closely related to the ovaries. If these women were in the reproductive years, some form of heat therapy rather than radiation was often preferred for these joints. The area was divided into a number of fields, treatment was given on alternate days or twice a week to each field in turn. The dose was formerly higher, but it was found that the incidence of leukaemia among these patients was 10 times higher than in the normal population. It was realised that perhaps too high a dose was being given to most of the red bone marrow and accordingly it was reduced. During treatment a blood count is obtained twice weekly and thereafter at every follow-up.

At follow-up appointments questions on pain, stiffness, respiratory or eye infections are asked. Many patients, since they have had the full course of radiation, require a non-steroidal anti-inflammatory drug if the disease is not controlled. Objective measurements of the disease are given by movements of the spine, chest expansion, the distance on bending between finger-tips and floor, E.S.R. and X-rays of the spine and affected joints.

In some patients radiation completely arrested the disease, in others it was slowed, while in the rest there was no apparent effect. Since it is a benign condition and there are now many anti-inflammatory drugs available, radiation was used less and less because of the risk of leukaemia. However the anti-inflammatory drugs are not entirely effective, and there is no doubt that patients did receive worthwhile palliation from radiation in the past, the whole question is therefore under review.

The nurse may be puzzled as to why so much higher doses are given to malignant conditions affecting the spine when the radiotherapist knows of the risk of leukaemia. This is essentially a matter of the gravity of the two conditions. Untreated the malignant lesion will result usually in death, the inevitable high radiation of the bone marrow has to be accepted.

Discontinued Treatment

Radiation was formerly employed to epilate skin affected by ringworm. The follicles were then easily penetrated by fungicides. Griseofulvin which can be given by mouth has made this treatment unnecessary, and in view of the number of patients who developed multiple skin carcinomata afterwards it would be unlikely that it would be revived. The use of radium for vascular naevi has also been abandoned, malignant change in the skin has followed its use. Acne and severe pruritus of the vulva or perineum are also examples of conditions which are no longer treated by radiation.

We can never be quite certain,
Which presents the problem,
Man or Nature,
Even less can we be sure
Which provides the answer.

27 Day-to-day Work

In this book we have discussed together the practice and theory of radiotherapy and chemotherapy together with the care of patients receiving radiation. It may not be possible for every reader to visit a unit and see these words translated into action, so in imagination we shall attempt to describe something of a working day in a ward, the treatment area, and the outpatient clinic.

We can begin in the ward and join the members of the unit on the weekly business round. They have reached the last patient in the men's ward. He is a middle-aged man who is looking very anxious. Bedclothes are held away from his legs by a bed cradle. He was referred by letter and has come into the ward straight from another hospital. He has not yet been seen in the clinic.

Sister introduces the patient and tells him who the consultant is. Before considering his case notes the doctor talks briefly to him and explains the identity of all the accompanying members of the radiotherapy team. He then asks for a summary of the history, previous treatment and illnesses, and present clinical findings. The account is short and given by the junior doctor who has already seen the patient. Apparently this man presented with severe pain in the back, weakness of the legs, some sensory loss and disturbance of micturition. Investigations at the referring hospital confirmed a provisional diagnosis of a collapsed vertebra with spinal-cord compression. A laminectomy was performed relieving the pressure, and histology of the biopsy taken showed this to be a secondary deposit from a carcinoma of the bronchus. There is still slight weakness in the legs, some loss of sensation, but sphincter control has returned, although pain still persists. The X-rays and scans are examined away from the bedside. Any teaching or general discussion on this type of lesion is given at the same time, so avoiding the patient hearing details of complications or other lesions which do not apply to him. Often a patient misinterprets these snatches of conversation or the facial expressions accompanying them and is unnecessarily worried.

On returning to the patient the consultant asks him how he feels and what progress he thinks he has made. Sister recognises her cue and says she feels he is worrying abot being away so long from his family. It is obviously more important to deal with this question than to go on straight away to physical examination. It is soon apparent that there is some underlying financial problem and the medical social worker is introduced. She promises to return later when the patient's wife is visiting. The consultant now explains the length of treatment, the planning which is to take place later in the day and promises to talk to the patient's wife. It is also made clear that the patient may have a longer discussion with the consultant in the clinic. Sister asks that the ward can be told in good time when he is to be taken to the department so that an analgesic can be given. The senior radiographer who is on the round promises this.

Finally the consultant makes a brief physical examination, and after introducing the physiotherapist, suggests the treatment he would like her to give. Before leaving the bedside, the occupational therapist is also asked to help. It is clear that the patient has an active mind and is fretting at his forced inactivity.

In the ward office the consultant explains that he is asking for a histology review of the last patient's biopsy specimen, depending on the result it may be decided to follow radiation with chemotherapy. A full discussion of all the patients takes place, prognosis, treatment and progress. Sister is able to give fuller details and any problems encountered by other members of the team are discussed. The medical social worker would like to know whether one patient will be able to go straight to convalescence, the two therapists ask if they can push the rehabilitation of another patient faster, and the speech therapist feels that family stress is impeding the progress of her patient. At the end of the discussion every member of the team knows the plan for each patient and is prepared. Sister is now more equipped to deal with the questions from relatives, the radiographer can arrange treatment schedules, the specialist therapists are briefed on the part they can play, and the medical social worker is ready for the further talks she must have with both patients and relatives. Although he is now in the care of a team, each member will spend time with our new patient individually and so enable him to discuss matters more freely than is possible with a large team present.

The consultant on leaving the ward passes through the treatment area, and this is a good opportunity to look at the machines, the mould room, the radioactive storage area and watch some of the patients being treated. In the first treatment room are the machines of lower energy, up to 140 kV. The lesions treated are superficial, from eczema to rodent ulcers. On the shelves are the applicators and various pieces of lead for making cut outs for irregular areas. The trolley with the eye-shield tray is also kept here. The patient coming in to be treated next is an elderly man with a rodent ulcer on the side of his nose. The radiographer soon makes friends with him and is able to take a paper tracing of the area marked for treatment. She transfers this to a piece of lead of the correct thickness and cuts out the marked area. This is bent over the nose and sellotaped in place. Protectors are slipped into the nostrils. When he is resting comfortably the machine is fitted with the correct applicator and brought down on to the lesion. The radiographer has already shown the patient how she is able to see him on the closed circuit television viewer. When she has satisfied herself that all is well, there is a last check of the treatment card, the timer is set, and the machine started. At the end of treatment the patient comes out and seems quite unconcerned.

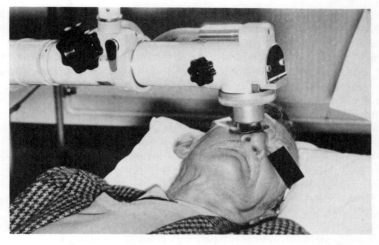

Fig. 27.1.   Low voltage machine, patient set up for treatment

Next door the control panel shows us the machine is working at a higher voltage. The patient being set up has had a mastectomy and is receiving post-operative radiation. She is at the end of her daily treatment and is having one of the glancing fields applied to the chest wall. Accurate alignment is ensured with the marked fields. After the radiation has been given, the radiographer enters up the day's record and tells the patient that she is to be seen in the clinic. It is a week since she started treatment and it is time for her routine check by the doctor. The machines in the next two rooms are of the same type. The patient being taken into one of them is on the Stryker frame and is having treatment to his spine. Although ordinary movement causes him pain, he can be turned easily without any spinal movement on this frame.

At the end of this section there are two machines. Neither treatment room is closed by a heavy door, but only by wooden gates. However to reach the machine we have to turn round a thick wall, this is protection by a maze device. In one room is a cobalt machine. The large metal ring enables the machine head to travel right round the treatment couch. This is fixed to the floor but the 'table top' can be moved up and down and to and fro mechanically. The patient being set up is having the larynx treated and is wearing a Perspex shell to hold his head in the correct position. The size of the field is set by altering shutters in the machine. A light shines through this field area and enables the radiographer to align the field correctly. The angle of the machine head is read off on a scale fixed to the machine. In the other room there is a linear accelerator. Here too the field size is defined by shutters and setting up is by a light device. The patient is having the para-aortic and iliac nodes treated. The kidneys are being shielded by protective blocks.

The betatron is housed in another building and on our way there we can look at the radioactive storage area and at the mould room. The radioactive storage safe is closed. It contains separate drawers for each size of needle and box. On the bench nearby the needles are prepared and threaded. The operator stands behind the thick protective blocks and uses long-handled instruments. Close by are the transport containers of various sizes.

The door of the physicist's office is open. He has an X-ray of an implant of the tongue on the viewing box. The implant was carried out earlier and today the calculations are being made to fix the exact time the needles must remain in place to deliver the required dose.

In the mould room a patient is waiting for his plaster impression to be taken. He has a lesion of the nasopharynx spreading into the ethmoid sinus and the area to be treated has been marked on the face. The patient's head is on the same-sized rest that will be used during treatment. His skin has been greased and small lint pads placed over his eyes. Wet plaster bandages are moulded over the face and down to the headrest. In a few moments the shell is firm enough to be sprung off and the patient is able to go. The technician fills the impression with plaster which when set gives a cast of the patient's head. Using a special machine

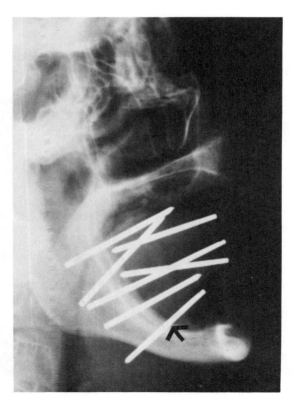

Fig. 27.2.   X-ray, implant of tongue

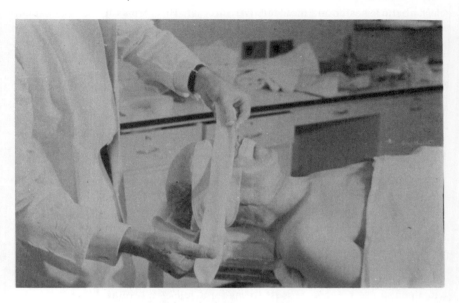

Fig. 27.3.   Applying plaster bandages to make a cast

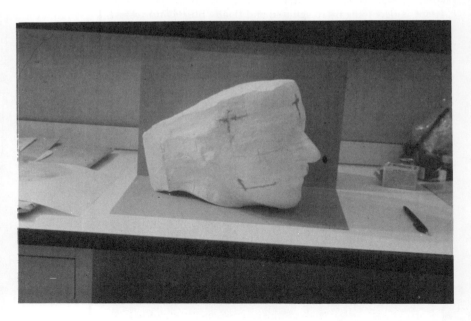

Fig. 27.4.   Completed plaster cast, treatment area marked

clear plastic is heated and moulded over this cast. This forms the shell the patient will wear during treatment.

In this building is housed the betatron. Here the observation window is a wide liquid-filled tank, the patient can be seen just as well as on the other machines. The radiographer is able to move this heavy machine or adjust the position of the table using finger-tip pressure on a series of buttons on a portable control panel. The patient being treated has a brain tumour and a special treatment shell has been prepared. To square up the surface of the head to receive the applicator the shell is double, the space between the two layers being filled with water. The treatment is nearly finished and the fields are sharply demarcated on the head by the loss of hair. The skin is dry and a dusky plum colour typical of the skin reaction to this type of treatment.

The consultant is now seeing the first patient in the clinic. This is a woman of 50 who has been referred from a gynaecologist. It is obvious that she is very nervous and frightened. Quietly the doctor asks her how she is feeling after her operation. She has had a total hysterectomy to remove a uterine carcinoma. Gradually her history is taken including details of her family life. It emerges that she has grown-up daughters still at home. Her husband is out at work all day and she lives not far from the hospital. She has been told that she had a tumour removed and that she needs treatment to follow her operation. While she is being examined, nurse prepares request forms for a full blood count. Chest X-ray was taken before operation. By this time the doctor is explaining the treatment to the patient. It is agreed that she may remain at home provided she rests and allows her family to look after her. There is obviously something wrong as the patient is becoming more agitated and finally bursts into tears. She says that one

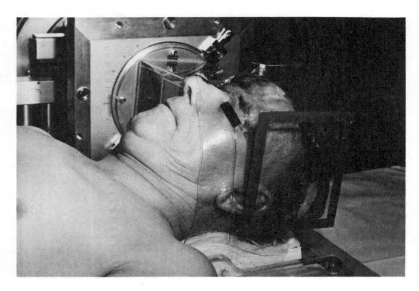

Fig. 27.5.   Patient wearing plastic shell, set up for treatment on the betatron machine

of her relatives died of cancer a short while ago and that she is afraid. Fortunately the histology report shows that the tumour was a very early one and was completely removed. It is possible to assure her that the operation was completely successful and that radiation is a precautionary measure. It would be unwise to subject her to any further delay and so it is arranged that she can start treatment at once. The physicist is asked to come in. The abdominal fields are marked and the physicist then takes a body contour and measurements of width and depth. He explains the reasons for this as he does it. While he makes the necessary calculations, the senior radiographer, who has joined the clinic team, takes the patient to meet the radiographer who will be treating her.

The next two patients have been sent down from the radiographer. The first is the woman we saw having treatment for a mastectomy. The doctor enters the dose reached on the notes, and asks her how she feels. Since her reply shows she feels very well, by a few seemingly casual questions he assures himself that she is not doing too much at home. The skin shows no erythema. She is told all is going well and that treatment will continue.

Next to come in is the man who is having treatment to the larynx. His voice is very hoarse and he looks tired. The record card shows that this was his last treatment. He complains of dysphagia and a slight dry cough. After examining the chest and the lymphatic areas of the neck, the radiotherapist makes a mirror examination of the larynx. The pharynx is erythematous. The vocal cords are oedematous but the right, which was roughened by growth, is now much smoother. It is explained that the soreness and dysphagia are a reaction to radiation and that this will improve. He is advised to rest his voice and told how to take steam inhalations. Although there are no physical signs in the chest and the cough is probably due to pharyngitis, an X-ray is requested. The patient is anxious to return to work, but he has a severe reaction and is a salesman needing to talk most of the day. The doctor suggests therefore that he comes back in a week and waits to make the decision, but he warns him that it will probably be a month before he can return to work.

Our new patient from the ward is now waiting and is brought in on the Stryker frame. He has had time to prepare his questions and is soon firing them off. He now seems less worried about his financial position since the medical social worker has seen him, but he is very anxious to know when he can go back to work. The doctor asks him whether he thinks he could do this now and the patient admits it is impossible. It is suggested to him that he must first have treatment before a date can be considered, meanwhile concentrating hard on physiotherapy. The area of the spine to be radiated is marked and the patient taken off for his first treatment. Later, when the consultant has had time for discussions with the referring hospital, the family doctor, and also to get to know the patient, his wife and family, there will come the first of many conversations on the nature of his illness.

The nurse brings in a doctor's letter with the next patient. He is a man in his early sixties who has had two rodent ulcers treated in the past. His doctor has requested an earlier follow-up appointment as he is worried about a fresh lesion at the edge of the lower lip. This has the appearance of a malignant tumour but the therapist knows he must have a biopsy, particularly since he suspects from the site that it could this time be a squamous cell carcinoma. He asks a nurse to have a biopsy set prepared in the small theatre attached to the department, for as one of the unit doctors is free it is possible for the biopsy to be done later in the morning. A telephone message has come from the ward saying that the wife of the new patient has just arrived. As her husband is having treatment now the doctor decides to go back to the ward and talk to her.

As we shall be coming back to the combined clinic in the afternoon we can take this opportunity to leave. Before doing so, we can look in on the nurse in the theatre and see how she sums up her work. To begin with she makes it clear it is not a post for a junior nurse. She is happy to teach junior nurses and feels there is much she has learned she can pass on, but she is sure that the pressures on her are too varied for the inexperienced to be able to cope.

All doctors have their own way of doing things, but it is important that she not only remembers these but also learns the approach to a patient that a particular doctor uses. She feels that by intelligent anticipation she can ensure the smooth running of a clinic. A patient or relative on the verge of volunteering important information can be completely put off by an unnecessary pause while some instrument or document is located.

The wife of a general practitioner who answers the telephone for her husband is sometimes unkindly called a protective dragon. Nurse smiles wryly as she says she must be just this. Telephone calls, unless urgent or from an outside doctor, should not be allowed to interrupt a clinic, and any staff who wish to speak to the doctor must be asked to wait for the interval between patients. There is nothing more calculated to destroy the confidence of the patient than a series of interruptions and enquiries about other patients, he begins to feel he is not receiving the doctor's full attention and that the clinic is like a railway waiting room. At all costs the impression of a factory conveyor belt must be avoided, however many patients are waiting there must be no feeling of pressure to speed up, and the nurse must accept the inevitable delays due to discussions with the patient or family, and indeed be prepared to create one by telling the doctor when relatives have accompanied a patient.

Many a nurse will at this point be thinking that a doctor can just as surely wreck this scheme. Although some delays are unavoidable due to ward emergencies, as part of the team a doctor also has his part to play in ensuring the smooth working of the clinic.

The size of clinics and the delays that occur can be a source of irritation to patients. Adequate staffing can help to minimise the problem. A consultation is not then held up because the nurse is busy elsewhere with a dressing or an injection. If a morning clinic is prolonged lunch times can be staggered so that the afternoon work can start on time. However experienced a receptionist is it is not always possible for her to judge how long it may take to see a particular patient. A nurse who has been in the clinic can indicate on the patient's slip whether the next appointment should be early in the list and if extra time is likely to be required. She can also make sure that there is no overbooking. This is important as any routine follow-up patient can unexpectedly present a problem and there must always be time for an emergency consultation.

While our conversation has been going on we have been able to note that there is equipment available for sudden emergencies. In particular there is suction apparatus and oxygen. In reply to a question nurse says that in an emergency, equipment is sometimes required for patients who collapse or are in respiratory difficulties.

Another nurse has come to take over and to assist at the biopsy. As we go we can see our nurse checking to see that X-rays and blood counts are available for the afternoon clinic, and making sure that forms are ready for those patients coming tomorrow who need X-rays or blood counts before being seen by the doctor.

In the afternoon we can attend the combined clinic. In addition to the radio-therapists, a surgeon, dentist and plastic surgeon are present. To this clinic come patients who are attending for follow-up after special surgery, or who have been referred for the joint planning of treatment. Our consultant has three patients on the appointment list.

He explains his first problem to his colleagues. The patient is a fit man of 55 who had a squamous cell carcinoma of the pinna treated two years pre-viously. Growth has now recurred, biopsy is positive, and there is a small mobile node just below the angle of the jaw. The patient is called in and the lesion and the neck examined by all the doctors. The surgeon asks for the latest chest X-ray, this is clear. The therapist explains that he has warned the patient that surgery is necessary. The man says that he is resigned to this but would like to know just what is involved. Somewhat to his surprise he gets no immediate answer but is asked to return to the waiting room while the doctors decide the best policy for him. Once he has left there is a lengthy discussion. It revolves round the extent of the surgery in view of the presence of the mobile node. Finally it is decided that the whole ear must be removed followed by block dissection of the neck if the node fails to regress on antibiotic therapy. As the therapist knows the patient so well it is he who sees him in another room. The reaction to the proposed treatment is a natural one, shock. It is some time before the doctor is able to convince him of its necessity and the fact that a prosthesis can be made for him. He agrees finally and is told that arrangements for admission will be made in two or three days. As the consultant is not happy about his emotional state he rings the family doctor and explains the position. He promises to look in on the patient later.

The consultant returns to the combined clinic and his next patient is shown in. She is coming up for the first time after discharge from the ward. Five years ago she had post-operative radiation following a mastectomy. A subsequent skeletal metastasis responded to oophorectomy, but after two years, further metastases developed and so she has been placed on an adrenal blocking drug. After checking on her general condition she is questioned specifically about her pain, this has improved. Her bone scan shows slight improvement so it is decided to postpone skeletal survey for a month and then to see her again. Although there are no symptoms of electrolyte imbalance she is sent for blood estimation.

Lastly our consultant tells his colleagues the history of the third patient. This is a young woman aged 20 who has been referred by an orthopaedic surgeon. This centre has specialised experience in treating bone tumours. The investi-gations and diagnosis are complete, but it is important that in this case there should be an agreed policy from the outset. The patient has an osteogenic sarcoma of the lower end of the right femur. Before she comes in everyone studies very carefully the chest X-rays, they are clear.

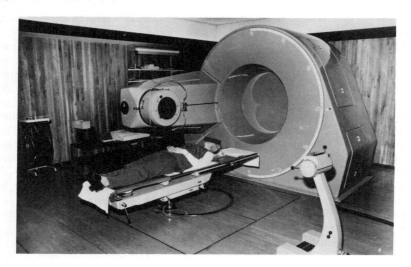

Fig. 27.6.   Linear accelerator

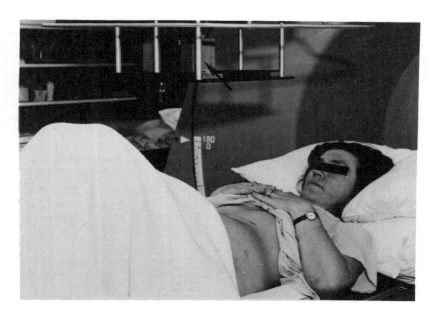

Fig. 27.7.   Preparation for treatment, note blocks to define the
treatment beam

After the consultation, discussion centres around the choice and timing of surgery and radiotherapy. Although the chest X-ray is at present clear, it is agreed that further investigations including CATscan are required. The leg is first to be given a radical course of radiation, followed by chemotherapy, and then, if the chest remains clear, amputation should be considered later. Our doctor leaves first to see the patient and explain the initial treatment, and then to have a full discussion with her husband. As she has a young child nurse can foresee family difficulties, and we see her ringing up the medical social worker to alert her she will probably be needed.

At the end of the day the notes are filed away but the problems cannot be shelved. Our nurse probably feels that she is by now qualified for service in the diplomatic corps, but at least she can never be bored.

> *If only I could retire to a quiet corner of the Earth,*
> *To pause, to think, to enjoy thinking.*
> *For I seem to enjoy my deepest thoughts*
> *When I think only of nothing.*

When we are born we are cast in the role of optimists,
Only if we believe that all problems can be solved
Can we dare to survive.
So within us there is always a dream,
A dream that one day the disease will no longer be a disease,
But that it will itself become for ever a dream.

28   The Future

During the months that I have spent revising this book, there have been many times when the contrast between the lines on the title page:

Cancer, created by life itself, exists within life,
Yet in the end makes life untenable,

and those at the head of this chapter, has struck me with great force. Nurses may have wondered whether they, or I, have any right to optimism, or whether we should hold only to the fatalism that 'Man is born unto trouble as the sparks fly upward'? I would rather say that the first lines are the present, but that there is every prospect of at least a partial fulfilment of our dream in the not too distant future.

Throughout the book we have discussed current promising lines of research, where else do we need to look, can we even define the problem we seek to solve? Watching my little granddaughter poring over a jig-saw puzzle, I realised that we are trying to do something similar. She would find a piece, decide that it belonged to a cat, and try to fit it into the picture that she was building up. Similarly we know many facts and make many discoveries, but we do not know either how they fit together or into the whole puzzle. My little girl has the picture on the box to guide her, we have no such advantage. Moreoever our jig-saw is constantly changing. The processes we explore react with, and are dependent upon, thousands upon thousands of other processes, all taking place simultaneously. Yet in the end it all revolves around D.N.A., the very stuff of life, infinitely variable, infinitely adaptable, and only by its expression enabling us to gaze inwards upon ourselves.

We must not forget however, that our patients cannot wait while we explore these fundamental issues. Our present treatments though they have been refined are essentially destructive. Nevertheless they do achieve a measure of success, and at the moment are all we have to offer. Our research must therefore be directed to refining and improving them, lessening their toxicity and increasing efficacy. We are also beginning to try and ameliorate the social and psychological effects of the disease on the patient and family, that is just a grand way of saying that we are all human beings, and so must try to understand and help the human problem. Nor should we leave the patient out of our reckoning, his hopes, fears, beliefs have an important part in determining his attitude, and can be harnessed to play a positive role in his treatment. In other words it is the whole man we treat.

Nor are the two lines of research divorced. As we discover the intracellular controls of aberrant development, so we may be able to design treatments which will strengthen those controls. The old gardeners knew that disease in cabbages could be attacked by liming the soil, tilting the balance in favour of the plant. Perhaps we can do the same. At present we are confronted by frank tumour, which biologically speaking is late in its development. At that stage it is probably too late to reverse it, and surgery, radiation, cytotoxics are all needed to remove it. If we could find it earlier, its removal could be less traumatic, less destructive, so research must also seek better, more refined methods of investigation. However even then, the conditions which induced the malignant change may still remain, or it may be impossible to eliminate the tumour completely. It is here that the strategy of strengthening natural controls could be of vital importance. Whether it will be through diet supplements, slight alterations in the environment, or even by introducing the necessary intracellular controls artificially, who knows? In the distant future we may even be able to map the genetic constitution of each individual and advise on a life style which could prevent the disease. Then just as I say now 'I remember when tuberculosis was dreaded, a taboo subject', some future author will say 'I remember when cancer . . .'

Very recently discussion on a trial of preventitive therapy has begun. It is proposed to administer the anti-oestrogen Tamoxifen to a large group of women with known high-risk factors for the development of breast carcinoma. Such a scheme has arisen out of earlier work monitoring hormone ratios. A significant reduction in the expected number of subsequent cancers would be a major advance. It must be stressed that as yet such a study is only proposed and much discussion is necessary before it begins.

Sometimes we try to force our pieces into a pattern into which they will not fit, because we are looking at them the wrong way round. The association of viruses and cancer has been long accepted, but our explanations were often involved and allocated the virus a very active role. Now we are beginning to see it in a different light, and realise that of itself the virus may do no more than alter the positioning of the genes on the chromosome, or add to the gene total. It is rather like the guest at a party who sits down between two people on a sofa thereby forcing them to behave differently, or who adds to the dust in the house by the mud he brings in on his shoes.

There is little doubt that as we fit together more of the puzzle we shall alter our previous concepts, not only in the field of cancer, but in the whole field of medicine. We know, at least in part, the initial difference between the normal and the cancer cell, but we do not yet understand why only some individuals develop overt tumour. We see that the cancer cell behaves almost like a unicellular organism. It no longer functions harmoniously in a communal whole, it regains activities which have long been suppressed and behaves like an individual. It grows, migrates, settles, as if it is almost autonomous. Yet it can be controlled, the focus of cancer cells can remain so small that it is never clinically manifest, carcinoma of the prostate is a prime example. Patients with quite advanced carcinoma can live in a kind of balance with their tumours, albeit an uneasy equilibrium. In yet other cases there have been well documented spontaneous remissions, not many, but enough to give pause for thought. So to our 'What is the difference?' we must add 'How is it maintained?' It is from the microscopic world of cellular biochemistry that our understanding of the whole process will come. Until that day, if we are honest, we must admit, that all our opinions, our theories, are no more than educated guesses based on observation. We do not know why this patient lives for many years with widespread disease, while another with every favourable prognostic indicator dies in a few months. When we do, why then of course we shall have our picture on the jigsaw puzzle box.

To return however to my central theme, in all the marvels of biochemistry, electronic gadgetry, sophisticated pharmacology, we must not lose sight of the patient. His needs are immediate, human, and because we too are human we can share them, understand them. We need compassion, not sentimentality, understanding as well as knowledge, and since we are all too human we shall fail at times, but fortunately our patients understand and forgive us. We may not be able to cure our cancer patient, but we can care for him.

> *There are no last words,*
> *No epitaph to be written,*
> *For the book is not yet finished,*
> *The life is not yet lived.*
> *The search for knowledge continues,*
> *Continues as long as Man himself.*
>
> Sempre, sempre io credo

Further Reading

There are many textbooks which will give the basic anatomy, physiology and bio-chemistry, and pathology. The whole field is both an expanding and changing one. To quote specific papers would be to refer to work which may shortly be superseded. Guidance should be sought from the hospital or postgraduate centre tutors and librarians. The following selection is of journals which are either wholly devoted to oncology, or from time to time carry relevant papers. In this way, a reader can keep abreast of current research and discussion.

Cancer
Cancer Research
Year Book of Cancer
(Year Book Medicine)
Clinical Radiology
The Lancet
The British Journal of
  Hospital Medicine
Medicine International
Journal of the Proceedings
of the Royal Society of Medicine

The Journal of the Americal
Medical Association
The New England Journal
of Medicine
Scientific American
Nursing Times
Clinics in Oncology
Progress against Cancer
The British Journal of Radiology
The British Medical Journal
Nature
Nursing Mirror

From time to time, new volumes appear in the *Recent Advances* series of books (Churchill Livingstone) and there is also a useful library of titles *Lecture Notes on* . . . . . . (Blackwell Scientific Publications Ltd).

I would, however, stress again that librarians and postgraduate tutors will be of the greatest help in suggesting up-to-date, relevant reading.

Index